Exposure Assessment in Environmental Epidemiology

Exposure Assessment in Environmental Epidemiology

SECOND EDITION

Edited by Mark J. Nieuwenhuijsen

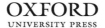

OXFORD
UNIVERSITY PRESS

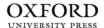

Oxford University Press is a department of the University of
Oxford. It furthers the University's objective of excellence in research,
scholarship, and education by publishing worldwide.

Oxford   New York

Auckland   Cape Town   Dar es Salaam   Hong Kong   Karachi
Kuala Lumpur   Madrid   Melbourne   Mexico City   Nairobi
New Delhi   Shanghai   Taipei   Toronto

With offices in

Argentina   Austria   Brazil   Chile   Czech Republic   France   Greece
Guatemala   Hungary   Italy   Japan   Poland   Portugal   Singapore
South Korea   Switzerland   Thailand   Turkey   Ukraine   Vietnam

Oxford is a registered trademark of Oxford University Press
in the UK and certain other countries.

Published in the United States of America by
Oxford University Press
198 Madison Avenue, New York, NY 10016

Cataloging-in-Publication data is on file at the Library of Congress
ISBN 978–0–19–937878–4

CONTENTS

CONTRIBUTORS

Ben Armstrong
London School of Hygiene and
Tropical Medicine
London, United Kingdom

Xavier Basagaña
Centre for Research in
Environmental Epidemiology
Barcelona Biomedical
Research Park
Barcelona, Spain

Rob Beelen
Institute for Risk Assessment
Sciences
Utrecht, the Netherlands

David Briggs
Department of Epidemiology
and Biostatistics School
of Public Health
Imperial College London
London, United Kingdom

Bert Brunekreef
Institute for Risk Assessment Sciences
Utrecht, the Netherlands and
Julius Center for Health Sciences
and Primary Care
University Medical
Center Utrecht
Utrecht, the Netherlands

John W. Cherrie
Heriot Watt University and
Institute of Occupational
Medicine
Edinburgh, United Kingdom

Payam Dadvand
Centre for Research in Environmental
Epidemiology
Barcelona Biomedical Research Park
Barcelona, Spain

Pierre Droz
Institute of Occupational Health
Services
Lausanne University
Lausanne, Switzerland

Melissa C. Friesen
Occupational and Environmental
Epidemiology Branch
Division of Cancer Epidemiology
and Genetics
National Cancer Institute
Bethesda, Maryland

John Gulliver
Department of Epidemiology
and Biostatistics
School of Public Health
Imperial College London
London, United Kingdom

Dick Heederik
Institute for Risk Assessment Sciences
Divisions of Environmental
Epidemiology and Veterinary
Public Health
Utrecht University
Utrecht, the Netherlands

Gerard Hoek
Institute for Risk Assessment Sciences
Utrecht, the Netherlands

Kees de Hoogh
Environmental Exposure and
    Health Unit
Department of Epidemiology and
    Public Health
Swiss Tropical and Public Health
    Institute
Basel, Switzerland

Patrick Levallois
Laval University
National Institute of Public Health of
    Québec (INSPQ)
Research Center of Québec Hospital
    University Center
Québec, Canada

Jérôme Lavoué
Department of Occupational and
    Environmental Health
School of Public Health
Université de Montréal
Montreal, Québec, Canada

Mark J. Nieuwenhuijsen
Center for Research in
    Environmental Epidemiology
Barcelona Biomedical
    Research Park
Barcelona, Spain

Marie Pedersen
Danish Cancer Research
    Society
Diet, Genes and Environment
Copenhagen, Denmark

Heike Schmitt
Institute for Risk Assessment
    Sciences
Divisions of Environmental
    Epidemiology and Veterinary
    Public Health
Utrecht University
Utrecht, the Netherlands

Sean Semple
Scottish Centre for Indoor Air
Division of Applied
    Health Sciences
University of Aberdeen
Aberdeen, Scotland

Helen H. Suh
Department of Health Sciences
Northeastern University
Boston, Massachusetts

Kay Teschke
School of Population
    and Public Health
University of British Columbia
Vancouver, British
    Columbia, Canada

Martie van Tongeren
Centre for Human Exposure
    Science
Institute of Occupational
    Medicine
Edinburgh, United Kingdom

Marc-André Verner
Department of Occupational and
    Environmental Health
School of Public Health
Université de Montréal
Montreal, Québec, Canada

Martine Vrijheid
Centre for Research in
    Environmental Epidemiology
Barcelona Biomedical Research Park
Barcelona, Spain

Cristina M. Villanueva
CREAL-Centre for Research in
    Environmental Epidemiology
Barcelona Biomedical
    Research Park
Barcelona, Spain

Frank de Vocht
School of Social and Community
    Medicine
University of Bristol
Bristol, United Kingdom

Clifford P. Weisel
Environmental and Occupational
    Health Sciences Institute
Rutgers University
Piscataway, New Jersey

SECTION I
Methods

1

INTRODUCTION TO EXPOSURE ASSESSMENT

Mark J. Nieuwenhuijsen

1.1 INTRODUCTION

Exposure is a substance or factor affecting human health, either adversely or beneficially. More precisely, in environmental epidemiology exposure to an environmental substance is generally defined as any contact between a substance in an environmental medium (e.g., water, air, soil) and the surface of the human body (e.g., skin, respiratory tract); after uptake into the body it is referred to as *dose*. Exposure assessment is the study of distribution and determinants of substances or factors affecting human health. It consists of three components; the design of the study, data collection, and the interpretation of the data. This chapter discusses briefly some of the basic issues, and introduces topics for the following chapters.

In environmental epidemiology, the focus is on chemical, biological, and physical substances in our everyday environment. In today's world risks associated with environmental exposure are generally small and therefore to detect a risk when there is truly a risk, the exposure assessment has to be very refined. This generally requires considerable effort and resources. Part of the exposure assessment process in environmental epidemiology is to optimize the exposure estimate with the aim of detecting a possible risk and/or optimizing the exposure–response relation in an epidemiological study. This can be achieved, for example, by optimizing the distribution of the variance of the exposure estimates. The main focus of this chapter is on chemical and biological substances, but the underlying principles will apply to other exposures as well.

Although the main focus is on environmental exposure assessment and epidemiology, we will also touch on occupational exposure assessment and epidemiology, which examines associations between work place exposure and disease, because the underlying principles and methods used are often very similar. Time and location (space) play an important role. The boundaries also become less clear when the exposure of interest occurs both in the environment and in the work place and through other pathways (e.g., mercury exposure for a subject with amalgam fillings working in a chloralkali plant, living in the vicinity of the plant, and eating fish). Traditionally exposure levels in the work place tended to be higher than in the general environment and the duration of exposure was generally shorter (approximately 8 hours per day vs. up to 24 hours per day). The higher exposure levels were often easier to measure than the lower environmental levels, and the work place provided a more defined environment in time and space than the general environment. In the work place the populations of interest are adults, whereas outside the work place there are also other (susceptible) groups such as children and the elderly with, for example, different behavioral patterns. Work place populations tend to be healthier than the general population. Finally, a number of those involved in occupational exposure assessment and epidemiology have moved to environmental exposure assessment and epidemiology or are involved in both.

1.2 EPIDEMIOLOGICAL STUDIES, DESIGNS, AND NEED FOR EXPOSURE INDICES

A major aim of environmental epidemiological studies is to determine if there is an association or not between a particular substance of interest, the exposure, and morbidity and/or mortality. If there is an association, it is desirable to be able to show an exposure (or dose)–response relationship, that is, a relationship in which the rate of disease increases as the level of exposure (or dose) increases. This will aid in the interpretation of such studies.

In recent years there has been increasing interest in the field of exposure assessment, causing it to develop rapidly. We know now more than ever to what, where, and how people are exposed, and improvements have been made to methods for assessing the level of exposure, its variability, and the determinants. New methods have been developed or newly applied throughout this field, including analytical, measurement, modeling, and statistical methods. The use of geographical information systems (GIS) for assessment of outdoor pollutants/factors has been essential. The use of remote sensing, personal sensors, and OMICS technologies is being explored to improve exposure assessment, and the concept of the exposome is re-energizing the field (see later). This all has led to a considerable improvement in exposure assessment in epidemiological studies, and therefore improvement in the epidemiological studies themselves.

In environmental epidemiology there are different study designs to assess the association between exposure and disease. The main study designs to obtain exposure–response relationships are as follows.

1. *Cohort study*, in which a group (i.e., cohort) of subjects are followed up over time to assess whether they develop the disease of interest or not. The subjects are classified by the level of exposure (e.g., yes/no, low, medium, and high) at entry to the study, but may be reclassified at a later stage. A risk estimate (e.g., relative risk or incidence rate ratio) is obtained by comparing the disease rate in subpopulations with different levels of exposure or external controls. The study can be prospective, that is, a cohort is assembled and followed up in the future, or retrospective, that is, the assembly date of the cohort and follow up was in the past. Prospective cohort studies have the advantage that the exposure can

be determined at the time of field work. Retrospective cohort studies require a reconstruction of historical exposure. They may need to go far back in time for diseases with a long latency time, which may make exposure assessment more difficult (see chapters 7).

2. *Cross-sectional study*, where at one point in time in a population subjects are classified by different levels of exposure (e.g., yes/no, none, low, medium, and high) and the frequency of disease is assessed for each level of exposure. A risk estimate (e.g., prevalence ratio) is obtained by comparing the disease frequencies in subpopulations with different levels of exposure or external controls.

3. *Case–control study*, in which the exposure of diseased subjects (cases) is compared with the exposure of (randomly selected) controls from the underlying sampling population. A risk estimate (e.g., odds ratio) is obtained by dividing the odds of exposure (in the past) for the cases by the odds of exposure (in the past) in the controls. A reconstruction of historical exposure may be required, going far back in time for diseases with a long latency time, which is often challenging. Recall bias, that is, bias in which cases are more likely to recall exposure in the past compared with controls, may be a particular problem. A case–control study could be nested within a cohort study, thereby reducing the effort required for the exposure assessment, given the smaller number of subjects, or improving the exposure assessment if the same effort is maintained, but for fewer subjects than in the full cohort.

4. *Time series study*, in which the day-to-day variability in exposure levels is correlated to the day-to-day variability in disease rate. Recently this approach has frequently been used in temperature and air pollution research, in which measurements from ambient air pollution monitoring stations have been linked to daily morbidity and mortality data. A specific issue is how well the ambient monitoring station results reflect the personal exposure of subjects in the population (see chapters 12 and 13).

Other study designs that have been used include case studies, ecological studies, and panel studies, but they are not discussed further.

All the study designs require exposure estimates or exposure indices to estimate the risk associated with the substance of interest, but they may differ depending on the study design. The design and interpretation of epidemiological studies are often dependent on the exposure assessment and therefore need careful consideration. Quantification of the relation between exposure and adverse human health effects requires the use of exposure estimates that are accurate, precise, and biologically relevant for the critical exposure period, and show a range of exposure levels in the population under study. Furthermore, there is also a general need for the assessment of confounders, that is, substances associated with both exposure and disease that may bias the study results. Assessment of confounders should be in as much detail as the assessment of exposure indices because measurement error in confounders may also affect the health risk estimates (see chapter 10).

1.3 SOURCE–RECEPTOR MODELS AND EXPOSURE ROUTE AND PATHWAYS

The physical course a pollutant takes from the source to a subject is often referred to as *exposure pathway*, whereas the way a substance enters the body is often referred to as *exposure route*. Source–receptor models include the routes and pathways of exposure and are helpful in understanding how people are exposed. In this kind of model it often becomes clear that humans create their own exposure by, for example, their activities and where they spend time, and that there is an interaction between the two. Figure 1.1 provides an example of a source–receptor model for air pollution. The source may be cars and air pollutants such as particles, carbon monoxide, and nitrogen dioxide, that are emitted from exhaust pipes. Dispersion will take place into the streets and beyond, leading to environmental concentrations. Dispersion takes place into so-called "micro-environments" such as houses, travel routes and modes, and work places where people come into contact with the pollutants and is now referred to as *exposure*. People will inhale the pollutants through the lungs, leading to whole-body uptake (dose), where it may react with the lung cells or it may be distributed to other parts of the body and may react with body tissue (biologically relevant dose). The reaction with the body tissue may have an impact on health.

In this case there is only one exposure route (inhalation). There are, however, three possible exposure routes for substances:

1. Inhalation through the respiratory system
2. Ingestion through the gastrointestinal system
3. Absorption through the skin

The exposure route(s) of a substance and the amount of uptake depends on, for example, the biological, chemical, and physical characteristics of the substances, location and activity of the person, and the persons themselves. Inhalation of particles through the respiratory system depends on the particle size or diameter (physical characteristic). Smaller particles are more often inhaled and penetrate deeper into the lungs. The inhalable dust fraction (particles with 50% cut-off diameter of

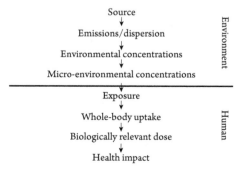

Figure 1.1 Source–receptor model for air pollutants.

100 μm) is the fraction of the dust that enters the nose and mouth and is deposited anywhere in the respiratory tract. The thoracic fraction (particles with a 50% cut-off diameter of 10 μm), often referred to as PM_{10}, is the fraction that enters the thorax and is deposited within the lung airways and the gas-exchange region. The alveolar fraction (particles with a 50% cut-off diameter of 2.5 μm), often referred to as $PM_{2.5}$, is deposited in the gas-exchange region (alveoli). The smallest fraction is ultrafine particulate, fraction which has a diameter of less than 100 nm. Furthermore, inhalation depends on the breathing rate of the subject: those doing heavy work may inhale much more air and more deeply (20 l/min for light physical activity versus 60 l/min for heavy physical activity) (activity of person). And, people move through different micro-environments with different particle concentrations (location).

Skin absorption can play an important role for uptake of substances such as solvents, pesticides, and trihalomethanes (see chapter 9). The volatile trihalomethanes are formed when water is chlorinated and the chlorine reacts with organic matter in the water. In this context there are a number of possible exposure pathways and routes (Fig. 1.2). The main pathway of ingestion is drinking tap water or tap water–based drinks (e.g., tea, coffee). Swimming, showering, bathing, and dish washing may all result in considerable uptake through inhalation and skin absorption and, for the former three, ingestion to a minor extent. Standing or flushing water in the toilet may lead to uptake via inhalation through volatilization of the trihalomethanes. The uptake of trihalomethanes may be assessed using the concentration measured in exhaled breath or serum (see chapters 16).

In the human body, the uptake, distribution, transformation, and excretion of substances such as trihalomethanes can be modeled using physiologically based pharmicokinetic (PBPK) models (see chapter 8). These models are becoming more sophisticated, although they are still rarely used in environmental epidemiology. They can be used to estimate the contribution of various exposure pathways and routes to the total uptake and model the dose of a specific target organ. For example, whereas trihalomethanes through ingestion may mostly be metabolized rapidly in the liver and not appear in blood, uptake through inhalation and skin increases the blood levels substantially. Furthermore, metabolic polymorphism may lead to different dose estimates under similar exposure conditions and this can also be

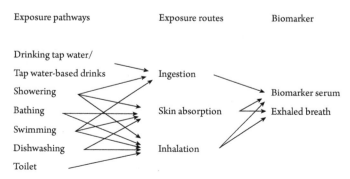

Figure 1.2 Examples of exposure pathways, routes, and biomarkers for trihalomethanes.

modeled. For a number of agents the level of external environmental exposure may either be reduced or increased depending on the capacity of Phase I (activation), Phase II (detoxification), and DNA-repair enzymes. In this approach genetic susceptibility markers (e.g., CYP1A1, CYP2E1, NAT1, NAT2, GSTM1, GSTT1, DNA repair capacity) are used as if they were internal personal protective equipment. For example, low capacity of activation enzymes (e.g., CYP1A1) and high capacity of detoxification (e.g., NAT2) and DNA repair enzymes would have higher protective functions than high capacity of activation enzymes and low capacity of detoxification and DNA repair enzymes, which may result in reducing cancer-causing doses of xenobiotics (Vineis, 1999).

1.4 EXPOSURE DIMENSIONS

Besides the actual nature of the exposure there are also three dimensions:

1. Duration (e.g., in hours or days)
2. Concentration (e.g., in mg/m^{-3} in air or mg/l^{-1} in water)
3. Frequency (e.g., times per week)

In the case of exposure through ingestion the dimensions are concentration, amount (e.g., litres), and frequency. Any of these can not only be used as an exposure index in an epidemiological study, but they can also be combined to obtain a new exposure index, for example, by multiplying duration and concentration to obtain an index of cumulative exposure. The choice of index depends on the health effect of interest. For substances that cause acute effects such as ammonia (irritation), the short-term concentration is generally the most relevant exposure index, whereas for substances that cause chronic effects such as asbestos (cancer), long-term exposure indices such as cumulative exposure may be a more appropriate exposure index. However, it is rarely used in environmental epidemiology, but mainly in occupational epidemiology.

For example, Hughes et al. (2001) carried out a nested case–control study to study the relationship between exposure to silica and the chronic disease silicosis in nine North American industrial sand plants. They found little association between

Table 1.1 The relationship between various silica exposure indices and silicosis in nine North American industrial sand plants

Employment duration (years)		Exposure concentration ($\mu g\,m^{-3}$)		Cumulative exposures ($\mu g\,m^{-3} \times years$)	
Index	Odds ratio	Index	Odds ratio	Index	Odds ratio
<16	1.0	≤100	1.0	≤700	1.0
16–22	1.0	>100	2.4	700 to ≤1800	2.5
22–27	0.7			>1800–5100	4.6
>27	2.6			>5100	5.2

employment duration (as proxy for exposure duration) and silicosis, some association between the concentration of silica and silicosis, but a strong association between cumulative exposure to silica and silicosis with a clear exposure–response relationship (Table 1.1).

1.5 EXPOSURE LEVEL AND VARIABILITY

The concentration of exposure varies temporally and spatially. Figure 1.3 provides the exposure levels of $PM_{2.5}$ (particulate matter with a 50% cut-off diameter of 2.5 μm), expressed as the number of particles, in a house during one day. Peak exposure levels, that is, exposure levels considerably higher than the overall average, are caused by someone smoking in the house. Furthermore, the measurements show that, although there appears to be a very good correlation between the $PM_{2.5}$ levels in the kitchen and the living room, the actual levels differ.

Exposure data often show a lognormal distribution, that is, the distribution of the measured or model data is skewed to the right. Figure 1.4 provides an example of the distribution of approximately 50 personal exposure measurements of $PM_{2.5}$. On the y-axis the number of measurements is shown and the x-axis shows the $PM_{2.5}$ concentration. As can be seen, the distribution is skewed to the right. Statistical tests can be carried out to assess if this is a lognormal distribution (e.g., Kolmogorov–Smirnov or Shapiro–Wilk tests).

The central tendency (i.e., the peak of the distribution) of a lognormal distribution is generally described by the geometric mean (GM), whereas the variability is described by the geometric standard deviation (GSD). They can be calculated as follows:

$$\mu = \frac{\Sigma \ln x}{n}, \quad \sigma^2 = \frac{\Sigma(\ln x - \ln \bar{x})^2}{n-1},$$
$$GM = \exp\mu, \quad GSD = \exp\sigma,$$
$$\text{Arithmetic Mean} = \frac{\Sigma x}{n}$$

where x is the concentration of the substance in a sample, n the number of samples, Σ the sum, ln the natural logarithm, μ the average of log transformed measurements, and σ^2 is the variance of log transformed measurements. The arithmetic mean (AM) provides the average of the exposure measurement. Besides the AM, GM, and GSD, the range, minimum, maximum, or 95% confidence intervals are also often reported.

The GM and GSD change with monitoring time, in contrast to the AM, which should be fixed, and approaches have been described to make them comparable for different monitoring times (Spear et al. 1986; Kumagai and Matsunaga 1994). The AM is commonly used to calculate an index of cumulative exposure (exposure intensity × exposure duration), although sometimes the GM is also used. The choice may depend on the shape of the exposure–response relationship as Seixas

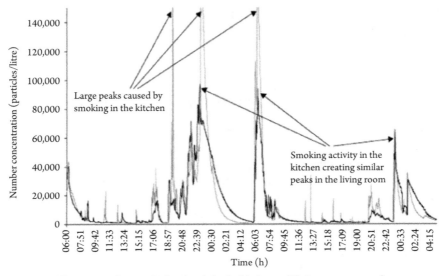

Figure 1.3 Variation in fine particulate levels in the kitchen and living room over a day.

et al. (1988) reported. They suggested that when adopting a linear exposure model, the AM is the appropriate measure. In other models, such as the linear-log (outcome proportional to logarithm of exposure), the GM would be more appropriate.

Where exposure concentrations are low, the amount of agent collected by the air monitor may be insufficient, not allowing detection by the laboratory analysis method; in other words, the exposure may be below the limit of detection (LOD) and the data are termed *censored* data. However, statistical analyses require that a number be assigned to these censored values. For accurate estimation of the mean and standard deviation, Hornung and Reed (1990) suggest using $LOD/\sqrt{2}$

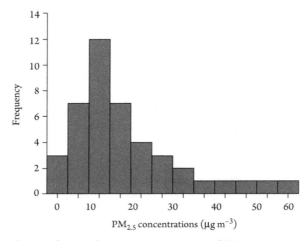

Figure 1.4 Distribution of personal exposure measurements of $PM_{2.5}$.

when data are not highly skewed, and LOD/2 when data are highly skewed (GSD approximately >3). Perkins et al. (1990) described a technique that uses the mean and standard deviation of the quantitated values and the number of censored values, in conjunction with a table to obtain the overall mean and standard deviation. Measurements below the detection limit can also be modeled by assigning a distribution to measurements between 0 and the detection limit and randomly assigning a value of this distribution to a value under the detection limit or by multiple imputation, all of which can influence the extent of bias that can be observed (Lubin et al. 2004).

Exposure generally varies from day to day for any given subject and from subject to subject, often referred to as the *within* and *between subject exposure variability*, respectively. The within and between subject variability can be estimated when repeated exposure measurements have been obtained using analysis of variance models (see chapter 5). Besides variability caused by subjects, there may be other determinants of exposure such as physical or meteorological conditions and these need to be identified to get a better understanding of what is causing the variability in exposure. (This is discussed further in chapters 5 and 13).

1.6 ECOLOGICAL VERSUS INDIVIDUAL EXPOSURE ESTIMATES

To obtain exposure estimate(s) for a population in an epidemiological study, two main approaches are available: (a) individual and (b) exposure grouping (Fig 1.5). In the first, exposure estimates are obtained at the individual level; for example, every member of the population is monitored either once or repeatedly. Information on individuals is gathered through a questionnaire (e.g., Environmental Tobacco Smoke (ETS), gas cooking, mold and damp) (Esplugues et al. 2013, Gehring et al. 2013), biological monitoring (e.g., PCBs, phthalates, phenols, metals) (Govarts et al. 2012; Llop et al. 2012; Gehring et al. 2013; Christensen et al. 2014), and smartphones and sensors (physical activity, air pollution, location) (de Nazelle et al. 2013; Nieuwenhuijsen et al. 2014) and estimates directly assigned to the subjects. In the second approach, the population is first split into smaller subpopulations, or more often referred to as exposure groups, based on specific determinants of exposure, and group or ecological exposure estimates are obtained for each exposure group. This approach is often used for outdoor exposures such as air pollution, noise, temperature, and green space. Geographical information systems (GIS) (see chapter 4) are used to allocate subjects, often their residences, and then assign exposure estimates based on routine monitoring stations (Wilhelm and Ritz 2005, Samoli et al. 2008), models (Beelen et al. 2014), land use characteristics such as green space (Dadvand et al. 2014) or remote sensing data (Kloog et al. 2012, Dadvand et al. 2014). More recently individual estimates for the residence are given (Beelen et al. 2014; see chapter 13) and used as an exposure index. In environmental epidemiological studies, exposure groups may be defined, for example, on the basis of distance from an exposure source (e.g., roads, factories, park). The underlying assumption is that

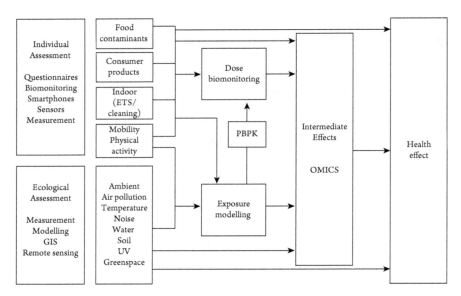

Figure 1.5 Individual versus ecological assessments.

subjects within each exposure group experience similar exposure characteristics, including exposure levels and variation. Exposure estimates can be assigned to the groups, for example, data from ambient air pollution monitors in the area in which the subjects live, or a model to predict the exposure. Alternatively, a representative sample of members from each exposure group can be personally monitored, either once or repeatedly. If the aim is to estimate mean exposure, the average of the exposure measurements is then assigned to all the members in that particular exposure group. However, this type of approach is generally not used in environmental epidemiology. Ecological and individual estimates can be combined, for example, in the case of chlorination by-products wherein routinely collected trihalomethane measurements providing ecological estimates are combined with individual estimates on actual ingestion, showering, and bathing (see chapter 16).

Intuitively, it is expected that the individual estimates provide the best exposure estimates for an epidemiological study. This is not often true, however, because of the variability in exposure and the limited number of samples. In general, in epidemiological studies individual estimates lead to attenuated, though more precise, health risk estimates than ecological estimates. The ecological estimates, in contrast, result in less attenuation of the risk estimates, albeit less precise. These differences can be explained by the classical and the Berkson-type error models (see chapter 10). The between-group, between-subject, and within-subject variance can be estimated using analysis of variance models (see chapter 5) and this information can be used to optimize the exposure–response relationship, for example, by changing the distribution of exposure groups as has been demonstrated in occupational epidemiological studies (Kromhout and Heederik 1995; Nieuwenhuijsen 1997; van Tongeren et al. 1997). In this case the aim is to increase the contrast in exposure between exposure groups, expressed as the ratio between the between-group variance and the sum of the between- and within-group variance, while maintaining reasonably precise exposure estimates of the groups (see chapter 5).

1.7 EXPOSURE CLASSIFICATION, MEASUREMENT, OR MODELING

Exposure can be classified, measured, or modeled and different tools are available for this, such as questionnaires, air pollution monitors, and statistical techniques, respectively. The methods are often classified as direct and indirect (Fig. 1.6).

The main aim of an exposure assessment is to obtain accurate, precise, and biologically relevant exposure estimates in the most efficient and cost-effective way. The cost of the exposure assessment increases with an increase in the accuracy and precision, and therefore the assessment is often a balancing act with cost on one side and accuracy and precision on the other (Armstrong 1996). The choice of a particular method depends on the aim of the study and, more often, on the financial resources available. Misclassification of the exposure can lead to attenuation in health risk estimates or loss of power in the epidemiological study, depending on the type of measurement error model (classical or Berkson), and should therefore be minimized (see chapter 10).

Subjects in an epidemiological study can be classified based on a particular substance and on an ordinal scale, for example, as exposed:

- Yes/no
- No, low, medium, high

This can be achieved, for example, by:

1. Expert assessment: For example, a member of the research team decides, based on prior knowledge, whether the subject in the study is exposed or unexposed, for example, lives in an area with highly contaminated soil or not.
2. Self-assessment by questionnaire, that is, the subject in the study is asked to fill out a questionnaire in which he or she is asked about a particular substance, for example, pesticides. Questionnaires are often used to ask a subject if she or he is exposed to a particular substance and also to estimate the duration of exposure.

Questionnaires can be used not only to ask the subject to estimate the duration of their exposure but also to obtain information related to the exposure, such as where people spent their time (time micro-environment diaries), work history including the jobs and tasks they carried out, what they eat and drink, and where they live (see chapter 2). These variables could be used as exposure indices in the epidemiological studies or translated into a new exposure index, for example, by multiplying the amount of tap water people drink and the contaminant level in the tap water to

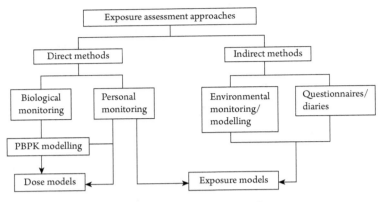

Figure 1.6 Different approaches to human exposure assessment.

obtain the total ingested amount of the substance. When used on their own they are often referred to as *exposure surrogates*.

Expert and self-assessment methods are generally the easiest and cheapest, but can suffer due to the lack of objectivity and knowledge and may therefore bias exposure assessment. Both experts and subjects may not know exactly what the subjects are exposed to or at what level and therefore may misclassify the exposure, whereas diseased subjects may recall certain substances better than subjects without disease (recall bias) and cause differential misclassification leading to biased health risk estimates (see chapter 10).

A more objective way to assess exposure, particularly concentration, is through measurement. Some examples:

1. Levels of outdoor air pollution can be measured by stationary ambient air monitors (i.e., ambient or environmental air monitoring). These monitors are placed in an area and they measure the particular substance of interest in this area. Subjects living within this area are considered to be exposed to the concentrations measured by the monitoring station. This may or may not be true depending on, for example, where the subject in the study lives, works, or travels. The advantage of this method is that it could provide a range of exposure estimates for a large population (see chapters 3, 4, and 12).

2. Levels of air pollution can be measured by personal exposure monitors or sensors (i.e., personal exposure monitoring). These monitors are lightweight devices that are worn by the subject in the study. They are often used in occupational epidemiological studies and are being used with increasing frequency in environmental epidemiological studies too. The advantage of this method is that it is likely to estimate the subject's exposure better than, for example, ambient air monitoring. The disadvantage is that it is often labor intensive and expensive (see chapter 5).

3. Levels of water pollutants and soil contaminants can be estimated by taking water and soil samples, respectively, and analyzing these for substance of interest in the laboratory. Often these need to be combined with behavioral factors such

as water intake, contaminated food intake, or hand-to-mouth contact to obtain a level of exposure.
4. Uptake levels of the substance into the body can be estimated by biomonitoring. Biomonitoring consists of taking biological samples such as urine, exhaled breath, hair, adipose tissue, or nails, for example, for the measurement of lead in serum. The samples are subsequently analyzed for the substance of interest itself or for a metabolite in a laboratory. Biomonitoring is expected to estimate the actual uptake (dose) of the substance of interest rather than the exposure (see chapter 6).

The measurement of exposure is generally expansive, particularly for large populations. Modeling of exposure can be carried out preferably in conjunction with exposure measurements either to help build a model and/or to validate a model. It is particularly important that the model estimates be validated.

Modeling can be divided into:

1. *Deterministic modeling* (i.e., physical) in which the models describe the relationship between variables mathematically on the basis of knowledge of the physical, chemical, and/or biological mechanisms governing these relationships (Brunekreef 1999). A deterministic model would be one in which indoor air particle concentrations are explained by including in the modeling, for example, the sources, volume of rooms, air exchange rate, and settling velocity of the particles (see chapter 3).
2. *Stochastic modeling* (i.e. statistical) in which the statistical relationships are modeled between variables. These models do not necessarily require fundamental knowledge of the underlying physical, chemical, and/or biological relationships between the variables. An example is the relation between land use characteristics such as road network, traffic density, altitude, population density, and green space and ambient air pollution levels, which is modeled using statistical regression techniques and a dataset of measurements (see chapter 13) and is often referred to as land use regression (LUR) modeling. Use of LUR modeling has recently gained strong interest in air pollution epidemiology because it is relatively cheap and provides air pollution estimates for many subjects.

It is extremely important to validate the modeled estimates and this is often not a trivial exercise; it requires substantial thought and resources but greatly increases the validity of the study (see chapter 13).

All these different approaches are not exclusive and often are combined to obtain the best exposure index. This involves some form of modeling. At times it may be difficult or impossible to measure the exposure to the actual substance of interest and therefore exposure to an "exposure surrogate" is estimated. This is often the case in environmental epidemiology, in which sample sizes may be large. It is important that the surrogate marker is as closely correlated as possible to the actual substance of interest. For example, the presence of a gas cooker or electric cooker could be a surrogate for the exposure to nitrogen dioxide (yes/no exposure). Living distance from a factory could be a surrogate for the emission of pollutants from the factory. However, there is some uncertainty in these cases regarding actual exposure; for example, the gas cooker may not actually be used often or the subject is out of the house while cooking takes place and therefore there should be some validation.

Figure 1.7 provides an overall view of the exposure assessment approaches that were most often used in environmental epidemiological research of birth cohorts in Europe (Gehring et al. 2013). Europe has more than 35 birth cohorts that examine the relationship between a range of environmental exposures and outcomes such as birth outcomes, growth/obesity, respiratory health, and cognitive development (Vrijheid et al. 2012).

A related issue is that people are often exposed to a number of pollutants simultaneously (a mixture), for example, to pesticides, solvents, air pollution, and disinfection by-products, although the levels may differ. Because not all the substances can be measured, a surrogate measure or exposure marker is chosen, for example, in the case of chlorination by-products in drinking water wherein trihalomethanes were used as a surrogate for other by-products (see chapter 16). Mixtures of exposure may cause problems in the epidemiological analysis, for example, when the effects of different pollutants need to be disentangled. A possible way around this is to choose study sites where the exposure levels of the individual pollutants in the exposure mixture differ substantially and where there is a gradient of exposure.

More recently to get away from studying one-exposure, one-health outcome associations, a new paradigm has been developed, the exposome (see chapter 14). The exposome encompasses the totality of human environmental (i.e., nongenetic) exposures from conception onwards, complementing the genome (Wild 2005; 2012). The exposome is composed of every exposure to which an individual is subjected from conception to death. Therefore, it requires consideration of both the nature of those exposures and their changes over time. For ease of description, three broad categories of nongenetic exposures may be considered: internal, specific external, and general external. First, the exposome comprises processes internal to the body such as metabolism, endogenous circulating hormones, body morphology, physical activity, gut microflora, inflammation, lipid peroxidation, oxidative stress, and aging. These internal conditions will all impinge on the cellular environment and have been variously described as host or endogenous factors. Second, there is the extensive range of specific external exposures, which include radiation, infectious agents, chemical contaminants and environmental pollutants, diet, lifestyle factors (e.g. tobacco, alcohol), occupation, and medical interventions. In the past these have been the main focus of epidemiological studies seeking to link environmental risk factors with cancer. Third, the exposome includes the wider social, economic, and psychological influences on the individual, for example: social capital, education, financial status, psychological and mental stress, urban–rural environment, and climate (Wild 2012). The dynamic nature of the exposome presents one of the most challenging features of its characterization. As a consequence, its myriad components need to be considered in relation to their temporal variation. In effect, at any given point in time, an individual will have a particular profile of

Topic	Biomonitoring	Measurements	Modelling	Questionnaire
Outdoor air pollution				
Water contamination				
Allergens & biological organisms				
Heavy metals				
Pesticides				
Persistent organic pollutants				
Emerging exposures				
Radiations				
Smoking and ETS				
Noise				
Occupation				

Figure 1.7 Predominant type of exposure assessment by exposure topic in European birth cohorts.

exposures. Therefore, to fully characterize an individual's exposome would require either sequential measures that spanned a lifetime, or a smaller number of measures that captured exposure over a series of extended periods (Wild 2012). Only because of the increase in new technologies including GIS, sensors, remote sensing, OMICS technologies, combined with more traditional approaches has it become possible to start assessing the exposome, and first attempts are being made in large European projects such as HELIX (Vrijheid et al. 2014), EXPOsOMICs, and HEALS.

1.8 VALIDATION STUDIES

In epidemiological studies, it is often not possible to obtain detailed exposure information on each subject in the study. For example, in a large cohort study it is not feasible to take measurements from each subject and administer a detailed exposure questionnaire. In this case it is desirable to carry out a small validation study on a representative subset of the larger population. Ideally this will be carried out before the main study begins and can utilize information from the literature. Questions in the questionnaire could be validated with measurements (see chapter 2) and some exposure models could be constructed (see chapter 5). The exposure assessment in the whole population could focus on key questions that have a major influence on the exposure estimates and thereby reduce the length of the questionnaire. Information on key determinants will also provide a better understanding of the exposure and how it may affect exposure–response relationships in epidemiological studies. Besides the validity, the reproducibility or reliability of various tools also can be evaluated in a subsample.

1.9 RETROSPECTIVE EXPOSURE ASSESSMENT

In epidemiological studies, when studying diseases with a long latency time, for example, cancer, it is not the current exposure that is of most interest for the study, but that in the past. A reconstruction of historical exposure is often referred to as *retrospective exposure assessment*. In occupational epidemiology, retrospective exposure assessment has a long tradition but less so in environmental epidemiology. An example is the study by Bellander et al. 2001 in Stockholm in which they modeled the exposure to a number of air pollutants coming from traffic and heating and then assigned them to the subject. Retrospective exposure assessment is often difficult because there are usually many changes over time, for example, changes in residences, in technologies of the pollution sources, and also changes in people's behavior (see e.g., chapters 2 and 16).

1.10 QUALITY CONTROL ISSUES

A well-designed and well-planned strategy carried out by well-trained personnel is essential for a successful exposure assessment. Issues such as cost, feasibility, accuracy, precision, validity, sample size, power, sensitivity, specificity, robustness, and reproducibility always need to be addressed (e.g., during sampling, storage, analysis) (Box 1.1), whereas feasibility and pilot studies need to take place before the actual study. Any form of bias (e.g., bias in sampling, selection, participation, monitoring, information, measurement error, exposure misclassification) should be avoided whenever possible, or if it cannot be avoided, should be well described.

Clear protocols for sampling, storage, and analysis, including quality control, should be written and available at any time and researchers in the study should be properly trained. Potential sources of bias should be addressed at every stage.

Control measurements, for example, filters that are not exposed but are otherwise treated as exposed filters, should be included (5%–10% of total samples), particularly when measurements are close to the detection limit.

Samplers can measure with differing accuracy, for example, over or under sampling the true level, and this should be addressed when different samplers are used in order to reduce or avoid bias. This can be done easily by comparative sampling, with adjustments for any difference observed.

Monitors and laboratory techniques measure with differing precision. Precision can be represented by the coefficient of variation (CV) and contributes toward the total variability observed in the measured exposure levels. However, this contribution is small compared to the environmental variability caused by factors such as differences in working practices and environmental conditions. An analysis by Nicas et al. (1991) suggests that the CV is in general 15% and that the GSD of the lognormal day-to-day environmental variability is in general 1.5, in which case the analytical variability contributes not more than 13% to the total variability observed in measuring a worker's shift-average exposure level. The greater the environmental variability, the less the collection and analytical variability contributes toward the total variability. Even CVs of around 25% contribute less than 20% to total variability as long as the GSD of environmental variability is larger than approximately 1.8.

1.11 CONCLUSION

This chapter provides a brief overview of the basic issues in the exposure assessment of environmental epidemiological studies. In the following chapters many

---

Box 1.1 Terminology used in measurement issues

Accuracy: The degree to which a measurement or an estimate represents the true value of what is being measured

Bias: Deviation of results or inferences from the truth, or processes leading to such deviation; any trend in the design, collection, analysis, interpretation, publication, or review of data that can lead to conclusions that are systematically different from the truth

Limit of detection (LOD): The minimum concentration of an analyte, in a given matrix and with a specific method, that statistically is significantly greater than zero, that is, the lowest concentration that can be measured with a certain degree of confidence

Precision: The degree of variability in a measurement or estimate, estimated, for example, by the standard error of measurements or the standard deviation in a series of replicate measurements

Power: The ability of a study to demonstrate statistically significant effects, which is determined by a number of factors including study design, magnitude of effect, and sample size

Reliability: The degree of stability exhibited when a measurement is repeated under identical conditions, that is, the degree to which the results obtained by measurement procedure can be replicated

Reproducibility/repeatability: A test or measurement is repeatable if the results are identical or closely similar each time it is conducted.

Robustness: A procedure is said to be robust if it is not very sensitive to departures from assumptions or variations in the conditions or practices under which it was set up.

Sensitivity: Is an index of the performance of a diagnostic tool, for example, for questionnaires: the proportion of truly exposed people in the population who are identified as exposed by the questionnaire. For measurement or analysis of exposure it refers to the response of the detector to a unit of analyte; the more sensitive, the more response, and hence a better detection limit.

Specificity: An index of the performance of a diagnostic tool, for example, for questionnaires: the proportion of truly nonexposed people in the population who are identified as nonexposed by the questionnaire. For measurement or analysis of exposure, it refers to the response of the detector to a particular analyte, that is, whether only the substance of interest is measured or also other substances.

Validity: An expression of the degree to which a measurement measures what it purports to measure

Source: Adapted from Last (1995).

---

are discussed in much greater detail. The focus is initially on some of the main methods and tools of exposure assessment, followed by newer tools such as PBPK modeling, which has rarely been used in this field but may provide a further refinement. The consequences of exposure misclassification and measurement error for epidemiological are discussed in great detail to show the importance of good exposure assessment and approaches to optimize it and the interpretation of epidemiological studies. The second section of the book discusses the more recent developments and research questions in exposure assessment of biological exposures, particulate matter, water contaminants, and radiofrequencies, and methods such as land use regression modeling, exposome research, and sensoring, including the consequences for and results of some epidemiological studies. These chapters show the great diversity and different levels of exposure assessment, but also the many commonalities. The following chapters attempt to describe the current status of the field, but are not meant to be exhaustive. They encourage the reader to think of how to improve exposure assessments. Exposure assessment is a relatively new field and further developments and refinements are still needed.

REFERENCES

Armstrong, B. (1996). Optimizing power in allocating resources to exposure assessment in an epidemiologic study. *American Journal of Epidemiology*, **144**, 192–197.

Beelen, R., Raaschou-Nielsen, O., Stafoggia, M., Andersen, Z. J., Weinmayr, G., Hoffmann, B., et al. (2014). Effects of long-term exposure to air pollution on natural-cause mortality: an analysis of 22 European cohorts within the multicentre ESCAPE project. *Lancet*, **383**, 785–795.

Bellander, T., Berglind, N., Gustavsson, P., Jonson, T., Nyberg, F., Pershagen, G., and Järup, L. (2001). Using geographic information systems to assess individual historical exposure to air pollution from traffic and house heating in Stockholm. *Environmental Health Perspectives*, **109**, 633–639.

Brunekreef, B. (1999). Exposure assessment. In *Environmental epidemiology: A text book on study methods and public health applications* (preliminary ed.). WHO, Geneva.

Christensen, K., Sobus, J., Phillips, M., Blessinger, T., Lorber, M., and Tan, Y. M. (2014). Changes in epidemiologic associations with different exposure metrics: A case study of phthalate exposure associations with body mass index and waist circumference. *Environment International*, **73C**, 66–76.

Dadvand, P., Wright, J., Martinez, D., Basagaña, X., McEachan, R. R., Cirach, M., et al. (2014). Inequality, green spaces, and pregnant women: Roles of ethnicity and individual and neighbourhood socioeconomic status. *Environment International*, **71**, 101–108.

De Nazelle, A., Seto, E., Donaire-Gonzalez, D., Mendez, M., Matamala, J., Rodriguez, D., et al. (2013). Improving estimates of air pollution exposure through ubiquitous sensing technologies. *Environmental Pollution*, **176**, 92–99.

Esplugues, A., Estarlich, M., Sunyer, J., Fuentes-Leonarte, V., Basterrechea, M., Vrijheid, M., et al. (2013). Prenatal exposure to cooking gas and respiratory health in infants is modified by tobacco smoke exposure and diet in the INMA birth cohort study. *Environmental Health Health*, **12**, 100.

Gehring, U., Casas, M., Brunekreef, B., Bergström, A., Bonde, J. P., Botton, J., et al. (2013). Environmental exposure assessment in European birth cohorts: Results from the ENRIECO project. *Environmental Health Health*, **12**, 8.

Govarts, E., Nieuwenhuijsen, M., Schoeters, G., Ballester, F., Bloemen, K., de Boer, M., et al.; OBELIX; ENRIECO. (2012). Birth weight and prenatal exposure to polychlorinated biphenyls (PCBs) and dichlorodiphenyldichloroethylene (DDE): A meta-analysis within 12 European Birth Cohorts. *Environmental Health Perspectives*, **120**, 162–170.

Hornung, R. W., and Reed, L. D. (1990). Estimation of average concentration in the presence of non detectable values. *Applied Occupational and Environmental Hygiene*, **5**, 46–51.

Hughes, J. M., Weill, H., Randos, R. J., Shi, R., McDonald, A. D., and McDonald, J. C. (2001). Cohort mortality study of North American industrial sand workers. II Case-referent analysis of lung cancer and silicosis deaths. *Annals of Occupational Hygiene*, **45**, 201–207.

Kloog, I., Melly, S. J., Ridgway, W. L., Coull, B. A., and Schwartz, J. (2012). Using new satellite based exposure methods to study the association between pregnancy $PM_{2.5}$ exposure, premature birth and birth weight in Massachusetts. *Environmental Health*, **11**, 40.

Kromhout, H., and Heederik, D. (1995). Occupational epidemiology in the rubber industry: Iimplications of exposure variability. *American Journal of Industrial Medicine*, **27**, 171–185.

Kumagai, S., and Matsunaga, I. (1994). Approaches for estimating the distribution of short-term exposure concentrations for different averaging times. *Annals of Occupational Hygiene*, **38**, 815–825.

Llop, S., Guxens, M., Murcia, M/, Lertxundi, A., Ramon, R., Riaño, I., et al.; INMA Project. (2012). Prenatal exposure to mercury and infant neurodevelopment in a multicenter cohort in Spain: study of potential modifiers. *American Journal of Epidemiology*, **175**, 451–465.

Lubin, J. H., Colt, J. S., Camann, D., Davis, S., Cerhan, J. R., Severson, R. K., Bernstein, L., and Hartge, P. (2004). Epidemiologic evaluation of measurement data in the presence of detection limits. *Environmental Health Perspectives*, **112**, 1691–1696.

Nicas, M., Simmons, B. P., and Spear, R. C. (1991). Environmental versus analytical variability in exposure measurements. *American Industrial Hygiene Association Journal*, **52**, 553–557.

Nieuwenhuijsen, M. J. (1997). Exposure assessment in occupational epidemiology: measuring present exposures with an example of occupational asthma. *International Archives of Occupational and Environmental Health*, **70**, 295–308.

Nieuwenhuijsen, M. J., Donaire-Gonzalez, D., Foraster, M., Martinez, D., and Cisneros, A. (2014). Using Personal Sensors to Assess the Exposome and Acute Health Effect. *International Journal of Environmental Research Public Health*, **11**, 7805–7819.

Perkins, J. L., Cutter, G. N., and Cleveland, M. S. (1990). Estimating the mean, variance and confidence limits from censored (<limit of detection), lognormally distributed exposure data. *American Industrial Hygiene Association Journal*, **51**, 416–419.

Samoli, E., Peng, R., Ramsay, T., Pipikou, M., Touloumi, G., Dominici, F., et al. (2008) Acute effects of ambient particulate matter on mortality in Europe and North America: Results from the APHENA study. *Environmental Health Perspectives*, **116**, 1480–1486.

Seixas, N. S., Robins, T. G., and Moulton, L. H. (1988). The use of geometric and arithmetic mean exposures in occupational epidemiology. *American Journal of Industrial Medicine*, **14**, 465–477.

Spear, R. C., Selvin, S., and Francis, M. (1986). The influence of averaging time on the distribution of exposures. *American Industrial Hygiene Association Journal*, **47**, 365–368.

van Tongeren, M., Gardiner, K., Calvert, I., Kromhout, H., and Harrington, J. M. (1997). Efficiency of different grouping schemes for dust exposure in the European carbon black respiratory morbidity study. *Occupational and Environmental Medicine*, **54**, 714–719.

Vineis, P. (ed.) (1999). *Metabolic polymorphisms and susceptibility*. IARC pub 148. IARC, Lyon, France.

Vrijheid, M., Casas, M., Bergström, A., Carmichael, A., Cordier S, Eggesbø, M., et al. (2012). European birth cohorts for environmental health research. *Environmental Health Perspectives*, **120**, 29–37.

Vrijheid, M., Slama, R., Robinson, O., Chatzi, L., Coen, M., van den Hazel, P., et al. (2014). The human early-life exposome (HELIX): Project rationale and design. *Environmental Health Perspectives*, **122**, 535–544.

Wild, C. P. (2005). Complementing the genome with an "exposome": The outstanding challenge of environmental exposure measurement in molecular epidemiology. *Cancer Epidemiology, Biomarkers & Prevention*, **14**, 1847–1850.

Wild, C. P. (2012). The exposome: From concept to utility. *International Journal of Epidemioiology*, **41**, 24–32.

Wilhelm, M., Ritz, B. (2005). Local variations in CO and particulate air pollution and adverse birth outcomes in Los Angeles County, California, USA. *Environmental Health Perspectives*, **113**, 1212–1221.

2

QUESTIONNAIRES

Mark J. Nieuwenhuijsen

2.1 INTRODUCTION

Questionnaires are frequently used in the exposure assessment of environmental epidemiological studies. Questionnaires may be the method of choice for assessing exposure because no other sources of information are available, or because they provide the most efficient study design, allowing a larger study size and greater statistical power than would be possible with other, more accurate measurement techniques. They may be used in combination with other methods, too. Information on presence of exposure (yes/no), duration, frequency, and pattern of exposure is often obtained by questionnaire or, to a much lesser extent, observation. Very few standardized questionnaires that have been validated are available in this area, which is a limitation, and further work needs to done. The design of new questionnaires often depends on the experience acquired with previous questionnaires.

Questionnaires are used and administered in a number of ways to obtain information (see later). At times it may not be possible to obtain information from the subject in the study because of death or disease, for example, Alzheimer's, and it may therefore be necessary to obtain the information from a so-called "proxy respondent" such as relative, friend, or colleague. This may require some modification of the questionnaire, but has been carried out quite successfully (Hansen 1996; Debanne et al. 2001). All the different forms of questionnaires require careful consideration of design and administration issues, including, for example, the length, detail of the required information, logistics, participation and completion rate, and costs involved (White et al. 2008). Questionnaires often tend to be too long and not all the information from the questionnaire is analyzed and/or used in the epidemiological study. One of the main questions the researchers should always ask themselves is "do we really require the answer of this question for our study aims?." If there is no justification for it, the question should be left out. An important issue is that the exposures of interest may have been in the past and subjects may not be able to recall these; this may lead to underreporting (Infante-Rivard and Jacques 2000). Furthermore, lack of understanding of the questions or knowledge of the exposure may bias the reporting. Recall bias, wherein those with disease are more likely to report certain exposures compared with those without disease even though there is no true difference, needs to be avoided and this requires careful consideration of the questions that are asked (Rothman and Greenland 1998).

2.1.1 Self-Administered Questionnaire

The self-administered questionnaire can be used to obtain information on present and past exposure. It is the easiest and cheapest; requires the least involvement from both subject and researcher; and can be handed out, sent to the subjects, or be computer administered (online). When sent out to the subjects it requires a valid address, because otherwise the subject may not receive it leading to a lower response rate. The response and completion rates in this method tend to be somewhat lower compared with other methods (Brogger et al. 2002). Monetary incentives can increase the response rate considerably (Edwards et al. 2002). The response rate can be improved by handing out the questionnaire, for example, for children at schools. Personal contact tends to increase response rates (Edwards et al. 2002). Recorded delivery may improve the response rate considerably, particularly if the subject actually lives at the address (Edwards et al. 2002). Mailed-out questionnaires can be easily discarded or forgotten and often require remailing to obtain a good response rate. The questionnaires cannot be too long because this is likely to lower the response and completion rates (Edwards et al. 2002). The subjects should be able to complete the questionnaire within about 30 to 60 minutes, preferably less. The questions need to be straightforward and easy to answer, otherwise lack of understanding by the subject may result in low completion rate or inappropriate answers. The advantage of a questionnaire is that it gives subjects the time to think about the questions, and if necessary obtain further information from elsewhere.

Finally, although the use of online questionnaires is increasing, there is little research in environmental epidemiology on how efficient they. From other fields there is evidence that web-based questionnaires could replace traditional paper questionnaires, with minor effects on response rates and lower costs (van de Looij-Jansen PM and de Wilde 2008, Hohwü et al. 2013).

2.1.2 Self-Administered Diary

The self-administered diary can be used (repeatedly) to obtain information on present exposures. They have been used frequently to obtain information on food and drink intake (Willett 1998) (Figure 2.1), and to a lesser extent in situations in which people spend their time in the form of micro-environment activity diaries, which are used to obtain information on, for example, exposure to air pollution (Künzli et al. 1997; Jantunen et al. 1998) (Figure 2.2). The collected information has at times been used to represent a much longer period than the actual observation period, and as validation for questionnaires. However, this requires careful interpretation of the data because there may be considerable differences in people's exposure over short periods, for example, differences between weekdays and weekends and seasonal

Date _____

(A) Cooking and washing up

	Duration (min)
Cooking involving boiling water	
Washing up by hand (excl. drying)	
Dishwasher running	

(B) Washing yourself

	Number	Duration (min)	Time spent in bathroom after bath/shower (min)
Shower			
Bath			

(C) Food and drink

	At home	At home/college	Elsewhere
Tap water (glasses)			
Boiled water (glasses)			
Tea (mugs)			
Coffee (mugs)			
Hot chocolate (mugs)			
Plain milk (glasses)			
Squash* (glasses)			

* including drinks made with powders

	At home	At home/college	Elsewhere
Soft drinks** (glasses)			
Beer (glasses)			
Wine (glasses)			
Spirits (glasses)			

** including fruits juices and fizzy drinks

	At home	At home/college	Elsewhere
Soups (bowls/mugs)			

(D) Swimming

	Length of session (min)
Swimming in a pool	

Seven-Day Water Diary

Please complete one page of the diary for each consecutive day of the week, including the weekend. Include ALL drinks and other liquids consumed. Give the required information on activities carried out EACH day. Please try to be as accurate as possible.

If you did not carry out a particular activity or did not consume a particular liquid please put a zero for duration or amount.

Remember to quote liquid consumption using the following guide (or a more precise measure if possible):

A 'glass' like the one pictured below is 200cc (so five glasses equals 1 litre), a mug equals one glass and a bowl equals two glasses.

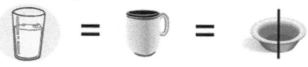

Figure 2.1 A section (introduction and one day) of a 7-day water diary to determine fluid intake, showering, bathing, and swimming among pregnant women.

Date: ______					Location									Activities		
Time		Briefly describe year activities	I am travelling by…					I am currently at…						I am…		Someone is smoking in the same room
			foot/ bike	motor-cycle	car/ taxi	bus	train	home		work		other		cooking	smoking	
								inside	outside	inside	outside	inside	outside			
6	0		○	○	○	○	○	○	○	○	○	○	○	○	○	○
	15		○	○	○	○	○	○	○	○	○	○	○	○	○	○
	30		○	○	○	○	○	○	○	○	○	○	○	○	○	○
	45		○	○	○	○	○	○	○	○	○	○	○	○	○	○
7	0		○	○	○	○	○	○	○	○	○	○	○	○	○	○
	15		○	○	○	○	○	○	○	○	○	○	○	○	○	○
	30		○	○	○	○	○	○	○	○	○	○	○	○	○	○
	45		○	○	○	○	○	○	○	○	○	○	○	○	○	○

Figure 2.2 Time micro-environment activity diary used by the EXPOLIS study.

differences. Further, the issue of the short observation period being representative of a longer period necessitates careful consideration of exposure determinants. The diary data can be used to estimate day-to-day variability within subjects and variability between subjects, and hence attenuation in risk estimates (see chapters 5 and 10) (Shimokora et al. 1998). The diaries need to be short and easy to fill out. The advantage of the diary is that it needs little, if any, recall, particularly if they are filled out as a routine process. Diary data can be combined with measurements to obtain improved exposure estimates. For example, Preller et al. (1995) administered a 14-day diary to pig farmers, in which they recorded their activities and factors related to endotoxin exposure, and measured the endotoxin exposure on two of the days. They used regression analysis to relate the measurements and diary data and build a model, which they then applied to the days without measurements to predict the endotoxin levels for a longer time period. The predicted estimates showed the least attenuated risk estimates when they modeled the relationship between endotoxin exposure and lung function decline (see chapter 5).

2.1.3 Face-to-Face Interview

Questionnaires used in face-to-face interviews have the advantage that an interviewer is present who can explain any question if necessary. Information can be obtained on present and past exposures. The interviewer can explain questions and explore the answers in more detail, if necessary. Particularly for a complex exposure situation, this may be an advantage. It requires a well-trained interviewer, particularly to avoid any interviewer bias and obtain the most relevant information. This method may result in more socially acceptable answers because an interviewer is present, and this needs careful attention. The questionnaire/interview can be of a longer duration than some of the other methods (1–2 hours). The logistics aspect is generally more difficult. Arranging face-to-face interviews at convenient times for both subject and interviewer can be difficult, particularly if they live far apart. Face-to-face interviewing can be very expensive and therefore is not used often in this field.

2.1.4 Telephone Interview

Questionnaires used in telephone interviews have the advantage that subjects can ask the interviewer to explain any question, if necessary. Information can be obtained on present and past exposures. The interviewer can explain questions and explore the answers in more detail, if necessary, although perhaps to a lesser extent than the face-to-face interview. As for the face-to-face interview, it requires a well-trained interviewer, particularly to avoid interviewer bias and obtain the most relevant information. The advantage compared to face-to-face interviews is that they are easier to organize and carry out because no visits are required; further, nowadays most people have a phone, so the costs involved are much lower. Subjects also may provide less socially accepted answers compared to the face-to-face interview. The interview duration needs to be much shorter, around 30 to 45 minutes. Telephone interviews facilitate direct entry into an electronic database, which reduces the time spent on data entry, although it is important to avoid mistakes by incorporating quality control checks. Interviews may need to be taped for quality control purposes. Examples of questions for self-administered, face-to-face, and telephone interviews are given in Figures 2.3 and 2.4.

2.1.5 Observation

Researchers may want to observe subjects to obtain information on exposure-related behavior, for example, the extent of hand-to-mouth contact among children, which may result in uptake of a particular substance (Freeman et al. 2001). The observation needs a questionnaire in the form of a checklist to be used by the researcher. Using a hand-held computer, the information can be linked to other information that is collected simultaneously such as measurement data. Observation is used to obtain information on present exposures. The observation period is thought to be representative of a much longer period when there is no observation, but the validity of this depends under what conditions the observation was carried out, that is, was it carried out under conditions representative of other periods and did the subject behave in the same way. This method may be more accurate and objective than some other methods, but it is also more time consuming and costly. At times it may be the only method to obtain exposure information because the subjects of interest, for example, young children, cannot provide the information by filling out questionnaires. The observation can take place in "real time" or video recordings can be made and analyzed later. The advantage of the method is that it requires little involvement from the subject and there is little problem with recall. However, it cannot be used for all subjects in an epidemiological study, only a subpopulation to obtain information for an exposure model or to validate a model.

2.1.6 Obtaining Information from Records

Researchers may want to obtain information from existing records, for example, for occupational information, job titles, and names of substances from company records. A questionnaire is needed to obtain the information in a systematic way and to note any problems with the information. The approach can be used to obtain information on past and present exposures. Although the information obtained from records may be at times more objective, it also has its limitations. The terminology used may differ over years and between companies (or other archives) and the organization of the information may not meet the needs of the study, for

1 **Were any home improvements such as decoration or painting made to your house just before or during the first 3 months of your pregnancy with *Childname*?**

    Yes

    No

    Don't know

1
2
3

Go to next section

Did this involve any of the following?

2 **Paint stripping?**

    Yes

    No

    Don't know

1
2
3

Go to Q5

3 **Did you yourself do any paint stripping?**

    Yes

    No

    Can't remember

1
2
3

Go to Q5

4 **Approximately how many hours did you spend paint stripping altogether?**

5 **Did the decoration involve painting?**

    Yes

    No

    Can't remember

1
2
3

Go to next section

6 **What kind of paint was used?**

    Gloss

    Emulsion

    Don't know

1
2
3

7 **Did you personally do any painting?**

    Yes

    No

    Can't remember

1
2
3

Go to next section

8 **How many hours did you spend painting altogether?**

Figure 2.3 Example of questions on painting the house in a reproductive study.

example, for payment purposes. In factories, most of the workers may be classified as production workers for payment purposes, and this may not be specific enough for epidemiological studies, for which more information is needed on the type of work that was actually done and the substances they worked with. Information may have been kept in books that have not been archived properly and may be difficult to read, therefore careful interpretation is needed. Questionnaires in this case can guide the researcher and enable the recording of the quality of the data, which can be analyzed at a later stage.

The next section is about work and hobbies.

1 **Were you employed during the first 3 months of
   your pregnancy with *Childname*?**

   Yes

   No

1	Go to next
2	section

*The following question will ask you details about your place of work. Please feel free not to answer
if you do not wish to identify your place of work.*

2 **What was the name and address of the
   company or organisation in which you worked?**

3 **In which department did you work?**

4 **What was your job title?**

5 **How many <u>hours per week</u> did you work
   in this job?**

6 **Until which week of your pregnancy with
   Childname did you continue to work?**

7 **Please state <u>your main tasks</u> at work and
   how many hours you spent at each task.**

Task	Number of hours per week

Figure 2.4 Example of questions on work in a reproductive study has its limitations. The terminology used may differ over years and between companies (or other archives) and the organization of the information may not meet the needs of the study, for example, for payment purposes. In factories, most of the workers may be classified as production workers for payment purposes, and this may not be specific enough for epidemiological studies, where more information is needed on the type of work that was actually done and the substances they worked with. Information may have been kept in books that have not been archived properly and may be difficult to read, therefore careful interpretation is needed. Questionnaires in this case can guide the researcher and enable the recording of the quality of the data, which can be analysed at a later stage.

2.2 THE DESIGN OF QUESTIONNAIRES

The aims of exposure questionnaire design are:

1. To obtain indices of exposure essential to the objectives of the study
2. To minimize errors in these indices
3. To create an instrument that is easy for the interviewer and subject to use, and for the researcher to process and analyze (White et al. 2008)

To keep the process on track, questionnaire design needs clear aims and objectives, a selection of items that need to be translated into questions, and a logical order. For example, when designing a questionnaire to study the exposure to chloroform, a by-product of the chlorination of drinking water taken up through ingestion, skin absorption, and inhalation during drinking, showering, bathing, and swimming, the aims and objectives can be defined as follows:

Aims
- To assess the duration of exposure to the primary chloroform-related water activities

Objectives
- At the end of the interview, we will have information on:
  The amount of ingested tap water
  The duration of showering
  The duration of bathing
  The duration of swimming

Each of the objectives can then be translated into questions, for example, for tap water ingestion:

How many glasses of tap water do you drink per day? ——glasses/day
How many cups of tea do you drink per day? ——cups/day
How many cups of coffee do you drink per day? ——cups/day

This information could subsequently be combined with information on the concentration of chloroform in tap water and some other factors to give an estimate for the actual intake of chloroform (see chapter 16). It is important to note that a number of uncertainties are introduced; for example, it is unclear how large a cup or glass is because people use different sizes. Assumptions would need to be made. Also there may be temporal variability in the number of glasses and cups. On the other hand, people cannot be asked how many (milli)liters of tap water they drink per day. It is difficult to provide a good estimate of variability over a long time period, particularly when going back far into the past. It will be very difficult for people to remember how many glasses of tap water they drank 20 years ago. Similarly, people tend to know reasonably well how often they shower, but they are not very good at giving an accurate estimate of the duration of a shower (in minutes) and it may not be useful to include the latter in a questionnaire.

2.3 ISSUES IN QUESTIONNAIRE DESIGN

Asking a question is one thing, getting a good answer another. It is extremely important to get a relevant answer of high quality to a question, because otherwise time and effort are wasted. There are a number of issues that need to be considered when designing a questionnaire (White et al. 2008). There is often a tendency to design a questionnaire that is too long and provides so much information that not all the answers to the questions can be used in the epidemiological analysis. The length of the questionnaire is dependent on the administration method (see earlier). A long questionnaire may reduce the response and completion rates considerably and therefore it is important to consider if each question contributes to the overall aims and objectives of the questionnaire. If it does not make a significant contribution then it should not be used. Also, it needs to be clear at this stage how the answer is going to be analyzed and how the answer relates to other answers in the study. Is useful new information obtained or does it repeat a previous question? High response and completion rates are essential for the success of a study (Rothman and Greenland 1998).

Avoid questions that go into too much detail and ask for information that the subjects cannot provide, or will provide but is not of good quality, particularly in the case of past exposures. The subject may remember that she used a pesticide a number of years ago and the broad category, but is unlikely to remember the name of the pesticide or the active ingredient (Engel et al. 2001). In certain situations it may be helpful to use more than one questionnaire, for example, a basic questionnaire and additional questionnaires such as a specific job questionnaire. The latter can be used for more in-depth questions on particular topics after the subject indicates in the former that these take place. This kind of approach has been used for occupational questions in community-based studies.

The longer the recall time, the less likely it is that the subject will give an answer of sufficient quality to be included in the analysis. The longer the recall period, the less detail can be expected from the subject. Complex exposure scenarios may occur, for example, where the subject is exposed to various substances over different time periods. This makes it difficult to design a simple and straightforward questionnaire and the complexity may overwhelm the subject and reduce the quality of the answers. In this case it is important to focus on key events. Rare events are likely to be remembered by the subjects only if they made a significant impact on their life or are somehow connected to other events.

There are still few, if any, standardized questionnaires for exposure assessment that have been validated. Many researchers therefore start from scratch, or base their design on previous experiences with questionnaire data. A critical evaluation of questionnaires that have been used in previous studies in the particular area, including how the answers were used in the analyses, will be very helpful in the design of a new questionnaire. At times it is advisable to use the same questionnaire as in the previous study, even though it could be improved, so that an exact comparison can be made with results of the previous study. Designing the questionnaire is often a very long process and many changes will be made along the way.

2.4 OPEN-ENDED OR CLOSED-ENDED QUESTIONS

Open-ended questions are questions without restrictions on the answers of the subjects, whereas closed-ended questions have restrictions in the form of a limited number of possible answers, for example, categories that subjects have to pick (Figures 2.3 and 2.4). Open-ended questions are used to record simple factual information such as name, weight, age, and occupational title. They are often used in occupational and environmental epidemiology, whereas closed-ended questions are often used in nutritional epidemiology, for example, in food frequency diaries (Willett 1998). The answer can be considerably different depending on whether the question is a closed- or open-ended question (Teschke et al. 1994). For closed-ended questions the answer may differ depending on the number of categories that are provided as a possible answer. However, most of the evidence comes from outside the field of environmental epidemiology and little research has been done specifically within this field. Open-ended questions need to be coded by a trained researcher before they can be analyzed, for example, subjects' occupation or tasks, and this may take a lot of time and careful interpretation of some of the answers and may itself introduce bias.

2.5 WORDING

The words used in the questionnaire should be understood by the subjects and they should neither be too difficult nor too simple (White et al. 2008). The questions should be clear, unambiguous, short, and to the point and the subject should not have to figure out what is actually being asked. There should be no unexplained or vague terms, jargon, or abbreviations. Only one question at a time should be asked and the questions should be unbiased. Questions cannot be too precise and the subject needs to be familiar with the topic of the question. In the case of closed-ended questions the answers need to be mutually exclusive. The answers should allow linkage to the aims and objectives of the questionnaire.

Here are some examples of questions that have problems:

"Do you drink tap water regularly?" This appears to be a straightforward question but it is unclear what is meant by "regularly." In this case it would be better to define what is meant by "regularly," for example, at least once a day or once a week.

"Do you take a shower and/or bath, and how often?" Here we have a number of questions in one question and these should be separated. For example:

- 1a. Do you take showers?
    - o Yes (go to question 1b)
    - o No (go to question to 2a)
- 1b. How many showers do you take per week? ——
- 2a. Do you take baths?
    - o Yes (go to question 2b)
    - o No (go to question 3)
- 2b. How many baths do you take per week? ——

It is also tempting to ask how long the person showers or bathes, but this is difficult for a person to know without timing the shower or bath. On the other hand, without timing the answer will be 5 or 10 minutes for a shower and it is questionable if this is the true duration, and it may not be very useful in any analyses because it is more or less the same for everyone. On the other hand it is unlikely to be far off the actual duration. In this case the frequency of showers is likely to be the more important factor when estimating the total duration of showering per week, and adding a question on the duration of showering that results in an inaccurate answer may be a waste of space.

"Where does your highest exposure to NO_2 take place?" Many subjects will not know what NO_2 is and even writing it down as "nitrogen dioxide" will not help. Furthermore, in general people will have little knowledge where nitrogen dioxide is present let alone where their highest exposure takes place. In this case surrogate questions should be used, for example, questions on the use of gas cookers and time spent near (busy) roads or in smoky places, which are all associated with nitrogen dioxide exposure.

"How many minutes per week are you exposed to traffic fumes?" This question may be too precise and the subjects will probably have to estimate first their duration each day and then add them up to get a total for each week, which may be too complicated in many cases. Also, subjects are unlikely to know exactly what they should count as traffic fumes. Are they exposed to traffic fumes when walking along a road, when they sit inside a car, when they live near a busy road, or in all three cases?

"Have you used any pesticides?" First, the time period is unclear in this question. Second, many subjects will not know what exactly is a pesticide and as such what they should count. Besides home and garden pesticides, do they include herbicides, shampoos against lice, pet collars against fleas, fly spray, mothballs, or bleach? Do they need to include both organic and nonorganic pesticides? This apparently simple question is unlikely to provide a satisfactory and easily interpretable answer, and should therefore be explained in more detail and broken up into a number of questions.

"Did you use any pesticides in 1973?" Besides the problems discussed previously, the additional problem in this case is the very precise time period, which is a long time ago. People are unlikely to remember this kind of detail. Introduction questions to aid their memory may help at times; for example, if interested in garden pesticides the researcher could ask if they had a garden in that particular year, followed by questions on particular pests they may have had.

2.6 FORMAT OF THE QUESTIONNAIRE

The format of the questionnaire is as important as the actual questions. Remember that it is easy for people to discard the questionnaire. In the case of paper questionnaires, long and complex looking ones do not encourage the subject to start filling them out. Make sure that the questionnaire looks nice, tidy, and appealing, but do not go over the top, and use a large enough letter type and easy-to-read font (White et al. 2008). Using different colors for different questionnaires can be helpful at times. Make sure to provide clear instructions on how to answer the questions, but do not make them too long because this will put off the subject. Use a logical order for your questions and start with some simple questions to get the subject going. Use the order in such a way that the subjects stay interested and that there is a natural flow. The former may be difficult when asking many exposure-related questions, particularly when a subject does not know how this relates to a particular disease or, in a case–control study, when asking controls. The response rate among controls often tends to be lower compared with the response rate among cases. Subjects are often not interested or do not know about, for example, chemicals, but they know about particular events (e.g., job, moving house, births) in their lives and this could be used in the questionnaire to obtain relevant information. Not only may these events be related to particular exposures, but they may also keep the subject interested and increase response rates (Edwards et al. 2002). Thank the subjects at the end and remind them what to do with the questionnaire.

Branching off, that is, going into more detail for particular questions is not easy with paper questionnaires because it will take up a lot of space on a page and a subject may get confused about what to answer. However, it is possible to use this with computer aids and in particular with telephone interviews, inputting data straight into the computer. This could be very useful and provide more specific information, for example, on occupational exposures (Stewart et al. 1998).

When asking for a job history the use of matrices can be very helpful at times, for example, with rows for each job and columns for job title, industry, tasks, and start and finishing date. A job title and the type of industry can provide substantial information about potential exposures, but the job titles used may vary in different companies. If possible, further information may need to be obtained about particular tasks that the subject carried out, particularly those that may be related to the exposure of interest (Stewart et al. 1998). Job history matrices can be coded and expressed as a job exposure matrix (see chapter 7), where the researcher codes the job information and relates it to certain exposures. For a good coding of occupation, it is generally necessary to have a few open-ended questions on company, job, and activities.

2.7 AIDS TO RECALL

As mentioned earlier, subjects may find it difficult to remember particular facts and need some help to answer questions. Multiple-choice questions or cards with alternative answers given by the researcher may be very helpful, particularly when there are a limited number of possible answers. A tiered approach can be very helpful; for example, when trying to estimate the exposure to a particular chemical at work, the questionnaire may ask, in this order:

- The employer the subject worked for
- The type of industry
- The job title
- The particular task that he or she carried out
- The type of chemicals that she or he worked with
- The name of chemicals that he or she worked with

This approach has a further advantage that even if the subject does not know the answer to the last question, answers from the previous questions could be used for some analyses in an epidemiological study, for example, disease in relation to the type of industry or the type of industry and job title. The information on the industry and job title can subsequently be coded by an expert (see chapter 7).

A calendar may also be used as an effective aid to recall. When studying risk factors of birth outcomes, a calendar could be helpful to determine where subjects lived or where they worked before conception and during different stages of various pregnancies. Pregnancies and everything around them are usually events that are clearly remembered.

In the case of the use of household pesticides, rather than asking the subjects directly if they used any flea sprays, which they may not directly recall, it may be useful to ask first if the subjects had:

- Any pets, followed by
- If they had any problems with fleas
- If they did do something about it
- If so, if they used a spray, collar, or other method
- If so, what the name was of the product

However, at times the subjects may not admit that they have had a flea problem, in which case the questions that follow will not be asked and the information is lost if they answered incorrectly.

Introducing these aids takes up more space in the questionnaire and there will always be a balancing act between space and the quality of the answers. In many circumstances, rather than asking for particular exposure to chemicals or other risk factors, surrogates are asked for. For example, in the case of indoor nitrogen dioxide exposure, the use of gas cookers.

2.8 CODING

Information from the questionnaire needs to be coded for analysis. In the case of closed-ended questions, this is straightforward, but it is more difficult for open-ended questions. It is important to formulate a coding scheme early on in the study, which helps to focus the analyses. Humans make mistakes, and therefore a good quality-control scheme needs to be carried out. Information may also need to be further translated, for example, in the case of a job history for which a job exposure matrix may be needed. Trained experts are required in this case to set up a job exposure matrix and carry out the coding, which may be a laborious task and provide mixed results (see chapter 7).

2.9 PILOT TESTING

Pilot testing is an extremely important part of questionnaire design, and sufficient time should be allocated for it (Sudman and Bradburn 1983). Before pilot testing the questionnaire on people who are representative of the target population, it should be evaluated by a number of other researchers, particularly those who have used similar questionnaires and used the answers in an epidemiological study. This may be followed by a sample of convenience, for example, relatives, friends, or colleagues. After this, the questionnaire should be tested on a sample of people representative of the target population. At this stage it may become clear if the intentions of the researchers are sufficiently understood by the subjects. In some cases it may take a number of pilot tests to get the questionnaire right, and at this stage researchers should be critical of their work and open to suggestions. The better the pilot testing, the fewer regrets there will be at the end of the study. Throughout the process written comments should be obtained that can be evaluated by a number of researchers.

During pilot testing the words and interpretations of questions are evaluated. At times this may be difficult to establish and it may need more in-depth discussion with the pilot subjects to determine how they interpreted the question and what they thought when giving an answer. Also, the researcher needs to evaluate how the answers can be interpreted and if they can be analyzed and used for the epidemiological study. This is extremely important at this stage, particularly because questions still can be changed. Simpler facts such as if all the questions were answered are easier to establish (White et al. 2008).

2.10 TRANSLATION

More and more, international multicenter studies are carried out, for example, in Europe, and this may require translation of questionnaires into different languages. Furthermore, the (large) influx of immigrants also requires translation of the questionnaire because they may not be sufficiently familiar with their new language to be able to answer any questions satisfactorily. In these cases the questionnaire should be translated and back translated, preferably by a number of experts familiar with the language and the topic. The researchers should be aware of cultural differences and take these into account in the questionnaire. After the translation has been carried out, the questionnaire should be pilot tested again to make sure that no information has been lost in the process and the questions are interpreted in the same way as the original questionnaire.

2.11 VALIDITY

A questionnaire may look good and the response to the questions may be good, but does the questionnaire actual measure what it needs to measure, that is, what is the validity of the questionnaire? Are those reporting longer exposure to environmental tobacco smoke (ETS) actually exposed to more ETS? Are the subjects working with solvents actually exposed to higher solvent levels? Do people who report drinking five glasses of tap water per day actually do so? Ideally all questions and answers should be validated, that is, compared to a gold standard. This could be done in a subset of the study population. However, often this is not possible. For example, because the questions relate to exposure in the past, there is no method to measure the substance of interest, or it is unclear what the gold standard is. Relatively few questionnaires have been validated.

Up to a certain extent, diaries can be used to validate a water ingestion questionnaire (Shimokura et al. 1998; Barbone et al. 2002), ETS exposure with personal exposure monitoring of nicotine (Coghlin et al. 1989; Eisner et al. 2001), or biomonitoring solvent metabolites (hippuric acid or methylhippuric acid) in urine in case of aromatic solvent exposure (Tielemans et al. 1999). The validation may only need to be carried out on a proportion of the population, and may provide invaluable information for the interpretation of the epidemiological study. The sensitivity, specificity, and predictive value of the various questions or the correlation between different questions from different methods can be determined, and therefore the extent of exposure misclassification, if any, and the effect on risk estimates (chapter 10).

Sensitivity is the probability of a positive answer when the exposure is truly present, whereas specificity is the probability of a negative answer when the exposure is truly absent (Figure 2.5). Positive predictive value is the probability that a person is actually exposed given that he or she gave a positive answer, and the negative predictive value is the probability that a person truly has no exposure given a negative answer.

Using a hypothetical example of a question validated with biomonitoring, it can be seen that in this case specificity is higher than sensitivity (Figure 2.5). In epidemiological studies, specificity has a stronger effect on the risk estimates compared to sensitivity and it is therefore important to keep the specificity as high as possible, even if this may reduce the sensitivity slightly (see chapter 10).

		Biomonitoring 'truth'			
		Yes	No		
Questionnaire	Yes	a (100)	b (70)	$a + b$ (170)	
	No	c (30)	d (800)	$c + d$ (830)	
		$a + c$ (130)	$b + d$ (870)		

$$\text{Sensitivity} = \frac{a}{a+c} = \frac{100}{100+30} = 77\%$$

$$\text{Specificity} = \frac{d}{b+d} = \frac{800}{70+800} = 92\%$$

$$\text{Positive predictive value} = \frac{a}{a+b} = \frac{100}{100+70} = 59\%$$

$$\text{Negative predictive value} = \frac{d}{c+d} = \frac{800}{30+800} = 96\%$$

Figure 2.5 Sensitivity, specificity, and predictive values

Tielemans et al. (1999) used biomonitoring to assess the validity of their various questionnaire methods and found sensitivity and specificity coefficients of around 0.30 to 0.55 and 0.77 to 0.92, respectively, when using a generic questionnaire for solvent exposure, whereas this increased to 0.40 to 0.70 and 0.75 to 0.93, respectively, when using a detailed, job-specific questionnaire that elicited details on occupational tasks, products, and frequency of activity. A population-specific job exposure matrix showed higher sensitivity (0.58) but lower specificity (0.73). The highest positive predictive value was found for the job specific questionnaire (0.52). Shimokura et al. (1998) compared questionnaire data and diary data for water-related activities and found that there was a good correlation between drinking water intake ($r = 0.78$) and for the time spent showering ($r = 0.68$), but found that the actual amount of reported drinking water intake was considerably higher when using the questionnaire compared with the diary (0.75 vs. 0.40 l/day^{-1}). The difference for showering was less (10.5 vs. 9.8 min day^{-1}). Eisner et al. (2001) found a moderate correlation ($r = 0.47$) between questionnaire reporting of ETS and personal measurements of nicotine, whereas Coghlin et al. (1989) found a much higher correlation ($r = 0.91$). A possible explanation of the difference may be the higher nicotine levels in the former study compared with the latter, which shows the importance of taking into account population characteristics. In a case control study by Engman et al. (2007) on the association between home environmental factors and asthma/allergy among children, 390 homes were visited by trained inspectors for ocular inspection of visible moisture damage and perceptions of moldy odor. Their observations were then compared with questionnaire reports collected 18 to 24 months earlier from the families. The questionnaire was a quite reliable source regarding technical parameters of the home but not for dampness problems. The questionnaire was better for predicting buildings without problems than detecting problems of moldy odor and visible indications of moisture. They suggested that to increase the validity of future questionnaires, simple drawings or information on critical spots for dampness could be used. Chodick et al. (2008) assessed how well participants' self-recorded time outdoors compared with objective measurements of personal ultraviolet radiation (UVR) doses. They enrolled 124 volunteers aged 40 and above. In a linear regression model, self-recorded daily time spent outdoors was associated with an increase of 8.2% (95% CI: 7.3–9.2%) in the personal UVR exposure with every hour spent outdoors. The amount of self-recorded total daily time spent outdoors was better correlated with the personal daily UVR dose for activities conducted near noon time compared with activities conducted in the morning or late afternoon, and for activities often performed in the sun (e.g., gardening or recreation activities) compared with other outdoor activities (e.g., driving) in which the participant is usually shaded from the sun. Their results demonstrated a significant correlation between diary records of time spent outdoors with objective personal UVR dose measurements. Yu et al. (2009) used self-administered, mailed questionnaires, test–retest responses to time-based and to activity-based approaches to evaluate sun exposure in 124 volunteer radiologic technologist participants from the United States: 64 females and 60 males 48 to 80 years of age. During childhood and adolescence the two approaches gave similar Intra Class Correlation (ICCs) for average numbers of hours spent outdoors in the summer. By contrast, compared with the time-based approach, the activity-based approach showed significantly higher ICCs during adult ages (0.69 vs. 0.43, $p = 0.003$) and over the lifetime (0.69 vs. 0.52, $p = 0.05$); the higher ICCs for the activity-based questionnaire were primarily derived from the results for females. Kütting et al. (2008) assessed whether a standardized questionnaire is a valid tool to identify exposure with acrylamide by relating the self-reported food and smoking history with a biomarker, namely hemoglobin-adduct levels of acrylamide. Smoking was significantly associated with adduct levels of acrylamide ($p < 0.0001$) and had a main contribution to the internal burden with acrylamide, but food intake did not. Self-reported data concerning smoking behavior were highly valid, whereas self-reported food intake was apparently not as useful for estimating food-related acrylamide exposure. Bergkvist et al. (2012) evaluated the relation between FFQ-based dietary PCB exposure, and serum PCB congeners, CB-118, CB-138, CB-153, CB-156, CB-170, and CB-180 in women (56–85 years of age, $n = 201$). The correlation between FFQ-based dietary PCB exposure and serum CB-153 was 0.41 ($p < 0.001$) for the concurrent (median 1.6 ng/kg body weight) and 0.34 ($p < 0.05$) for the past (median 2.6 ng/kg body weight) exposure assessment. Long-term validity of FFQ-based PCB estimates and the six serum PCB congeners ranged from 0.30 to 0.58 ($p < 0.05$). Teschke et al. (1994) found differences in the performance in questionnaires depending on whether they were closed- or open-ended questions (Teschke et al. 1994). The former generally showed higher sensitivity, although slightly lower specificity.

Besides the validity, there is the repeatability of the questionnaire, that is, are the answers reproducible, do we always get the same answer when we administer the questionnaire repeatedly (at times the term reliability is used here too). This can be assessed by administering the questionnaire twice to a proportion of subjects in the target population, and estimate, for example, the correlation between the answers (van de Gulden et al. 1993; Westerdahl et al. 1996; Farrow et al. 1996; Künzli et al. 1997; Barbone et al. 2002, Wu et al. 2013). The question raised often is whether the reproducibility of the questionnaire is measured or the variability in exposure. The interval between the two occasions should be long enough to provide independent observations, but not too long to avoid true variation in exposure. Some researchers tried to assess the reproducibility of a questionnaire, but used different methods of administration, for example, mailing and telephone or self-administered questionnaire and a face-to-face interview. This may introduce additional variation into the process and should be avoided. Künzli et al. (1997) used a number of different questionnaires to assess long-term ambient ozone exposure and found some differences in the reproducibility, showing the importance of assessing different questionnaire methods. Barbone et al. (2002) found good reproducibility for their questionnaire to assess tap water-related activities ($r = 0.6–0.9$). Fortes et al. (2009) investigated the reliability of reported lifetime household pesticide exposure through repeated administration of a standardized questionnaire. A questionnaire including detailed questions about lifetime frequency and duration of pesticide use in nonoccupational circumstances was administered on two occasions to 163 cutaneous melanoma cases and 113 controls. They investigated the agreement between the two measurements taken on average 12 months apart and studied the association between differences in the two measurements and a set of explanatory variables. The agreement for duration and frequency of use of pesticides outdoors was 89.5% (Cohen's kappa = 0.48) and 92.0% (Cohen's kappa = 0.40), respectively, whereas duration and frequency of use of pesticides indoors agreement was 75.4% (Cohen's kappa = 0.32) and 77.4% (Cohen's kappa = 0.28), respectively. The agreement was higher for duration (97.4%; Cohen's kappa = 0.72) and use of pesticides on domestic animals (86.4%; Cohen's kappa = 0.68). Overall, there was a good reproducibility in self-reported exposure to pesticides. Slusky et al. (2012) assessed the reliability of self-reported household use of pesticides and potential differences in reliability by case-control status, and by socio-demographic characteristics. The reliability was based on two repeated in-person interviews. Kappa statistics ranged from 0.31 to 0.61 (fair to substantial agreement), with 9 out of the 12 tests indicating moderate agreement. The percent positive agreement ranged from 46% to 80% and the percent negative agreement from 54% to 95%. Reliability for all pesticide types as assessed by the three reliability measures did not differ significantly for cases and controls as confirmed by bootstrap analysis. For most pesticide types, Kappa and percent positive agreement were higher for non-Hispanics than Hispanics and for households with higher income versus lower income. They suggested that reproducibility of maternal-reported pesticide use was moderate to high and was similar among cases and controls, suggesting that differential recall is not likely to be a major source of bias. Wu et al. (2013) constructed a sunlight exposure questionnaire for use in the Chinese population based on extensive literature review and item suitability for measuring lifetime exposure. 650 population-based Chinese women completed the sunlight exposure questionnaire through telephone interview. To assess the questionnaire reliability, 94 women were re-interviewed after 2 weeks. The questionnaire also had a good test–retest reliability (ICC: 0.59–0.93; κ: 0.51–1.00) and was found to be adequate for measurement of lifetime sunlight exposure among Hong Kong Chinese women.

2.12 CONCLUSION

This section shows that relatively few validation and repeatability studies have been done and that in general the questionnaires measure reasonably what they are supposed to measure but that measurement error does occur and should be addressed in any study. Quantification of the extent of measurement would certainly inform the interpretation of epidemiological study results.

REFERENCES

Barbone, F., Valent, F., Brussi, V., Tomasella, L., Triassi, M., Di Lieto, A., et al. (2002). Assessing the exposure of pregnant women to drinking water disinfection byproducts. *Epidemiology*, **13**, 540–544.

Bergkvist C, Akesson A, Glynn A, Michaëlsson K, Rantakokko P, Kiviranta H, et al. (2012). Validation of questionnaire-based long-term dietary exposure to polychlorinated biphenyls using biomarkers. *Molecular and Nutritional Food Research*, **56**, 1748–1754.

Brogger, J., Bakke, P., Eide, G. E., and Gulsvik, A. (2002). Comparison of telephone and postal survey modes on respiratory symptoms and risk factors. *American Journal of Epidemiology*, **155**, 572–576.

Chodick, G., Kleinerman, R. A., Linet, M. S., Fears, T., Kwok, R. K., Kimlin, M. G., et al. (2008). Agreement between diary records of time spent outdoors and personal ultraviolet radiation dose measurements. *Photochemistry and Photobioliology*, **84**, 713–718

Coghlin, J., Hammond, S. K., and Gann, P. H. (1989). Development of epidemiologic tools for measuring environmental tobacco smoke in pregnant women. *American Journal of Epidemiology*, **130**, 696–704.

Debanne, S. M., Petot, G. J., Li, J., Koss, E., Lerner, A. J., Riedel, T. M., et al. (2001). *Journal of the American Geriatrics Society*, **49**, 980–984.

Edwards, P., Roberts, I., Clarke, M., DiGuiseppi, C., Pratap, S., Wentz, R., and Kwan, I. (2002). Increasing response rates to postal questionnaires: systematic review. *British Medical Journal*, **324**, 1183–1192.

Eisner, M. D., Katz, P. P., Yelin, E. H., Hammond, K., and Blanc, P. (2001). Measurement of environmental tobacco smoke among adults with asthma. *Environmental Health Perspectives*, **109**, 809–813.

Engel, L. S., Seixas, N. S., Keifer, M. C., Longstreth, W. T. Jr., and Checkoway, H. (2001). Validity study of self-reported pesticide exposure among orchardists. *Journal of Exposure Analysis and Environmental Epidemiology*, 11, 359–368.

Engman, L. H., Bornehag, C. G., and Sundell, J. (2007). How valid are parents' questionnaire responses regarding building characteristics, mouldy odour, and signs of moisture problems in Swedish homes? *Scandinavian Journal of Public Health*, 35, 125–132.

Farrow, A., Farrow, S. C., Little, R., and Golding, J. (1996). The repeatability of self-reported exposure after miscarriage. ALPAC study team. Avonmouth study of pregnancy and childhood. *International Journal of Epidemiology*, 25, 797–806.

Fortes, C., Mastroeni, S., Boffetta, P., Salvatori, V., Melo, N., Bolli, S., and Pasquini, P. (2009). Reliability of self-reported household pesticide use. *European Journal of Cancer Prevention*, 18, 404–406.

Freeman, N. C., Jimenez, M., Reed, K. J., Gurunathan, S., Edwards, R. D., Roy, A., et al. (2001). Quantitative analysis of children's microactivity patterns: The Minnesota Children's Pesticide Exposure Study. *Journal of Exposure Analysis and Environmental Epidemiology*, 11, 501–509.

Hansen, K. S. (1996). Validity of occupational exposure and smoking data obtained from surviving spouses and colleagues. *American Journal of Industrial Medicine*, 30, 392–397.

Hohwü, L., Lyshol, H., Gissler, M., Hrafn Jonsson, S., Petzold, M., and Obel, C. (2013). Web-based versus traditional paper questionnaires: A mixed-mode survey with a nordic perspective. *Journal of Medical Internet Research*, 15, e173.

Infante-Rivard, C., and Jacques, L. (2000). Empirical study of parental recall bias. *American Journal of Epidemiology*, 152, 480–486.

Jantunen, M. J., Hänninen, O., Katsouyanni, K., Knöppel, H., Kuenzli, N., Lebret, E., et al. (1998). Air pollution exposure in European cities: The "Expolis" study. *Journal of Exposure Analysis and Environmental Epidemiology*, 8, 495–518.

Künzli, N., Kelly, T, Balmes, J., and Tager, I. B. (1997). Reproducibility of retrospective assessment of outdoor time activity patterns as an individual determinant of long-term ambient ozone exposure. *International Journal of Epidemiology*, 26, 1258–1271.

Kütting, B., Uter, W., and Drexler, H. (2008). The association between self-reported acrylamide intake and hemoglobin adducts as biomarkers of exposure. *Cancer Causes Control*, 19, 273–281.

Preller, L., Kromhout, H., Heederik, D., and Tielen, M. J. (1995). Modeling long-term average exposure in occupational exposure–response analysis. *Scandinavian Journal of Work Environment and Health*, 21, 504–512.

Rothman, K. J., and Greenland, S. (1998). *Modern epidemiology* (2nd ed.). Lippincott-Raven Publishers, Philadelphia.

Shimokura, G. H., Savitz, D., and Symanski, E. (1998). Assessment of water use for estimating exposure to tap water contaminants. *Environmental Health Perspectives*, 106, 55–59.

Slusky, D. A., Metayer, C., Aldrich, M. C., Ward, M. H., Lea, C. S., Selvin, S., and Buffler, P. A. (2012). Reliability of maternal-reports regarding the use of household pesticides: Experience from a case-control study of childhood leukemia. *Cancer Epidemiology*, 36, 375–380.

Stewart, P. A., Stewart, W. F., Siemiatycki, J., Heineman, E. F., and Dosemeci, M. (1998). Questionnaires for collecting detailed occupational information for community-based case-control studies. *American Industrial Hygiene Association Journal*, 59, 39–44.

Sudman, S., and Bradburn, N. M. (1983). *Response effects in surveys. A review and synthesis.* National Opinion Research Center Monographs in Social Research, Aldine, Chicago.

Teschke, K., Kennedy, S. M., and Olshan, A. F. (1994). Effect of different questionnaire formats on reporting of occupational exposures. *American Journal of Industrial Medicine,* **26,** 327–337.

Tielemans, E., Heederik, D., Burdorf, A., Vermeulen, R., Veulemans, H., Kromhout, H., and Hartog, K. (1999). Assessment of occupational exposures in a general population: comparison of different methods. *Occupational and Environmental Medicine,* **56,** 145–151.

Van de Gulden, J. W., Jansen, I. W., Verbeek, A. L., and Kolk, J. J. (1993). Repeatability of self-reported data on occupational exposure to particular compounds. *International Journal of Epidemiology,* **22,** 284–287.

van de Looij-Jansen, P. M., and de Wilde, E. J. (2008). Comparison of web-based versus paper-and-pencil self-administered questionnaire: Effects on health indicators in Dutch adolescents. *Health Services Research,* **43,** 1708–1721.

Willett, W. (1998). *Nutritional epidemiology* (2nd ed.). Oxford University Press, New York.

Westerdahl, J., Anderson, H., Olsson, H., and Ingvar, C. (1996). Reproducibility of a self-administered questionnaire for assessment of melanoma risk. *International Journal of Epidemiology,* **25,** 245–251.

White, E., Armstrong, B. K., and Saracci, R. (2008). *Principles of exposure measurement in epidemiology.* Oxford University Press, Oxford.

Wu, S., Ho, S. C., Lam, T. P., Woo, J., Yuen, P. Y., Qin, L., and Ku, S. (2013). Development and validation of a lifetime exposure questionnaire for use among Chinese populations. *Scientific Reports,* **30, 2793.**

Yu, C. L., Li, Y., Freedman, D. M., Fears, T. R., Kwok, R., Chodick, G., et al. (2009). Assessment of lifetime cumulative sun exposure using a self-administered questionnaire:reliability of two approaches. *Cancer Epidemioly and Biomarkers Prevention,* **18,** 464–471.

3

ENVIRONMENTAL MEASUREMENT AND MODELING
INTRODUCTION AND METHODS USING GEOGRAPHICAL INFORMATION SYSTEMS

John Gulliver, David Briggs, and Kees de Hoogh

3.1 INTRODUCTION

Exposure assessment in environmental epidemiology often relies on environmental measurement and modeling, as opposed to personal exposure measurement and modeling (chapter 5), in contrast to occupational epidemiology wherein the opposite occurs. This is partly due to the differences in the size of study populations, which can be very large for environmental epidemiological studies and makes only environmental modeling and monitoring feasible. Examples of environmental pollutants and their main exposure pathways and routes are:

1. Everyday indoor and outdoor air pollutants such as particulate matter, NO_2, CO, and volatile organic compounds (VOCs), from sources such as traffic, gas cooking, and (passive) smoking, with uptake through inhalation
2. Water contaminants such as arsenic, nitrate, and nitrite; pesticides and chlorination by-products from geological sources; and agriculture and water treatment, respectively, with uptake mainly through ingestion, and sometimes skin absorption and inhalation (e.g., trihalomethanes)
3. Soil contaminants such as pesticides, metals, dioxins and VOCs from agriculture, industry, and landfills, with uptake through ingestion (including hand-to-mouth contact) and inhalation
4. Food contaminants from deposition of air pollutants, uptake from soil, with uptake through ingestion

Environmental measurements and models may not take into account differences in ingestion, inhalation, and skin absorption rates and differences in pathways of subjects and may therefore under- or overestimate personal exposure or uptake, but there may still be a good correlation between environmental and personal exposure estimates, which is essential for epidemiological studies (see chapter 10). Validation studies should be carried out to examine these issues. Chapters 3 and 4, however, focus entirely on external exposures and do not cover effective or actual biological dose.

Exposure assessment in environmental epidemiological studies often makes use of temporal and spatial variability in environmental levels of exposure. Traditionally, studies have used crude proxies like distance from a source such as an industrial point source, radio and TV transmitters, roads, or landfill (Dolk et al. 1997, 1999; Elliott et al. 2001; Hoek et al. 2002), but with more advanced methods and more detailed source data becoming available, more sophisticated exposure measures are being developed.

The main focus of this chapter and the next is on geographical approaches to estimating pollution dispersion and exposure assessment. The focus throughout this chapter is on the principles of geography and exposure, and the use of measurements and developing models using geographical information systems (GIS) to undertake exposure assessment.

3.2 GEOGRAPHY AND EXPOSURE

3.2.1 Basic Principles

The fact that a geographical approach to exposure assessment can be taken is based on a simple assumption: that environmental exposures show geographic variation. In fact, usually more is needed than this in order to estimate exposures with any degree of confidence. There is also a need for this geographical variation to be reasonably systematic (rather than random) and at a sufficiently coarse scale to enable the detection of these variations with the tools that are available. Systematic variation is important, because it enables the prediction of variations in exposure. This means that exposures do not have to be measured everywhere, but can be estimated on the basis of other factors. The scale of variation is important both because the methods of exposure assessment are inevitably only approximate, and because people are not static but move around in the environment. If levels of pollution vary dramatically over very short distances, we may therefore end up with serious errors in the exposure estimates. This may not matter much if, in the study design, population groups or areas with large differences in average exposure still can be identified—in those circumstances any association with health will be diluted but should not be removed. It matters much more when we are seeking effects of quite subtle variations in exposure, for in those cases we may not be able to reliably distinguish different levels of exposure within our population.

Fortunately, in many cases these requirements can be satisfied. Many forms of pollution do show considerable systematic spatial variation. This occurs because most pollution derives from specific sources (often associated with some form of human activity), from which it disperses into the environment. During dispersion, it inevitably tends to spread out and concentrations become progressively diluted. The simple fact that the emission sources are geographically distributed (and often clustered) in some way nevertheless means that levels of pollution vary. The pathways of dispersion in the environment are also strongly constrained, so that dispersion is limited. As a result—unfortunately for those who live in more polluted environments but luckily for epidemiologists (who usually don't)—levels of exposure vary geographically. Indeed, like many other phenomena, pollution tends to conform to what has been dubbed Tobler's *first law of geography*: that all things are related to everything else, but near things are more related than those far apart (Tobler 1970).

3.2.2 Geographic Approaches and Methods

Based on Tobler's law, many different geographical approaches and techniques can be used to assess levels of exposure to environmental pollution. Classifying these different methods in any rigid way is difficult, for they tend to overlap and increasingly they are often used in combination. One important factor that distinguishes between them, however, is whether they are based on monitored pollution (or exposure) data, or whether they derive estimates from data on source activities. Another factor is their level of sophistication—essentially the extent to which they take account of local variation in exposures and in human activity.

Whatever method of assessment might be used, it is important to remember that we need to deal with exposures, not only pollution. It is not enough, therefore, simply to estimate patterns of pollution in the environment. These also need to be related to the population of interest. At some stage, therefore, geographic approaches to exposure assessment have to combine information on the environment and population. With new tools, such as GIS, this is becoming relatively easy. One of the main factors that limits the reliability of many exposure measures, however, is this link. People are not distributed evenly across the world. Even within an urban area, major variations in population density occur. Further, the socioeconomic characteristics of the population also vary geographically. Since these socioeconomic factors may themselves affect health, they also need to be taken into account in epidemiological studies, and often we need to control for their potential confounding effects. Therefore, just as much attention needs to be paid to the population that is studied as to the environmental patterns of pollution.

These different approaches to exposure assessment can also be applied within different epidemiological study designs. The most obvious application is in what are often called *ecological* or group designs, in which comparisons are made between whole groups of people, usually based on where they live. In these cases, data are not available on individual exposures (or other relevant characteristics), but everyone in each area is treated as if they were the same. Exposures are therefore averaged across an entire area, such as a city or administrative district. Equally, aggregate estimates of this type are often used in time-series studies. In these, the focus of attention is on changes in exposure and their associations with health outcome over time (e.g., from day to day). Spatial variations (e.g., differences in exposure between one area and another on any one day) are ignored. But geographic techniques may equally be applied to estimate exposures at the individual level, for example, by predicting the pollutant concentration at the place of residence of each participant. This allows them to be used in other study designs, such as case–control, cohort, or panel studies. Indeed, with some of the newer techniques that are now being developed, we can even model exposures as people move through the environment, as can be seen in chapter 4.

3.2.3 Data Needs and Availability

As mentioned before, measurements, or direct measurements of exposures, are thought to be the ideal method to be used for exposure assessment, either by measuring levels of pollutants in urine or blood (biomonitoring) or levels of pollutants in air, soil, or water. However, when taking measurements isn't possible or the measurements are too sparse, then information on source emissions and/or a model of the processes of pathways and routes to exposure is needed. To consequently estimate exposures, detailed information on geographic and possibly temporal patterns of the population is needed. To be able to do this, geographic methods of exposure assessment are needed. Frustratingly in many cases, one of the most serious challenges that these methods face is also lack of data. Three types of data are generally required: monitored concentrations (or exposures) for the pollutants of interest; data on the distribution and characteristics of the sources from which they are derived; and information on the target population. With some methods (e.g., dispersion modeling), a wide range of other data may also be required, for example, on meteorological conditions. Because geographic methods generally need to be used over large study areas, and often retrospectively, these data can rarely be collected using purposively designed monitoring or sampling campaigns. Instead, for the most part, they have to be acquired from existing, often routine sources. Because these have usually been set up for reasons other than exposure assessment or epidemiological research, they tend to be far from optimal.

Some indication of the problems that can be faced may be given by considering the sorts of data sets that might be needed for a study on air pollution in Great Britain. The number of monitoring stations for most of the pollutants of interest is small: There are only about 109 automatic monitoring sites as part of the Automatic Urban and Rural Network for NO_2 or PM_{10}, to represent an area of some 250,000 km^2 and a population of around 63 million people. The number of monitoring sites for other pollutants, such as VOCs and ozone is considerably fewer. Emission data are available for several pollutants, including PM_{10}, NO_x, SO_2, and VOCs, on a 1-km grid across the country, categorized by source. But these provide estimates only of average annual emissions and give no indication of short-term variations, which in many cases are substantial. Data on crucial meteorological factors, such as wind speed and wind direction, are available for only about 100 monitoring stations, and many of these tend to be clustered in coastal or relatively rural areas. Detailed population data are provided on a routine basis by the decennial census. For 2001 and 2011 these were reported for output areas, which cover about 125 households. In urban areas output areas are small; in the countryside, however, they may be anything up to 10 km² or more in extent. Intercensual estimates are provided only for local authority districts, which cover areas of several hundred square kilometers. Using any of these data for exposure assessment thus poses serious challenges; and in many cases even the best data become limited by the worst when they have to be linked and combined. All this pertains to probably the best-served area in terms of pollution, namely air pollution. With other media, such as drinking water quality, soil pollution, or noise, the available data are even more restricted. Great Britain, of course, is extremely rich in data compared to many other countries, especially in the developing world. It is not surprising that exposure assessment is often seen as an attempt to squeeze as much information as possible out of inadequate and imperfect data sets.

   Where there is little measured data, modeling becomes important and there are a number of different approaches. In the following sections (3.3 and 3.4) measurements, GIS methods, and the combination of measurements and models in GIS are discussed, and a number of examples are provided. Chapter 4 discusses the use source-dispersion and micro-environmental models for exposure assessment.

3.3 OVERVIEW OF METHODS

As mentioned in the beginning of this chapter, due to the size of the population, population-based studies often cannot rely on personal monitoring and monitoring, but need to perform environmental monitoring and modeling to estimate the exposures of the study population. As mentioned earlier, air pollution is relatively well measured through routine monitoring networks (e.g., UK-National Air Quality Archive, AIRBASE EU) and as such can be used in exposure modeling. Other environmental pollution, such as electro-magnetic fields and noise, however, either are not routinely or rarely measured.

3.3.1 Measuring Environmental Exposures

Epidemiological study designs for outdoor air pollution such as the time-series studies have related temporal (day-to-day) variation in air pollution to day-to-day variability in morbidity and mortality (Katsouyanni et al. 1995; Dockery and Pope 1997). Other studies such as the "Six Cities Study" have used the spatial differences in air pollution to define the exposure index (Dockery et al. 1993; Dockery and Pope 1997). The environmental measurements for most of these studies were obtained from stationary ambient monitoring stations that routinely measure the air pollution levels at one or more points in the area where the subjects lived. Specific monitoring campaigns can be conducted to measure environmental exposure levels, but only for current exposure, and these are often thought to be too expensive.

An important issue is how well these environmental measurements represent the subjects' actual exposure; this is discussed in chapter 10.

Epidemiological studies of water contaminants such as chlorination disinfection by-products have used water treatment practices or routinely collected trihalomethane levels in a water zone or distribution network as their exposure index. Occasionally these environmental measurements have been combined with personal data on ingestion, showering, or swimming obtained by questionnaire to obtain more specific exposure indices (see chapter 16).

Where routine measurements are used it is important to ensure that a quality control program is in place to evaluate the quality of the measurements, to avoid any bias as a result of differences in the measurement methodology and interpretation of results.

Certain areas within environmental epidemiology rely less on routinely collected data. For example, epidemiological studies of the effects of environmental tobacco smoke have often used questionnaires (e.g., whether spouse is smoking or not) or biomonitoring (e.g., cotinine) to obtain exposure estimates. The latter only indicates recent exposure, but can be used to validate questionnaire data (Etzel 1997; Wu 1997). Biomonitoring (e.g., blood benzene) has also been used frequently in studies on the effect of benzene exposure (Manuela et al. 2012). Studies on radon and electromagnetic fields have relied on a mixture of questionnaire data, expert knowledge, environmental measurements, and modeling of determinants (Brownson and Alavanja 1997; Savitz 1997, Röösli et al, 2010). Studies examining house dust for metals, house dust mite allergen, or pesticide residues have their own specific methods; adapted vacuum cleaners clean a specified area (e.g., $1/m^2$) for a specific time period (e.g., 2 minutes) (Keegan et al. 2002). Similarly, soil sampling involves the collection of multiple samples (e.g., $n = 20$) of top soil (e.g., 0–5 cm) at specific locations in the study area (Keegan et al. 2002). The information can be combined with information on hand-to-mouth contact or consumption of vegetables grown in the soil (and uptake of contaminant into vegetables) to obtain more specific exposure indices.

Issues involved in the measurement of environmental exposure such as what and where to measure, for how long and how many measurements to take, and how to assess the variance components and exposure determinants are discussed in the chapter on personal monitoring and modeling (chapter 5). Many of the issues involved are fairly similar; however, there are some differences. For example, stationary ambient monitors can be larger than personal monitors and can collect more material for further analysis and measure lower levels because of the larger volume of air sampled.

3.3.2 Introduction to Exposure Modeling

What is clear though is that measurements are not appropriate for large populations in some instances and that where personal measurements can't be done on large

Table 3.1 Exposure methods applied in air pollution epidemiological studies

Approach	Procedure	Method	Study	Exposure metric
Proximity based	Point-in-polygon	Data from monitoring sites attributed to whole city/study area	Moolgavkar (2000)	Average daily concentrations of PM_{10}, CO, SO_2, NO_2, and O_3
	Distance	Linear distance measured between place of residence and monitoring site to produce exposure distance "bands"	Ostro et al. (2010)	Monthly average concentrations of fine particulates and elemental composition
	Buffering	Exposed populations are assumed to be those who live within the specified distance of the emission source.	Harrison et al. (1999)	Residence <100 m from a major road
	Distance	Linear distance is measured between place of residence/ school and emission source (motorway).	Brunekreef et al. (1997)	Distance from homes and schools to the motorway
Spatial Interpolation	Kriging	Pollutant concentrations interpolated from monitored data, using universal kriging	Künzli et al. (2005)	Long-term mean ambient concentrations of $PM_{2.5}$
	Inverse distance weighting	Pollutant concentrations interpolated from monitored data based on inverse distance	Hoek et al. (2001, 2002)	Weighted average of regional, urban, and local concentrations of NO_2 and BS

(continued)

Table 3.1 Continued

Approach	Procedure	Method	Study	Exposure metric
Land Use Regression		Empirically derived LUR models developed for each study area	Gehring et al. (2010); Raaschou-Nielsen et al. (2013)	Mean annual concentrations of NO_2, NO_x, PM_{10}, $PM_{2.5}$, and soot
Dispersion modeling		Using AIRVIRO	Nyberg et al. (2000)	Long-term (1960s–80s) concentrations of NO_2 and SO_2
		Using CALINE4	Wu et al. (2009)	Trimester specific NO_x and $PM_{2.5}$ concentrations
Hybrid modeling		Dispersion model output combined in an LUR approach with other predictor variables.	Wilton et al. (2010)	Long term NO_2 and NO_x concentrations

numbers of individuals, then modeling is used. A number of different methods/ techniques to model the spatial and temporal variation of traffic-related air pollution exposures, for example, have been applied to small areas or address locations in epidemiological studies. The introduction of GIS has greatly extended the range of models available for exposure assessment (Nuckols et al., 2004). Both Jerrett et al. (2005) and Briggs (2007) reviewed and evaluated intra-urban air pollution models used in epidemiological studies. They broadly categorised models as: proximity-based, spatial interpolation, land use regression, dispersion modeling, and hybrid models in which two or more of the techniques described above are combined; for example, outputs from dispersion modeling have been included as variables in LUR (Wilton et al., 2010). Table 3.1 summarizes epidemiological studies by the type of method and exposure metric that has been used.

The remainder of this chapter introduces GIS techniques used to undertake exposure assessment. This is preceded with an introduction on the principles of GIS and a description of GIS data and software. There are separate chapters on dispersion modeling (chapter 4) and land use regression modeling (chapter 13).

3.4 GEOGRAPHICAL INFORMATION SYSTEMS AS A TOOL FOR EXPOSURE ASSESSMENT

3.4.1 What Are Geographical Information Systems?

Geographical approaches to exposure assessment are not new. They are often (although perhaps with some generous reinterpretation of history) traced back to the classic study of cholera in London, by John Snow in the mid-nineteenth century (Snow 1855). For many years, however, the right tools have been needed. Traditional cartographic techniques could be used in a relatively simple way to describe and display patterns of pollution and show simple associations with population distribution or with health, but the instruments required to analyse these data in any rigorous way were lacking. Since the 1980s, these have become available in the form of GIS.

In simple terms, GIS are computerized mapping systems. As such, they comprise a computer, software, data, and whatever other devices are needed to capture and display the data (e.g., scanner, plotter, printer). However, GIS can do more than simply map data. They also provide the capability to integrate the data into a common spatial form, and to analyse the data geographically. It is these capabilities that give GIS their special power in relation to exposure assessment. The ability to integrate the data implies that they can be used to bring together data on the environment, population, and health—all of which may have been collected in very different spatial formats (e.g., as points, lines, or areas, at different spatial scales)—and convert them into a common geography. This allows them to be linked, combined, and compared. The analytical functions available in GIS enable these data then to be queried and manipulated in many different ways. They can be used, for example, to examine the spatial associations between different features (e.g., people, sources of pollution, and pollution monitoring sites) and to determine how closely these are connected in space. They can be used to explore spatial patterns in the same features, and fit models that summarize the patterns that are found. We can then use these models to interpolate between our sample points, and hence to estimate conditions at locations for which we do not have data. In addition, we can use GIS in combination with other models (e.g., dispersion models) to simulate the ways in which pollutants propagate in the environment, and the exposures that occur thereby.

Although many methods of exposure assessment (see also chapter 1) are now being used in environmental epidemiology, in truth some studies still use relatively simple techniques. Sometimes there is rightful suspicion about technologies such as GIS. They may be powerful, and GIS are certainly persuasive, but that does not always mean that the answers they provide are right. Some degree of scepticism is certainly merited with any method of exposure assessment, and in most cases we would be wise to validate our estimates against independent data. For this reason geographical methods do not stand apart from other techniques, such as personal monitoring, but are complementary. Few of the techniques we will consider in the following sections also depend entirely on GIS. Many can be applied in other ways.

But the use of GIS undoubtedly makes them more practicable and above all provides the capability to extend them to larger areas or populations with relative ease.

3.4.2 Geographical Information Systems Software

Until recent years most leading GIS software (e.g., ESRI's ArcGIS,[1] MapInfo[2]) was only commercially available. There are, however, a growing number of freely available, *open-source* GIS offering a broad range of functionality. GRASS[3] (Geographic Resources Analysis Support System) GIS, for example, originally developed by the US military in the 1980s for environmental planning and land use management, now has over 350 modules covering a wide range of GIS capabilities, with particular strengths in raster analysis and image processing; GRASS is endorsed by the Open Source Geospatial Foundation.[4] An increasingly common feature of open-source GIS is their integration with freely available mathematical and statistical software (e.g., Matlab,[5] R[6]) for geo-statistical modeling (e.g., Kriging). GRASS GIS also offers support for PostgreSQL,[7] allowing integration with powerful databases. PostgreSQL, also freely available, also offers its own GIS functionality (PostGIS),[8] which is particularly good at dealing with GIS analysis of very large datasets. Commercially available GIS like ArcGIS nonetheless remain widely used by many organisations because they offer a large range of functionality for data manipulation and analysis.

3.4.3 Geographic Data and Geographic Information Systems

There are some problems in acquiring the data needed to carry out geographic methods of exposure assessment. In using these techniques another issue comes to the fore: All the data that are used must be *georeferenced*. This means that it must be possible to relate every data point or observation to a geographic location, defined in terms of its two-dimensional (or, where height is also important, three-dimensional) geographic coordinates. Georeferencing can be done in several different ways. Sometimes it is direct. For example, pollution monitoring sites or places of residence may be referenced by their latitude and longitude or x,y coordinates (e.g., in meters from a specified origin). In other cases, georeferencing is more indirect. Populations might only be available for census districts, or whole cities or regions, so their spatial connection is only to an area. It is this area that is then formally georeferenced, usually by digitally encoding its boundaries (e.g., by digitizing them onto a base map within the GIS).

Georeferencing of the data serves several vital functions. First, it enables every feature to be fixed in space and thus to be mapped. Second, it allows the features to be linked geographically, and in this way matched to a common geography. Third, it provides information on the *topology* of these features. We can tell, for example, which administrative areas are adjacent to each other, where two roadlines intersect, or where a power line passes through a housing estate. This enables us to make stronger inferences about the relationships between the features we have mapped, and the possible pathways and processes of exposure that might exist. It is important to realize, however, that the way in which we conceptualize space is highly fluid. The entities and objects that we recognize in the world, and which we may then try to map, are not always so clear-cut, but to a large extent are constructs of our minds. A roadway, for example, can be seen as a continuous feature in its own right, or just as a rather irregular gap between houses. In particular, the way in which we conceive of any feature depends upon the scale of analysis we use. A feature such as a landfill site might be seen as an area at one scale, but effectively represented as a point at another. How we conceive of, and georeference, features in a GIS therefore depends on circumstances and need. We do, however, have to be aware of the implications of representing space in these different ways, for when we change the form of spatial representation, we may also change the implied topology. When represented as part of a continuous network, for example, stream water, monitoring sites are connected in a very specific way. If represented as unconnected points, the topological connections are lost. If we used these two different constructs to model, say, the distribution of the pollution within the river network, we might obtain very different results.

3.5 DISTANCE AND PROXIMITY MEASURES

The simplest model of exposure is based on proximity and assumes that people living near an emission source (e.g., traffic) are more highly exposed than people living further away, following the previously mentioned Tobler's law (1970). For example, Brunekreef et al. (1997) found an association between reduced lung function in schoolchildren living near motorways and density of truck traffic. Many studies looking at air pollution and health have used nearest monitoring site to assign exposures to populations. This can be done in two ways: using distance (i.e., a NEAR analysis) or by creating so-called "Voronoi" or "Thiessen polygons." The first studies looking at an association between adverse health effects and air pollution depended on data from sparse monitoring networks. Thus the Six Cities Study by Dockery et al. (1993), mentioned earlier, used air pollution data measured at six centrally located monitoring sites to estimate exposures for the six communities involved. However, nearest air pollution monitoring station has been shown to be a poor marker for air pollutant exposures in complex urban environments (Gulliver et al. 2011).

In this context, Tobler's law might seem to apply. If things that are closer together tend to be more similar, equally, levels of pollution might be expected to decline with distance from source. Distance from, or proximity to, the sources of pollution thus appears to offer a useful and easily applicable measure of exposure. All GIS offer automated functions for measuring distance between different types of features used to represent pollution sources and population (points, lines, areas). It is certainly an approach that has been used widely, especially in the context of air pollution. Many studies of traffic-related air pollution, for example, have classified exposures in terms of the distance to the nearest main road, the road traffic volume on the nearest road, etc. Buffering is another often-used method in exposure assignment; buffers are concentric circles around points or distance bands following shapes of lines (e.g., roads) or areas. Multiple buffers may be used to define different zones (i.e., concentric circles) of exposure (i.e., low to high) related to different distances from pollution source (e.g., 0 m–200 m, >200 m–400 m, >400 m–600 m).

An example of where buffering has been used is in a study of congenital anomalies around landfill sites in Great Britain (Elliott et al. 2009). In this case, the rationale for using a simple distance measure to define exposed and unexposed groups was based on several considerations. One was the relatively poor quality of the data on landfill sites: Exact boundaries of these were rarely known, and most were identified only by a point location (usually the gateway). More importantly, neither the exact pollutants being emitted from the landfill sites, nor the pathways of dispersion (e.g., by air or groundwater) were known. For both these reasons, the use of sophisticated models was not considered worthwhile. On the other hand, what little work had been done previously clearly suggested that exposures, by any route, were likely to be confined close to the sites, and certainly within a kilometer or two. At the same time, the large number of sites that had to be considered (some 8804 in all including 607 sites that handled special hazardous wastes), and their often close clustering, meant that many people lived within a few kilometers of a number of different landfill sites. Without real knowledge about the spatial variation in exposures, however, the cumulative risks from these multiple sites could not be reliably assessed. In consequence, it was decided to use a simple threshold distance (2 km) to distinguish between "exposed" and "unexposed" populations. Using buffering techniques in a GIS, therefore, circles 2 km in radius were drawn around each of the landfill sites, and these were then intersected with postcode coordinates of over 10 million births (136,821 congenital anomalies), 1983–1998 (Figure 3.1). A landfill exposure index was developed to weight postcode locations in the exposed group based on whether they fell within one or more buffers around landfill sites. Based on this, the birth of every child between 1983 and 1998 could be allocated an exposure index for the exposed group (index of 1, 2, 3, 4, etc.) and unexposed group (index of 0). Postcode locations were subsequently intersected with a 5 × 5 km grid and linked to data on births and congenital anomalies. It is often the case that the size of geographical unit

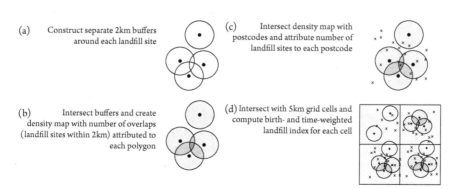

Figure 3.1 Buffering around landfill sites and intersection with postcodes and a 5-km grid holding data on births and congenital anomalies.

for analysis in epidemiological studies is governed by the geographical density of cases, hence the reason in this study for using a minimum grid size of 5-km squares.

Using this exposure measure, the authors found that there was a weak association between the geographic density of (special) hazardous waste sites and certain congenital anomalies at the level of 5×5 km grid squares.

Some problems with these relatively simple source-based measures also need to be recognized. Implicit within them, for example, is that pollution spreads uniformly away from its source. This is clearly not always the case: wind direction determines the dispersion of air pollution; slope angle may constrain the spread of pollution in the soil; in networks, such as rivers or drinking water supply systems, pollutants will be channelled along specific and complex pathways; in other systems, such as the food supply chain, distance is likely to be an extremely poor proxy for dispersion. Because they are inherently nonspecific (they do not relate to a particular pollutant nor exposure pathway), they can also be difficult to interpret. They might suggest that people living in certain areas suffer increased health risks, but they do not tell us why. It is perhaps partly for this reason that the health risks from both types of sources (road traffic and landfill sites) remain only poorly assessed and controversial. Almost certainly, we need more specific and more powerful measures of exposure if we are to detect and measure these risks reliably, against the large background of "noise" with which we have to contend in epidemiological studies.

3.6 INTERPOLATION METHODS

Tobler's (1970) first law of geography implies that in things geographical, distance is the key. In so far as this is true, it means that two people who live close to each other are likely to have more similar exposures than two people who live further apart. Where data on pollution levels are available from a number of sampled locations (i.e., measurements), spatial interpolation techniques can be used to model the pollution surface and thereby estimate conditions at unsampled locations simply on the basis of their relative proximity to the sampling points.

Commonly used techniques include simple point-in-polygon operations, trend surface analysis, inverse distance weighting (IDW) (Hoek et al. 2001, 2002), and kriging (Künzli et al. 2005). Trend surface analysis is an inexact interpolator, in that a smooth surface is fitted to measurement data using regression techniques and the surface created does not necessarily reproduce the values at measurement locations. Inverse Distance Weighting is a local interpolation technique to estimate values at unsampled locations as a function of values at sampled locations within a specified zone of influence (e.g., radius). The weighting (or influence) of surrounding locations is usually a function of inverse distance. Kriging is based on the principle that spatial variation can be broken down into three distinct elements: systematic trend (or drift), local trend (spatially correlated random variation), and noise (spatially uncorrelated random variation). Kriging focuses on estimating the second of these components by examining the relationship of distance between pairs of sample points and their difference in terms of the monitored concentrations. By intersecting the resulting map of pollution concentrations with the population distribution, an assessment of exposures can then be made. Explicitly or implicitly, these principles are commonly used as a basis for exposure assessment in many different fields.

3.6.1 Point in Polygon Techniques

Interpolation is something we carry out intuitively—so much so, in fact, that we often do not realize that we are doing it. It is simply the art of estimation on the basis of the evidence that surrounds us. It is a technique that is used almost universally in epidemiological studies, for rarely if ever do we have complete data on pollution levels or exposures, either over time or space. We therefore have to fill in the gaps by interpolation.

Geographically, probably the simplest way in which this is done is by point-in-polygon techniques. Essentially this involves taking data from a single sample point and extending it to its surrounding area. This methodology is so simple that it does not need sophisticated mapping tools. It is done routinely in many time-series studies of air pollution, merely by assigning populations to the monitoring stations within their city. Daily concentrations from the monitoring stations are then computed (e.g., by averaging data from all the available sites within a city) and assigned to everyone living within that city. Associations may then be sought between this averaged pollution concentration and health outcome (e.g., mortality or numbers of hospital admissions) from day to day. The same technique can also be used for studies of long-term exposures and chronic health effects. It was used, for example, in the seminal "Six Cities Study" in the United States (Dockery et al. 1993). This study compared rates of respiratory illness, including mortality, across six cities with contrasting levels of pollution, each city being classified by averaging long-term data from the available monitoring stations. A strong gradient was found for several health outcomes, especially with particulates (PM_{10}) and SO_2, and results from this study have become the foundations of many of the air quality guidelines adopted across the world.

This approach to exposure assessment is evidently very naïve, in that it takes no account of spatial variations in exposure: Everyone within each area is assumed to get the same exposure. Slightly more sophistication can be introduced, however, by allocating different areas to different monitoring or measurement stations. This raises the question of which stations get assigned to which areas. One way of doing this is by simple proximity: Each area is considered to be represented by its closest monitoring station. A GIS technique known as Thiessen (or Voroni) tessellation is useful for this purpose: This can be used to create polygons around each monitoring station so that every location in the city is associated with its nearest station (Figure 3.2). Populations can thus be assigned to, and represented by, their nearest monitoring site.

3.6.2 Trend Surface Analysis

The simple methods described earlier are clearly a very crude approximation of reality. If we look at the pollution surfaces that they produced, we would find that they consisted of flat areas, within which the pollution levels are assumed to be the same,

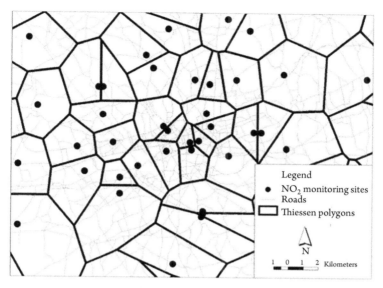

Figure 3.2 Thiessen polygons around NO_2 monitoring sites in London.

separated by abrupt changes. In the real world, of course, pollution surfaces tend to be much smoother. In order to model these more realistically, therefore, methods need to be used that treat the pollution field as a continuously varying surface, not as a set of discrete blocks.

Spatial interpolation is a group of methods that are used to create continuously varying surfaces. In broad terms, interpolation methods may be categorised as *local* or *global*. Global methods fit a single model or mathematical function (i.e., fixed parameters) to sample locations, whereas in local interpolation model parameters vary depending on the values of measurements in the area surrounding measurements locations. Trend surface analysis is a global, "inexact" (i.e., the values of sample locations are not necessarily maintained in the resulting surface) interpolation method, defined by a mathematical regression function (a polynomial), which fits a relatively smooth surface through sample point locations. There are a number of different polynomials that can be applied to the data depending on the complexity of the underlying surface, as shown in Eqs. 3.1 to 3.3.

Linear:

$$z = \beta_0 + \beta_1 x + \beta_2 y \qquad\qquad \text{(Eq. 3.1)}$$

Quadratic:

$$z = \beta_0 + \beta_1 x + \beta_2 y + \beta_3 x^2 + \beta_4 y^2 + \beta_5 xy \qquad\qquad \text{(Eq. 3.2)}$$

Cubic:

$$z = \beta_0 + \beta_1 x + \beta_2 y + \beta_3 x^2 + \beta_4 y^2 + \beta_5 xy + \beta_6 x^2 y + \beta_7 xy^2 + \beta_8 x^3 + \beta_9 y^3 \qquad \text{(Eq. 3.3)}$$

where $\beta_0, \beta_1, \ldots, \beta_n$ are the coefficients of the regression (i.e., polynomial), and z is the predicted exposure at location x, y.

Trend surfaces may be useful, for example, in creating maps of ambient temperature from data collected at meteorological stations because temperatures tend to change gradually over relatively large distances, but would not be appropriate for creating outdoor air pollution surfaces in urbanised countries because these often change rapidly and unevenly around irregularly distributed sources.

3.6.3 Inverse Distance Weighting

Some methods are essentially deterministic, and model surfaces as a function of the inverse distance between the monitoring sites. The user determines what type of function to apply, and the software then calculates the estimated pollution level at each location based on the distance from, and measured pollution levels at, each of the surrounding monitoring sites. This approach thus rigorously applies Tobler's law in assuming that nearer monitoring sites are likely to provide better estimates of pollution levels at any location than those further away. In some cases a simple linear function of distance is used $(1/d)$, but more commonly some form of inverse power function is used, on the principle that the "influence" of more distant sites declines more than proportionally to distance. Probably the most common is an inverse square $(1/d^2)$. Eq. 3.4 is used to apply IDW. The "weights" (λ) for measurements from each sampled location (i.e., those included up to the maximum distance being considered around each unsampled location) are calculated using Eq. 3.5.

$$z_j = \sum_{i=1}^{n} \lambda_i z_i \qquad \text{(Eq. 3.4)}$$

where z_j is the estimated exposure at location j, and λ are the weights applied to each measurement value (z) at a series of sampled locations (i).

$$\lambda_i = \frac{1/d_i^p}{\sum_{i=1}^{n} \frac{1}{d_i^p}} \qquad \text{(Eq. 3.5)}$$

where d_i is the distance between unsampled location j and each sampled location i, and p is the power function for distance (e.g., $1/d^2$).

Application of IDW is either to a series of "receptor" point locations (e.g., address locations in an epidemiological study) or to create a continuous surface (i.e., which can in turn be used to derive exposures for different geographical units) using a "moving window." Moving window techniques are relatively simple and essentially deterministic. The "window" is typically a square or circular area that is moved across the map, centring on each location in turn. The pollution concentration at that location is then determined by taking the inverse distance-weighted average of all the monitoring sites that fall within the window. The size (and shape) of the window is selected by the user, and should be chosen to ensure that it contains enough monitoring sites to provide a reliable estimate for each location, but not so many that it ends up oversmoothing the surface.

IDW methods have the advantage that it is relatively easy to apply and require no data other than the, for example, monitored pollution concentrations and locations of each monitoring site, and are available as standard functions in almost any GIS. They nevertheless have some disadvantages. First, the results they produce depend upon decisions made by the user (e.g., the choice of inverse distance function and—in the case of the moving window methods—the window size). They also work effectively only where there is a reasonably dense network of monitoring or sample sites; otherwise, areas tend to occur within which the estimates may be highly generalized and unreliable.

In practice, they have also had surprisingly little use in environmental epidemiology. This is partly, perhaps, because the data available usually do not meet the requirements of the techniques: Monitoring stations are often too sparse or too clustered. More generally, however, it may be because epidemiologists are not always aware of the existence of these techniques. Certainly they should not be ignored, for by providing area-weighted estimates of pollutant concentrations, rather than simple averages, they can undoubtedly improve exposure assessment and allow some of the local spatial variation in exposures to be taken into account.

3.6.4 Geostatistical Techniques

As already mentioned, one of the problems with deterministic techniques such as inverse distance weighting is their dependence on decisions of the user—decisions that in many cases are inevitably not always well informed. In general, it would therefore seem more justifiable to use stochastic methods of surface modeling, which allow the data to decide. One such approach, which is increasingly being used, is geostatistics. Geostatistical techniques include a wide range of different methods, among which kriging is the best known. Various forms of kriging are now available as a standard function in a number of GIS, including ArcGIS and freely available statistical software that can couple with GIS (e.g., R).

Kriging comprises a varied suite of techniques, all based on the same underlying assumptions, namely that spatial variation in the phenomena of interest can be subdivided into three main components: systematic variation (or drift); random but spatially correlated variation; and random, spatially uncorrelated variation (or noise). Kriging models the components of variation by examining spatial patterns in the available data. Generically, kriging thus attempts to solve Eq. 3.6.

$$z_i(x) = m(x) + j(x) + \varepsilon \qquad\qquad (Eq. 3.6)$$

where $z_i(x)$ is the estimated value of the variable z_i at location x; $m(x)$ is a measure of the systematic variation (i.e., trend or drift) at x; $j(x)$ is a stochastic, locally varying component of variation at x, and ε is the residual variation or noise.

Under the simplest forms of kriging (ordinary kriging), $m(x)$ is assumed to be zero—that is, there is assumed to be no systematic variation or trend. The spatially correlated random component of variation then becomes the focus of attention, and this is modeled by analysing the association between the difference in the measured values at each pair of sample points and their distance apart (or lag). This is done by measuring the semi-variance, which is defined in Eq. 3.7.

$$\gamma(h) = \frac{1}{2}n\sum_{i=1}^{n}(Z_{xi} + Z_{xi} + h)^2 \qquad\qquad (Eq. 3.7)$$

where γ is the semi-variance with respect to distance between pairs of locations, h is the distance between the n pairs of sites, and $Z(xi)$ is the value of variable Zi at site x.

Different models may then be fitted to the data (e.g., spherical, exponential, Gaussian), and the optimum one chosen using cross-validation techniques or other methods. The resulting semi-variogram (Figure 3.3) typically shows two diagnostic features: a small "nugget" effect, where the model intersects with the y-axis (reflecting the residual error or noise), and a relatively steep rising limb to a "sill," where it then levels off. The distance to the sill is referred to as the range and shows the distance from each point within which the spatially correlated variation is effective. In other words, it indicates the area around each location from which sample points may be drawn to make estimates.

Ordinary kriging, as described, provides a relatively straightforward way of modeling pollution levels in areas where there is a reasonably dense network of sample points and no strong trend or drift. If a regional trend is present, however, it can lead to biased estimations, especially where monitoring stations are relatively far apart. Systematic trend (or drift) between the sample locations is usually assessed as a precursor step to creating a model for the semi-variogram. The trend component can also be modeled either globally (i.e., a single trend across the whole data set as per trend surface analysis described in section 4.2.2) or locally (by generating a local surface for the subset of surrounding points): In the latter case the user has to determine how many local points (i.e., what percentage of data points) should be used. The semi-variogram is specified on the residuals from the trend analysis, and then the trend and residuals are summed before ordinary kriging is applied.

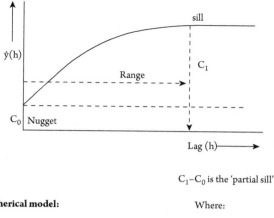

$C_1 - C_0$ is the 'partial sill'

Spherical model:

Where:

$$\gamma(h) = \begin{cases} \dfrac{3h}{2a} - \dfrac{1}{2}\left(\dfrac{h}{a}\right)^3 & \forall h < a \\ 0 & \forall h \geq a \end{cases}$$

h: lag distance
a: range
$\gamma(h)$: semi-variance

Figure 3.3 A typical semi-variogram with a spherical model used to define the relationship of distance between pairs of sampled locations to be applied in kriging.

Ordinary kriging can be applied without considering trend, but trend is often considered as a prior stage to developing the semi-variogram. Ordinary kriging with trend removal is not the same as universal kriging. In universal kriging, both components (trend + stochastic) are fitted simultaneously. There are several other types of kriging: block, disjunctive, indicator, probability, and kriging with external drift (see Webster and Oliver 2007).

Once computed, the model is then applied to all the unsampled locations within the study area. This is done by passing a filter (moving window) across the map, visiting each location in turn. The pollutant concentration at each location is then computed based on the model derived from the sample data. The size of the moving window is defined by the user, either by setting minimum and maximum numbers of sample points (monitoring stations) to be used for each computation, or by delimiting a search radius. The search radius is usually set to be at least equivalent to the "range" defined by the semi-variogram, in order to ensure that it captures all the relevant information from the surrounding monitoring sites.

Kriging techniques attracted attention in the earth sciences relatively early—they originated from geology and quickly spread into applications such as soil mapping (Burrough and McDonnell 1998). They are being used for pollution mapping and exposure assessment, and under some circumstances they have proved to be highly effective. Liu and Rossini (1996), for example, used ordinary kriging to assess short-term ozone concentrations in Toronto. Cressie (2000) illustrates its use to model daily PM_{10} concentrations in Pittsburgh, and Künzli et al. (2005) used universal kriging to model long-term ambient concentrations of $PM_{2.5}$ in Los Angeles. Järup (2000) also describes the application of ordinary kriging to model the distribution of cadmium in moss, in Mönsterås, Sweden, as a basis for assessing associations with urinary cadmium.

In all cases one of the key strengths of kriging is that it not only provides an approximation of the pollution surface, but also yields estimates of its standard error at each location. This enables the reliability of the modeled surface to be examined, and exposure estimates to be weighted accordingly. An important recent extension to geostatistical analysis is Bayesian kriging, which provides a rigorous assessment of model uncertainty (i.e., error) in addition to surfaces of exposure estimates. Vicedo-Cabrera et al. (2013), for example, used Bayesian universal Kriging to predict long-term concentrations of sulphur dioxide (SO_2) and nitrogen dioxide (NO_2) as markers of children's air pollution exposure for different regions of Italy. Nevertheless, kriging does have its limits. Like other methods of interpolation, it works best when the monitoring sites are evenly and densely spread. It is also less effective when the pollution surface shows complex structural variations (e.g., associated with local emission sources) that are not well represented by the monitoring stations. It is thus constrained by the available monitoring data, and as we have seen this is often severely limited.

3.7 CONCLUSION

The GIS-based methods of exposure assessment clearly have a great deal to offer in environmental epidemiology. When monitored data are sparse, they provide a range of methods for estimating pollution levels at unsampled sites and constructing maps of pollution. They also provide the means to link these estimates of pollution to population distribution, and thereby assess exposures either for individuals or for population groups.

Geographical exposure assessment equally offers a way of translating established dose–response functions into measures of health risk—that is for health impact assessment. By estimating the distribution of exposures across the population, they allow the attributable health risk, or the overall burden of disease, from a specified pollutant or source activity to be estimated. This is important for policy, for it is often on the basis of calculations such as this that issues are prioritized and the decision for action made. Just as important are the visualization capabilities of GIS. Maps are persuasive, and their ability to make maps of exposure or health risk more-or-less to need, and then to interrogate them interactively, means that GIS are especially powerful tools. Yet models and maps can also lie. So in using these techniques, we have to be careful. We need to remember that they are only approximations of reality. We need to recognize that few, if any, of the techniques we use are wholly neutral or objective: In various ways, sometimes explicitly, often implicitly, we make choices and decisions that influence the results we obtain. These results are also subject to uncertainty, so we should always try to check them by validation against independent data, such as personal monitoring. Above all, we should use and interpret them cautiously. Together with a little imagination and insight, these techniques can certainly help us to generate new and exciting hypotheses. But if we want to use them as part of a process of hypothesis testing, or as a basis for intervention and policy, we must at all times be guided by what is both environmentally and biologically plausible. Geography is thus just one of the sciences that we need to employ in pursuing questions about the effects of environmental pollution on health, or what we should do about them.

NOTES

1. http://www.esri.com/software/arcgis
2. http://www.mapinfo.com
3. http://grass.osgeo.org/
4. http://osgeo.org/
5. http://www.mathworks.co.uk/products/matlab/
6. http://www.r-project.org
7. http://www.postgresql.org
8. http://postgis.net

REFERENCES

Briggs, D. J. (2007). The use of GIS to evaluate traffic-related pollution. *Occupational and Environmental Medicine*, **64**(1), 1–2.

Brownson, R. C., and Alavanja, M. C. R. (1997). Radiation I. Radon. In *Topics in environmental epidemiology* (eds. K. Steenland and D. Savitz), 314–349. Oxford University Press, New York.

Brunekreef, B., Janssen, N. A. H., de Hartog, J., Harssema, H., Knape, M., and van Vliet, P. (1997). Air pollution from truck traffic and lung function in children living near motorways. *Epidemiology*, **8**, 298–303.

Burrough, P. A., and McDonnell, R. A. (1998). *Principles of geographical information systems*. Oxford University Press, Oxford.

Cressie, N. (2000). Geostatistical methods for mapping environmental exposures. In *Spatial epidemiology. Methods and applications* (eds. P. Elliott, J. C. Wakefield, N. G. Best, and D. J. Briggs), 185–204. Oxford University Press, Oxford.

Dockery, D. W. and Pope, C. A. (1997). Outdoor air I: Particulates. In *Topics in environmental epidemiology* (ed. K. Steenland and D. Savitz), 119–166. Oxford University Press, New York.

Dockery, D. W., Pope III, A., Xu, X., Spengler, J. D., Ware, J. H., Fay, M. E., et al. (1993). An association between air pollution and mortality in six US cities. *The New England Journal of Medicine*, **329**, 1753–1759.

Dolk, H., Elliott, P., Shaddick, G., Walls, P., and Grundy, C. (1997). Cancer incidence near high power radio and TV transmitters in Great Britain: II. All transmitter sites. *American Journal of Epidemiology*, **145**, 10–17.

Dolk, H., Thakrar, B., Walls, P., Landon, M., Grundy, C., Suez Lloret, I., et al. (1999). Mortality among residents near cokeworks in Great Britain. *Occupational and Environmental Medicine*, **56**, 34–40.

Elliott, P., Briggs, D., Morris, S., de Hoogh, C., Hurt, C., Kold Jensen, T., et al. (2001). Risk of adverse birth outcomes in populations living near landfill sites. *British Medical Journal,* **323**, 363–368.

Elliott, P., Richardson, S., Abellan, J. J., Thomson, A., de Hoogh, C., Jarup, L., and Briggs, D. J. (2009). Geographic density of landfill sites and risk of congenital anomalies in England. *Occupational and Environmental Medicine,* **66**, 81–89.

Etzel, R. A. (1997). Environmental tobacco smoke. I: Childhood diseases. In *Topics in environmental epidemiology* (eds. K. Steenland and D. Savitz), 200–226. Oxford University Press, New York.

Gehring, U., Wijga, A. H., Brauer, M., Fischer, P., de Jongste, J. C., Kerkhof, M., et al. (2010). Traffic-related air pollution and the development of asthma and allergies during the first 8 years of life. *American Journal of Respiratory and Critical Care Medicine,* **181**, 596–603.

Gulliver, J., Vienneau, D., Fecht, D., de Hoogh, K., and Briggs, D. (2011). Comparative assessment of GIS-based methods and metrics for estimating long-term exposure to air pollution. *Atmospheric Environment,* **45**(39), 7072–7080.

Harrison, R. M., Leung, P.-L., Somerville, L., Smith, R., and Gilman, E. (1999). Analysis of incidence of childhood cancer in the West Midlands of the United Kingdom in relation to proximity to main roads and petrol stations. *Occupational and Environmental Medicine,* **56**, 774–780.

Hoek, G., Fischer. P., van den Brandt, P., Goldbohm, S., and Brunekreef, B. (2001). Estimation of long-term average exposure to outdoor air pollution for a cohort study on mortality. *Journal of Exposure Analysis and Environmental Epidemiology,* **11**, 459–469.

Hoek, G., Brunekreef, B., Goldbohm, S., Fischer, P., and van den Brandt, P. A. (2002). Association between mortality and indicators of traffic-related air pollution in the Netherlands: A cohort study. *Lancet,* **360**, 1203–1209.

Järup, L. (2000). The role of geographical studies in risk assessment. In *Spatial epidemiology: Methods and applications* (eds. P. Elliott, J. C. Wakefield, N. G. Best, and D. J. Briggs), 415–433. Oxford University Press, Oxford.

Jerrett, M., Arain, A., Kanaroglou, P., Beckerman, B., Potoglou, D., Sahsuvaroglu, T., et al. (2005). A review and evaluation of intraurban air pollution exposure models. *Journal of Exposure Analysis and Environmental Epidemiology,* **15**, 185–204.

Katsouyanni, K., Zmirou, D., Spix, C., Sunyer, J., Schouten, J. P., Ponka, A., et al. (1995). Short-term effects of air-pollution on health—a European approach using epidemiologic time-series data—the Aphea Project—background, objectives, design. *European Respiratory Journal,* **8**, 1030–1038.

Keegan, T., Hong, B., Thornton, I., Farago, M., Jakubis, P., Jakubis, M., et al. (2002). Assessment of environmental arsenic levels in Prievidza District. *Journal of Exposure Analysis Environmental Epidemiology,* **12**, 179–185.

Künzli, N., Jerrett, M., Mack, W. J., Beckerman, B., LaBree, L., Gilliland, F., et al. (2005). Ambient air pollution and atherosclerosis in Los Angeles. *Environmental Health Perspectives,* **113**, 201–206.

Liu, L. J. S., and Rossini, A. J. (1996). Use of kriging models to predict 12-hour mean ozone concentrations in Metropolitan Toronto—a pilot study. *Environment International,* **22**, 677–692.

Manuela, C., Francesco, T., Tiziana, C., Assunta, C., Lara, S., Nadia, N., Barbara, S., Maria, F., Carlotta, C., Valeria, D.G., Pia, S.M., Gianfranco, T., and Angela, S. (2012). Environmental and biological monitoring of benzene in traffic policemen, police drivers and rural outdoor male workers. *Journal of Environmental Monitoring*, **14**(6), 1542–1550.

Moolgavkar, S. H. (2000). Air pollution and daily mortality in three US counties. *Environmental Health Perspectives*, **108**, 777–784.

Nuckols, J. R., Ward, M. H., and Jarup, L. (2004). Using geographic information systems for exposure assessment in environmental epidemiology studies. *Environmental Health Perspectives*, **112**(9), 1007–1015.

Nyberg, F., Gustavsson, P., Järup, L., Bellander, T., Berglund, N., Jakobsson, R., and Pershagen, G. (2000). Urban air pollution and lung cancer in Stockholm. *Epidemiology*, **11**, 487–495.

Ostro, B., Lipsett, M., Reynolds, P., Goldberg, D., Hertz, A., Garcia, C., et al. (2010). Long-term exposure to constituents of fine particulate air pollution and mortality: Results from the California teachers study. *Environmental Health Perspectives*, **118**, 363–369.

Raaschou-Nielsen, O., Andersen, Z. J., Beelen, R., Samoli, E., Stafoggia, M., Weinmayret, G., et al. (2013). Air pollution and lung cancer incidence in 17 European cohorts: prospective analyses from the European Study of Cohorts for Air Pollution Effects (ESCAPE). *Lancet Oncology*, **14**, 813–822.

Röösli, M., Frei, P., Bolte, J., Neubauer, G., Cardis, E., Feychting, M., et al. (2010). Conduct of a personal radiofrequency electromagnetic field measurement study: proposed study protocol. *Environmental Health*, **9**, 23.

Savitz, D. A. (1997). Radiation II: Electromagnetic fields. In *Topics in environmental epidemiology* (eds. K. Steenland and D. Savitz), 295–313. Oxford University Press, New York.

Snow, J. M. (1855). *On the mode of communication of cholera* (2nd ed.). Churchill Livingstone, London.

Tobler, W. R. (1970). A computer movie simulating urban growth in the Detroit region. *Economic Geographer*, **46**, 234–240.

Vicedo-Cabrera, A. M., Biggeri, A., Grisotto, L., Barbone, F., and Catelan, D. (2013). A Bayesian kriging model for estimating residential exposure to air pollution of children living in a high-risk area in Italy. *Geospatial Health*, **8**(1), 87–95.

Webster, R., and Oliver, M. (2007). *Geostatistics for environmental scientists* (2nd ed). Hoboken, NJ, Wiley.

Wilton, D., Szpiro, A., Gould, T., and Larson, T. (2010). Improving spatial concentration estimates for nitrogen oxides using a hybrid meteorological dispersion/land use regression model in Los Angeles, CA and Seattle, WA. *Science of the Total Environment*, **408**, 1120–1130.

Wu, A. H. (1997). Environmental tobacco smoke II: Lung cancer. In *Topics in environmental epidemiology* (eds. K. Steenland and D. Savitz), 200–226. Oxford University Press, New York.

Wu, J., Ren, C., Delfino, R. J., Chung, J., Wilhelm, M., and Ritz, B. (2009). Association between local traffic-generated air pollution and preeclampsia and preterm delivery in the south coast air basin of California. *Environmental Health Perspectives*, **117**(11), 1773–1779.

4

ENVIRONMENTAL MEASUREMENT AND MODELING
SOURCE DISPERSION AND MICRO-ENVIRONMENTAL MODELS

Kees de Hoogh, David Briggs, and John Gulliver

4.1 INTRODUCTION

There are a number of techniques for exposure assessment, including those that can be undertaken within a geographical information system such as proximity methods and spatial interpolation (chapter 3). This chapter deals with models of the exposure pathway between source and receptor by defining the sources of contamination, describing the transport and transformation of the contaminant through the environmental media, and calculating concentrations of the contaminant at the location of a receptor, which can vary in time and space (e.g., people move through the environment and are as such not only exposed at the home address, but also at work, during their commute, at different times of the day). The focus of this chapter is mainly on different methods simulating the dispersion of air pollution illustrated with a few examples of applications in environmental epidemiological studies. One additional example shows the development and application of a propagation model outside the air pollution theme, describing an exposure model of electromagnetic fields (EMF) radiation around mobile phone masts.

4.2 LAND USE REGRESSION MODELING

Land use regression (LUR) was first developed and applied in the Small Area Variations in Air quality and Health (SAVIAH) study, in which it was used to estimate exposures to traffic-related air pollution for Huddersfield, Amsterdam, and Prague (Briggs et al., 1997). Since then it has been widely used in epidemiological studies for exposure assessment (Hoek et al., 2008).

The use of LUR modeling extends the principles of proximity-based methods (see chapter 3) to model the contribution (i.e., as a proxy for source emissions and sinks) of different geographical variables (e.g., land cover, transport networks, topography) to spatial variability in air pollution concentrations.

Typically, monitoring data at a relatively small number of monitoring sites (40–120) are combined with explanatory variables that are extracted using circular buffers of variable distance, representing the area of influence of each source type, at each measurement site within a geographical information system (GIS). Regression analysis is used to determine the coefficients (i.e., weights) of the set of variables that explain the highest proportion of variation in measured concentrations. Then LUR models can be used to estimate long-term air pollution concentrations at unmonitored locations in the same study area. Recent studies have shown that pollution surfaces created by LUR models generally remain spatially stable over time (Gulliver et al., 2013; Wang et al., 2013), thus making LUR a potentially powerful tool for assessing historic exposures (see also chapter 13).

Land use regression (LUR) modeling uses data from a "training" set of monitoring stations to develop regression-based models of the associations between pollution levels and relevant environmental variables. These models are then applied to each location within the study area to develop an exposure estimate. The approach was used by Briggs et al. (1997), for example, to model NO_2 concentrations in Huddersfield, Amsterdam, and Prague. In each case, passive samplers (Palmes tubes) were deployed at up to 80 sampling locations for periods of 2 weeks, on four occasions throughout the year. Using GIS techniques, a range of potential covariates were then extracted, including data on road traffic density (e.g., traffic volume, road length), land use (e.g., areas of industrial, urban, residential land), and altitude in the surrounding area. Slightly different models were developed in each city because of differing availability of data. In Huddersfield, however, NO_2 concentrations were found to be effectively predicted by a model comprising three variables: a measure of road traffic volume (vehicle kilometres) in the surrounding 40- and 300-meter buffer zones, a measure of the area of intensively built-up land in the surrounding 300-meter buffer zone, and altitude. This was used to map NO_2 concentrations across the study area, at a resolution of 10 meters. The map was also validated against independent data from additional monitoring sites.

Subsequently, the model was further adapted and applied to model NO_2 concentrations in three other cities, as well as in Huddersfield for a later year (Briggs et al. 2000). Again, validation showed that it gave reliable estimates of air pollutant concentrations, with a standard error of estimate of only 5 to 10 $\mu g/m^{-3}$ (<20% of the mean concentration). In more recent years LUR has been widely adopted in epidemiological studies. Its popularity is likely due to its inherent simplicity, relatively low data demands, and preference over dispersion modeling, in which there is a lack of information to characterize pollution emissions, especially in national studies in which detailed emissions inventories are rarely available. Certainly LUR is the most widespread method used in air pollution exposure assessment and has generally seen good performance in model validation studies. For this reason chapter 13 focuses on the development and application of LUR in exposure studies.

4.3 SOURCE DISPERSION MODELING

Whenever we have better understanding of the environmental systems involved, we can use more sophisticated models to simulate both the processes and pathways of pollutant propagation in the environment, and thereby begin to obtain more realistic and dynamic estimations of exposures. One way of doing this is through the use of dispersion (or pollutant propagation) models.

Although some dispersion models are fully integrated within a GIS environment, the basic proprietary software is usually standalone. This section describes the basic principles of dispersion modeling and describes some of the available dispersion models. The next section (4.4) then shows a few examples of these methods in environmental epidemiological studies.

In general terms, dispersion models consist of mathematical representations of the processes that generate pollutants and control their movement, dilution, and fate in the environment. Dispersion modeling is far more firmly established in the field of air quality than in other areas. Most of the applications for exposure assessment have thus tended to focus on atmospheric pollution. Atmospheric dispersion models (mostly) use Gaussian equations to model the transport of gaseous pollutants through the atmosphere and predict ground level concentrations. They were originally developed as a tool for regulatory compliance modeling and are traditionally used in environmental impact assessment. They require detailed input data on emissions (for industrial sources: stack height, stack diameter, emission rate, temperature of exit gas; for traffic: flow, composition, speed), and meteorological parameters (a minimum of wind direction, wind speed, ambient temperature, cloud cover). Advanced dispersion models like ADMS-Urban (Advanced Dispersion Modeling System) (McHugh et al., 1997) and AERMOD (Paine et al., 1998) have rarely been used in epidemiological studies, possibly because of their demanding data requirements. Dispersion models are solely used for air pollution, whereas the other methods described in these sections can also be applied to other pollutants/contaminants.

Examples include Nyberg et al. (2000), who used the AIRVIRO model to map concentrations of NO_2 and SO_2 between the 1960s and 1980s in Stockholm. Exposures were then estimated for *c.* 1000 cancer cases and 2000 controls by dropping the place of residence onto the pollution maps within a GIS. When adjusted for confounding by smoking, the results showed a small, but statistically significant, increased risk of lung cancer for exposures to NO_2, though not to SO_2. Because NO_2 is largely generated by road traffic, whereas SO_2 tends to come from stationary combustion sources such as domestic heating systems, the implication was that this risk is primarily a function of traffic-related air pollution. Examples of using dispersion modeling for short-term averaging periods include Wu et al. (2009), who modeled trimester-specific NO_x and $PM_{2.5}$ concentrations for a study on air pollution and preterm delivery in California.

So long as the processes are sufficiently well understood and can be simulated by the available data, propagation models can also be applied to other forms of pollution. One example is noise pollution. High levels of exposure to road traffic have been associated with increased risk for cardiovascular conditions and risk factors including hypertension (Stansfeld and Matheson, 2003), but results have not been consistent across population groups (Bluhm et al., 2007; de Kluizenaar et al., 2007; Floud et al., 2011; van Kempen and Babisch, 2012). Nonetheless, exposure to environmental noise is ubiquitous and increasing in terms of road traffic noise and the reduction of the night time quiet period. Despite limited evidence of association between noise and health, traffic-related noise is said to account for over 1 million healthy years of life lost annually to ill health and may lead to a disease burden that is second only in magnitude to that from air pollution (WHO-JRC, 2011). Noise is, however, understudied compared to air pollution. Recent years have seen the development of sophisticated GIS-based noise models (e.g., SoundPlan,[1] CadnaA[2]), which have more recently been used to assess noise level exposures in studies of noise and health (Ko et al., 2011; Gan et al., 2012).

The ability to use dispersion/propagation modeling for exposure assessment—and, indeed, the reliability of these models—depends primarily on the availability of the necessary input data. As chapter 3 shows, these data requirements are often demanding, and far beyond the capabilities of many epidemiological studies. In air pollution modeling, for example, as noted earlier, detailed data may be needed not only on the characteristics of the emission source (e.g., traffic volume, composition, speed, emission control technologies, percentage of cold starts), but also on meteorological conditions (wind speed, wind direction, mixing height, etc.), surface topography, and building characteristics. Approximation of these data inputs (e.g., by using proxy data or data from other areas) is sometimes feasible and, but for the occasionally overzealous concerns of modeling experts, might be done more frequently. Nevertheless, it also carries risks of reducing both the reliability and the acceptability of the results. As with interpolation techniques, therefore, data availability represents an important limitation.

One solution to this dilemma is to try to make use of all the data available, and to combine both source-based and monitoring information. A number of methods have been developed with this in mind. New Bayesian approaches, for example, aim to combine outputs from air pollution models with information from monitoring sites (site type, season, day of the week) to provide space and time varying exposure assessments (de Nazelle et al., 2010; Blangiardo et al., 2011).

Hybrid modeling combines two or more modeling approaches or models and measurement data: for example, dispersion modeling for explicitly defined sources such as traffic and significant point source (i.e., industry) combined with other predictor variables representing diffuse sources (e.g., housing, light industry, minor roads) (Wilton et al., 2010). Meteorology has sometimes been combined with LUR models to predict short-term exposures to air pollutants (Arain et al., 2007).

4.3.1 Mass Balance Model for a Well-Mixed Box

The first type of model we will briefly describe provides an understanding of the physical and chemical processes that control the spatial and temporal variability of a pollutant concentration in the environment. It is important that these should be understood before designing any modeling or even measurement-based exposure assessment study.

We first consider the simplest possible case of a box containing a certain volume of the environment, within which the pollutant of interest can be considered to be well mixed, with constant concentration everywhere in the box. The rate of increase of the amount of pollutant in the box is given by the sum of the sources minus the sum of the sinks of that pollutant.

The mass balance equation (Eq. 4.1) can be written as:

$$\frac{\partial C}{\partial t} = P_{ADV} + P_E + P_{CH} - L_{ADV} - L_{DEP} - L_{CH} \qquad \text{(Eq. 4.1)}$$

where the left hand side describes the change in time t of the concentration of a pollutant C with respect to time, and the right hand quantifies the production P and the loss L due to advection (ADV), emission (E), deposition (DEP), and chemical transformation (CH) (Gryning and Schiermeier, 1996).

Eulerian and Lagrangian models are examples of mass-balance models. In Eulerian models the boxes are located in a three-dimensional grid and air moves from one box to the other based on atmospheric conditions, whereas Lagrangian models follow the trajectory of the box as it moves through the atmosphere.

4.3.2 Plume Modeling

The consideration of air pollution in the previous section has omitted one of the most important processes that occur at short range in the atmosphere. That is the spreading of pollution horizontally and vertically, perpendicular to its direction of average movement. In the atmosphere, the spreading is caused by turbulence. If we are sure that chemical sources and sinks, and sinks due to deposition, are small over the distances of interest (in the atmosphere, typically up to about 50 km), a plume model provides a lot more information about the distribution of pollutant concentrations in the environment downwind of the source, more easily than any Eulerian or Lagrangian box modeling approach. Consequently, it is plume models that have most often been used in emission-based exposure modeling, alongside the more empirical methods that rely on environmental measurements (e.g., statistical modeling).

The simplest case for movement of pollution through the atmosphere is emissions from a single point in a homogeneous body of air. On average, the random nature of the spreading causes the concentration to assume a Gaussian distribution, just as any other random process (such as measurement error) causes a Gaussian distribution around an average value. The maximum concentration is found directly downwind of the source, with steadily decreasing levels of the pollutant being found as one moves perpendicular to the direction of the average wind away from the line of maximum concentration.

The Gaussian plume model will be briefly described here. The Gaussian plume model is appropriate when modeling in the near field (0–100 km). In this model, the plume has a Normal (Gaussian) distribution of concentration in the vertical (z) and lateral directions (y). The concentration χ at any point is given by Eq. 4.2:

$$\chi = \frac{Q}{2\pi \bar{u} \sigma_y \sigma_z} exp\left(-\frac{y^2}{2\sigma_y^2} \right) \times \left[exp\left(-\frac{(z-H)^2}{2\sigma_z^2} \right) + exp\left(-\frac{(z+H)^2}{2\sigma_z^2} \right) \right] \qquad \text{(Eq. 4.2)}$$

where Q is the pollutant mass emissions rate ($\mu g/s$); $\bar{u}$ is the wind speed (in m/s); x, y, and z are the along-wind, cross-wind, and vertical distances (in meters), respectively; and H is the effective stack height (the height of the stack + the plume rise [in m]). The parameters σ_y and σ_z measure the extent of plume growth, and are the standard deviations of the horizontal and vertical concentrations in the plume (in m) (Figure 4.1).

At plume centerline, $y = 0$, and ground level, $z = 0$, the equation (Eq. 4.3) reduces to give ground level concentration below the plume centerline such that

$$\chi = \frac{Q}{\pi \bar{u} \sigma_y \sigma_z} exp\left(-\frac{H^z}{2\sigma_z^2} \right) \qquad \text{(Eq. 4.3)}$$

1. Concentrations are directly proportional to emission rate Q, as in the box model
2. Unless the source is at ground level, the maximum concentration will occur at a point some distance downwind from the stack

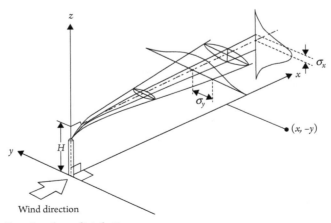

Figure 4.1 Gaussian plume distribution.

3. The distance to the maximum concentration increases with increasing effective stack height
4. The maximum concentration will decrease with increasing effective stack height

The effective stack height is determined by plume buoyancy (if it is warmer than the surrounding air), or momentum (if it is released at a high velocity). To model a point source, data is needed on stack height and diameter, exit velocity or volume flow rate, temperature, and emission rate of each pollutant in grams per second; suitable topographical and meteorological data are also necessary.

The Gaussian model for line sources (Figure 4.2 and Eq. 4.4) is similar to the one for point sources. The concentration C from a finite crosswind line source Ls is given by:

$$C(x,y,z) = \frac{QS}{2\sqrt{2\pi}\,\sigma_z(x)U} exp\left(-\frac{(z-z_p)^2}{2\sigma_z^2}\right)$$

$$\times \left[erf\left(\frac{y+L_s/2}{\sqrt{2\sigma}\,y}\right) - erf\left(\frac{y-L_s/2}{\sqrt{2\sigma}\,y}\right)\right] + \text{reflection terms} \qquad \text{(Eq. 4.4)}$$

where most of the terms are similar as in the previous equation, with the difference that z_p is the height of the plume above the ground (m); U is the wind speed at plume height (m/s) (see also Figure 4.2).

4.4 EXAMPLES

An example of a plume dispersion model is ADMS, which was developed by Cambridge Environmental Research Consultants in the United Kingdom. In

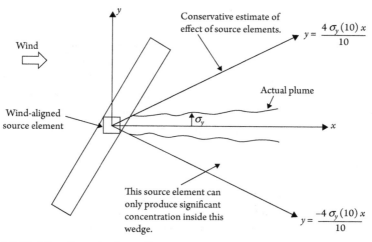

Figure 4.2 Modeling dispersion from a line source.

contrast to earlier Gaussian plume modeling systems, which use discrete categories to describe the stability of the atmospheric boundary layer, and which assume Gaussian distributions in all stabilities as described earlier, ADMS uses two parameters to describe the state of the atmospheric boundary—boundary layer depth and Monin–Obukhov length. The vertical concentration distribution is Gaussian in neutral and stable conditions, but is a skewed Gaussian in convective conditions. Gaussian distribution is assumed in the crosswind horizontal direction for all stabilities. ADMS is a so-called "second-generation" Gaussian-type plume model, with other examples including the USEPA's AERMOD.

4.4.1 Point Source Modeling

A recent study by Ashworth et al. (2013) describes an example of dispersion modeling around a point source; ADMS was used to compare atmospheric dispersion modeling and distance from source as an exposure assessment method for pollutants released from municipal solid waste incinerators (MSWIs). The two MSWIs included in the study; Crymlyn Burrows in Wales and Marchwood in England, were built to operate according to the most recent European Waste Incineration Directive (2000/76/EC). Crymlyn Burrows and Marchwood MSWIs were licensed to throughput respectively 52,500 and 210,000 tons per year. For each MSWI, detailed data were obtained from the Environment Agency for input in ADMS, including stack characteristics (height, diameter, flue exit velocity and flow rate, flue exit temperature etc) and emissions data (daily emissions for particulate matter). Hourly meteorological data (wind direction, wind speed, cloud cover, and temperature) was obtained from the Meteorological Office. For Crymlyn Burrows, which is situated in hilly terrain, altitude data were extracted from the Ordnance Survey PANORAMA Digital Terrain Model (DTM). Horizontal resolution is 50 meters; vertical resolution ranges from 2 meters in urban lowlands to 3 meters in hilly rural areas. To determine the surface roughness and Monin-Obukhov lengths, land cover data was extracted from the CORINE Land Cover Map 2000 (EEA, 2005).

Figure 4.3 shows the annual average ground-level concentration of PM modeled around Marchwood MSWI plotted against distance away from the MSWI at postcode centroid. Please note that the predicted PM concentrations are extremely low compared with, for example, existing annual mean ambient urban background concentrations of PM (+/– 20 µg/m^3 in the United Kingdom in 2013). In this study the estimated concentrations are therefore used as an indicator of other, more harmful pollutants, like dioxins and furans. The two main features of the concentration are:

1. The maximum of concentration is not immediately adjacent to the plant because the pollution does not disperse vertically downward from the elevated source.
2. The concentration falls off rapidly with distance from the source, decreasing to about 7% of the maximum at 10 km away.

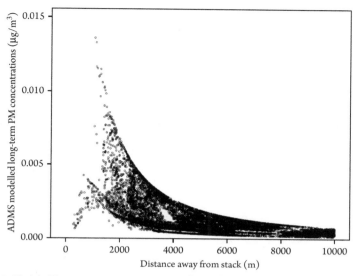

Figure 4.3 Modeled long-term PM concentrations ($\mu g/m^3$) plotted against distance away from the Marchwood MSWI at postcode centroid.

This figure does not show that the concentration bands are not circular, but are stretched along the main prevalent wind directions (highest concentrations are generally found north-east, opposite of the prevalent wind direction blowing south-west).

4.4.2 Line and Grid Source Modeling

A recent study compared several dispersion model estimates with land use regression–generated exposure estimates in multiple study areas across Europe (de Hoogh et al. 2014). In the Bradford study area, LUR model estimates were compared to NO_2 exposure concentrations estimated by ADMS-Urban, a dispersion model that contains a line source (i.e., roads) model. The model comparison was performed at 20,919 address locations of the Born in Bradford birth cohort.

Data on traffic flows, emission inventory, altitude and meteorological parameters were obtained for the Bradford area. Digital road data was obtained from the UK national mapping agency's (Ordnance Survey) Meridian 2 (2009) product, which has an accuracy of approximately 1 meter. Traffic count data for all major roads in Bradford were obtained from the City of Bradford Metropolitan District Council for 2009 and consisted of a combination of manual and automatic counts at numerous locations in the Bradford study area. Seasonal conversion factors were used to extract annual average daily traffic for total and heavy goods vehicles. Traffic data at unmonitored road links were estimated based on the surrounding monitored links. The traffic data were linked to the road network by linking points to the correct road links based on road names or, if not available, on distance. Emission rates for the roads were subsequently generated in ADMS-Urban. Emission data for all other sources were extracted from the UK National Atmospheric Emission Inventory at a 1×1 km scale. Hourly meteorological data (temperature, wind speed, wind direction, cloud cover) were obtained from the nearest national meteorological station.

The road traffic data were imported into ADMS-Urban as *line sources*, whereas the other emission sources, representing, for example, domestic heating, industry, agriculture were imported as *area sources* (see Figure 4.4).

Annual average NO_2 concentrations were estimated for 2009 for all cohort addresses. These estimates were then compared to annual mean NO_2 concentrations

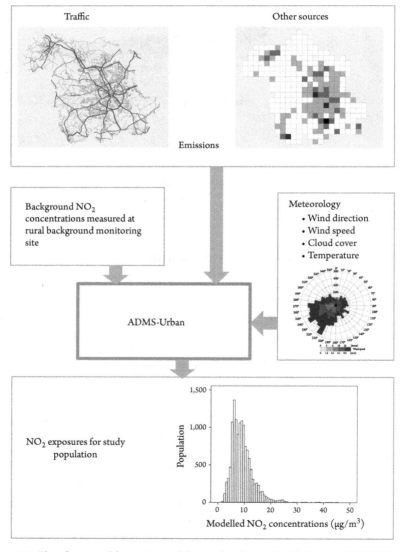

Figure 4.4 Flow diagram of dispersion modeling undertaken in Bradford using ADMS-Urban.

estimated using the NO_2 LUR model, as developed in the ESCAPE project (Beelen et al. 2013). The comparison between dispersion and LUR model estimates showed a high correlation (Pearson R = 0.67), a result that was also found in most of the other study areas, which implies that both methods may be useful for epidemiological studies of small-scale variations of outdoor combustion related air pollution, typically from road traffic (de Hoogh et al., 2014).

4.4.3 Models for Indoor Micro-environments

This kind of modeling approach can also be used at a smaller scale for micro-environments. One example of this type of model is INDEX, which is a simple spreadsheet-based formulation of a mass-balance model to simulate indoor concentrations of particulates (and other inert pollutants) based on outdoor concentrations. The INDEX model produces probabilistic distributions for each target location (http://www.integrated-assessment.eu/resource_centre/index_indoor_exposure_model, accessed 15-08-2014) and was developed by researchers at Imperial College London.

Based on a detailed review of previous experimental and observational studies, INDEX was developed by adapting and parameterising standard mass-balance equations. It focuses especially on particulates, but can be adapted for other pollutant species if the relevant pollutant-specific characteristics (e.g., settling velocities) are known.

Required model input is the average (and standard deviation) of ambient concentration at the building facade or nearby monitoring site and the wind speed frequency. Other optional input data include building/room characteristics (e.g., dimensions of room, window/doors area, porosity, both artificial and natural); pollutant characteristics (e.g., diameter, density, deposition velocity, filtration efficiency); meteorological conditions (e.g., wind speed, wind direction, surface roughness, vertical wind speed coefficient); and analytical conditions (time resolution, monitoring height).

The main equation (Eq. 4.5) used in the model is:

$$C_i(s,t)=C_o(s,t)*(1-F(s))*X(t,i)/(D_r(s)+X(t,i)) \qquad \text{(Eq. 4.5)}$$

where:

- $C_i(s,t)$ = modeled indoor concentration of pollutant s at time t ($\mu g/m^3$)
- $C_o(s,t)$ = measured concentration of pollutant s, at time t, at ambient monitoring station or at the façade of the residence ($\mu g/m^3$)
- $F(s)$ = Filtration efficiency, proportion of incoming pollutant s that is filtered during ingress (e.g., by adsorption onto curtains, surfaces)
- $X(t,i)$ = Frequency of complete air exchange via wall i, in time t
- $D_r(s)$ = deposition rate. Number of times per hour that pollutant s would be totally lost via deposition from air, at monitoring height, via deposition (per hour)

The model has been coded in an Excel spreadsheet, downloadable without charge, and also includes a comprehensive manual with more detailed information about the model. There are a couple of factors the model does not take into account that could have a substantial effect; room occupancy—so no allowance for re-suspension caused by human activities inside the room—and releases from static indoor sources such as heating or cooking devices. Field validation has also shown that (as with all such models) performance is highly dependent on the accuracy of estimation of the ambient concentrations and meteorology: Estimates are likely to be more reliable when these are based on a nearby monitoring site, or can be modeled for the building facade.

4.4.4 Modeling Electro-magnetic Fields

The following example shows the development and application of a propagation model outside the air pollution theme. It describes the development and field validation of a GIS-based exposure model (Geomorf) used in a study investigating the possible health effects of EMF radiation around mobile phone masts in the United Kingdom (Elliott et al. 2010; Briggs et al. 2012). This study is a good example of an exposure assessment for which no existing measurement data or modeling approach was available. Moreover, the difficulties in exposure modeling were exacerbated both by the complexity of the propagation processes and the need to obtain estimates for large study populations, in this case national level. Thus reliable measures of exposures needed to be obtained because any health effects are likely to be small, whereas exposures show a high level of variability over short distances depending upon where people live in relation to the emission sources. Similar to the Gaussian plume model in section 4.3.2, this model uses a Gaussian formulation to simulate the spatial variations in power densities surrounding mobile phone masts, based on power output, antenna height, and tilt of the mobile phone mast and information about the propagation environment (e.g., obstruction by terrain). Model calibration was done using field data from 151 measurement sites (1510 antenna-specific measurements) around a group of masts in a rural location, and 50 measurement sites (658 antenna-specific measurements) in an urban area. Different parameter settings were found to be necessary in urban and rural areas to obtain optimum results. The calibrated models were then validated against independent sets of data gathered from measurement surveys in rural and urban areas.

The full Geographical Model of Radio-Frequency exposures (Geomorf) is described in Eq. 4.6:

$$E_{ij} = 10 \log_{10} \left[\frac{1000 \times P_j}{4\pi \times D_{ij}^2} \times Ld_{ij} \times Lt_{ij} \times Fs_{ij} \right] \qquad \text{(Eq. 4.6)}$$

(a)

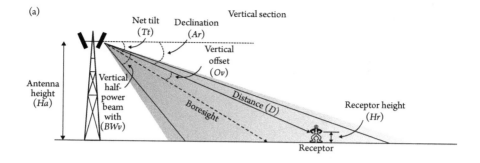

(b)

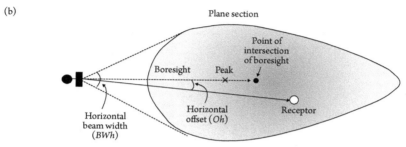

Figure 4.5 Schematic diagram of power density from a directional RF antenna.

where:

- E_{ij} is power density (dBm/m^2) at receptor i, attributable to antenna j.
- P_j is the radiated power output (W) from antenna j.
- D_{ij} is the linear distance of site i from antenna j (metres).
- Fs_{ij} is the shielding factor for site i from antenna j (from 1, unshielded, to 0, fully shielded).
- Ld_{ij} is distal direction and Lt_{ij} is transverse direction for site i from antenna j (metres)

A schematic diagram of this model is shown in Figure 4.5.

4.5 TIME–SPACE MODELS

Strictly speaking, all the methods outlined previously are essentially measures of pollutant concentrations, rather than exposure, in that they take no direct account of where people are. Exposures are assessed usually by dropping the place of residence of the individual participants onto the resulting pollution map, or by computing some form of population-weighted average across an area. Notably, in all these situations people are seen as static and tied to their home. As we all know, this is rarely the truth. Most of us spend a considerable part of the day outside the home, often in far-flung places. Indeed, there are several anomalies in doing exposure assessment in this way. We are likely to be at our home, for example, mainly at night. In many cases, however, the times of greatest environmental pollution are during the day, when road

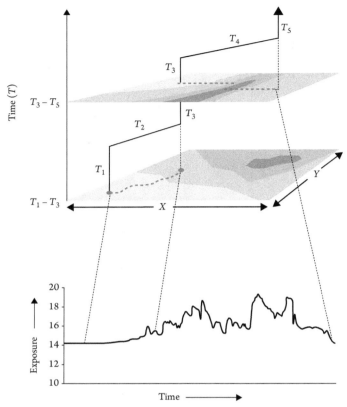

Figure 4.6 Idealized exposure assessment of outdoor air pollution.
Gulliver, J., and Briggs, D. J. (2005). Time-space modelling of journey-time exposure to traffic-related air pollution using GIS. *Environmental Research*, **97**(1), 10–25.

traffic and industry are most active. The geographies we use to estimate pollution and population distributions are therefore curiously mismatched. To make matters worse, when we are at home we tend to be indoors. Yet—in studies of air pollution especially—we tend to use estimates of *outdoor* pollution as the basis for our exposure measure. Sometimes it seems quite surprising that studies using these types of exposure estimation find anything at all! Yet it is also these associations between health and outdoor pollution levels that are then used as a basis for setting pollution standards and guidelines in many cases. If we are to obtain more realistic estimates of exposure, we clearly need to move away from this rather naïve view of the world. We need to recognize that people move, and that they do not spend all their time at home (but outdoors). This requires a far more sophisticated type of exposure model—one that takes account of human time–activity patterns and pollution levels in the sorts of micro-environments (e.g., bedroom, kitchen, living room, commuting to work, work, and pub) in which they spend their time. Thus in Eq. 4.7:

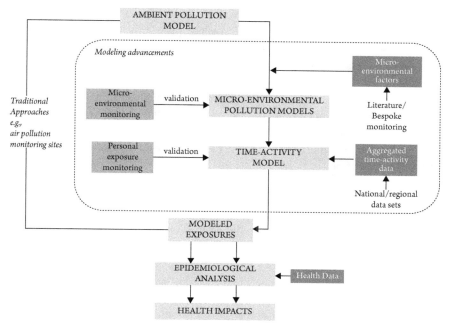

Figure 4.7 Comparison of traditional and new approaches (inside the dashed box) in air pollution exposure assessment.

$$E = \sum_{i=1}^{n} (t,C)_{ij} \qquad \text{(Eq. 4.7)}$$

where E is the amount of exposure for periods $i = 1, \ldots, n$; t_{ij} is the amount of time during period i spent in micro-environment j; and C_{ij} is the pollutant concentration in micro-environment j during period i.

In applying this approach, we thus wish to model the exposures of individuals, or groups of individuals, as they move through a changing pollution field (Figure 4.6).

The principles of accounting for space–time and micro-environmental (i.e., indoor locations; transport modes) variations in air pollution concentrations in exposure assessment (Figure 4.7) have been demonstrated (Jensen et al., 2001; Gulliver and Briggs, 2005), but so far have been assessed by few epidemiological studies. Developing "dynamic" models of exposures is, though, a major undertaking, not least because detailed information on population travel and occupancy patterns is scarce in most areas, and where available it has often been collected in limited surveys, thus raising issues about its generalizability. Notwithstanding improvements in GIS techniques for handling space–time population data, dynamic exposure models are still emerging technologies.

Recently, Beevers et al. (2013) have embarked on developing a dynamic exposure model for air pollution exposure assessment in London. The model integrates detailed population geographies (small areas, postcodes, addresses) with a rich dataset on travel and occupancy patterns of the population of London, and uses these data with network analysis routines in GIS to model the spatial and temporal patterns of population exposures. Micro-environmental models are also proposed to account for indoor air pollution exposures (homes, work, in-cabin transport modes). An important aspect of the development of such methods in an epidemiological context is that once validated, they could be used to quantify misclassification of exposures related to traditional methods of exposure modeling that rely on maps of outdoor air pollution, and use only residential address to define the geography of the population.

4.6 CONCLUSION

If the wrong spatial resolution or averaging time is used, gross exposure misclassification can occur. Many studies produce information that is a lot less useful than it should be, because of failure to take into account the basic science that controls the spatial and temporal variability of the pollutants of interest, and this problem becomes most acute when trying to compare the results of studies of different pollutants, where it is vital to know how and why two pollutants might have different spatial and temporal variability.

To date, although some studies rely on relatively simple methods, increasingly more sophisticated methods are being used in epidemiological studies such as dispersion modeling described in this chapter. In most cases, however, little account has been taken of population dynamics; instead, exposures are usually in relation to the place of residence. These simplifications are often justifiable because of the general nature of the hypothesis being tested, uncertainties about the specific toxic agent involved, or the poor quality of the health data. But they do not need to be so. With the help of GIS techniques it is now feasible to develop far more realistic models of exposure, including time–activity patterns of people.

NOTES

1. http://www.soundplan.eu/english
2. http://www.datakustik.com/en/products/cadnaa

REFERENCES

Ashworth, D., Fuller, G. W., Toledano, M. B., Font, A., Elliott, P., Hansell, A. L., and de Hoogh, K. (2013). Comparative assessment of particulate air pollution exposure from municipal solid waste incinerator emissions. *Journal of Environmental and Public Health*, **2013**, Article ID 560342, 13 pages. doi:10.1155/2013/560342.

Arain, M. A., Blair, R., Finkelstein, N., Brook, J. R., Sahsuvaroglu, T., Beckerman, B., et al. (2007) The use of wind fields in a land use regression model to predict air pollution concentrations for health exposure studies. *Atmospheric Environment*, **41**, 3453–3464.

Beelen, R., Hoek, G., Vienneau, D., Eeftens, M., Dimakopoulou, K., Pedeli, X., et al. (2013). Development of NO2 and NOx land use regression models for estimating air pollution exposure in 36 study areas in Europe—the ESCAPE project. *Atmospheric Environment*, **72**, 10–23.

Beevers, S., Kitwiroon, N., Williams, M., Kelly, F., Anderson, H.R., and Carslaw, D.C. (2013). Air pollution dispersion models for human exposure predictions in London. *Journal of Exposure Science and Environmental Epidemiology*, **23**, 647–653.

Blangiardo, M., Richardson, S., Gulliver, J., and Hansell, A. (2011). A Bayesian analysis of the impacts of air pollution episodes on health in the Greater London area. *Statistical Methods in Medical Research*, **20**(1), 69–80.

Bluhm, G., Berglind, N., Nordling, E., and Rosenlund, M. (2007). Road traffic noise and hypertension. *Occupational and Environmental Medicine*, **64**, 122–126.

Briggs, D., Beale, L., Bennett, J., Toledano, M. B., and de Hoogh, K. (2012). A geographical model of radio-frequency power density around mobile phone masts. *Science of the Total Environment*, **426**, 233–243.

Briggs, D. J., Collins, S., Elliott, P., Kingham, S., Fisher, P., Lebret, W., et al. (1997). Mapping urban air pollution using GIS: A regression-based approach. *International Journal of Geographical Information Science*, **11**, 699–718.

Briggs, D. J., de Hoogh, C., Gulliver, J., Wills, J., Elliott, P., Kingham, S., and Smallbone, K. (2000). A regression-based method for mapping traffic-related air pollution: application and testing in four contrasting urban environments. *Science of the Total Environment*, **253**, 151–167.

de Hoogh, K., Korek, M., Vienneau, D., Keuken, M., Kukkonen, J., Nieuwenhuijsen, M. J., et al. (2014). Comparing land use regression and dispersion modelling to assess residential exposure to ambient air pollution for epidemiological studies. *Environment International*, **73**, 382–392.

de Nazelle, A., Arunachalam, S., and Serre, M.L. (2010). Bayesian maximum entropy integration of ozone observations and model predictions: An application for attainment demonstration in North Carolina. *Environmental Science & Technology*, **44**, 5707–5713.

de Kluizenaar, Y., Gansevoort, R. T., Miedema, H. M., and de Jong, P. E. (2007). Hypertension and road traffic noise exposure. *Journal of Occupational and Environmental Medicine*, **49**, 484–492.

Elliott, P., Toledano, M. B., Bennett, J., Beale, L., de Hoogh, K., Best, N., and Briggs, D. J. (2010). Mobile phone base stations and early childhood cancers: case-control study. *British Medical Journal*, 340:c3077

European Environment Agency. (2005). CORINE Land Cover (CLC 2000), http://www.eea.europa.eu/publications/COR0-landcover.

European Council. Directive 2000/76/EC of the European Parliament and of the Council of 4 Decmber 2000, on the incineration of waste, Annex V. Official Journal of the European Communities. European Union. 2000. http://eur-lex.europa.eu/legal-content/EN/TXT/PDF/?uri=CELEX:32000L0076&from=EN

Floud, S., Vigna-Taglianti, F., Hansell, A., Blangiardo, M., Houthuijs, D., Breugelmans, O., et al. (2011). Medication use in relation to noise from aircraft and road traffic in six European countries: results of the HYENA study. *Occupational & Environmental Medicine*, **68**(7), 518–524.

Gan, W. Q., McLean, K., Brauer, M., Chiarello, S. A., and Davies, H. W. (2012). Modeling population exposure to community noise and air pollution in a large metropolitan area. *Environmental Research*, **116**, 11–16.

Gryning, S. E., and Schiermeier F. A. (1996) *Air pollution modeling and its application XI*. Plenum Press, New York.

Gulliver, J., and Briggs, D. J. (2005). Time-space modelling of journey-time exposure to traffic-related air pollution using GIS. *Environmental Research*, **97**(1), 10–25.

Gulliver, J., de Hoogh, K., Hansell, A., and Vienneau, D. (2013). Development and back-extrapolation of NO2 land use regression models for historic exposure assessment in Great Britain. *Environmental Science & Technology*, **47**(14), 7804–7811.

Hoek, G., Beelen, R., de Hoogh, K., Vienneau, D., Gulliver, J., Fischer, P., and Briggs, D. (2008). A review of land-use regression models to assess spatial variation of outdoor air pollution. *Atmospheric Environment*, **42**, 7561–7578.

Jensen, S. S., Berkowicz, R., Hansen, H. S., and Hertel, O. (2001). A Danish decision-support GIS tool for management of air quality and human exposures. *Transportation Research Part D*, **6**, 229–241.

Ko, J.E., Chang, S. II., and Lee, B.J. (2011). Noise impact assessment by utilizing noise map and GIS: A case study in the city of Chungju, Republic of Korea. *Applied Acoustics*, **72**, 554–550.

McHugh, C. A., Carruthers, D. J., and Edmunds, H. A. (1997). ADMS-Urban: An air quality management system for traffic, domestic and industrial pollution. *International Journal of Environment and Pollution*, **8**, 666–674.

Nyberg, F., Gustavsson, P., Järup, L., Bellander, T., Berglund, N., Jakobsson, R., and Pershagen, G. (2000). Urban air pollution and lung cancer in Stockholm. *Epidemiology*, **11**, 487–495.

Paine, R. J., Lee, R. F., Brode, R., Wilson, R. B., Cimorelli, A. J., Perry, S. G., et al. (1998). *Model evaluation results for AERMOD, RTP NC 27711*. Washington, DC, US EPA.

Stansfeld, S. A., and Matheson, M.P. (2003). Noise pollution: Non-auditory effects on health. *British Medical Bulletin*, **68**, 243–257.

van Kempen, E., and Babisch, W. (2012). The quantitative relationship between road traffic noise and hypertension: a meta-analysis. *Journal of Hypertension*, **30**(6), 1075–1086.

Wang, R., Henderson, S. B., Sbihi, H., Allen, R. W., and Brauer, M. (2013). Temporal stability of land use regression models for traffic-related air pollution. *Atmospheric Environment*, **64**, 312–319.

Wilton, D., Szpiro, A., Gould, T., and Larson, T. (2010). Improving spatial concentration estimates for nitrogen oxides using a hybrid meteorological dispersion/land use regression model in Los Angeles, CA and Seattle, WA. *Science of the Total Environment*, **408**, 1120–1130.

World Health Organisation and Joint Research Council (WHO/JRC). (2011). *Burden of disease from environmental noise. Quantification of health life years lost in Europe*. Copenhagen, Denmark, 2011a. Available at: http://www.euro.who.int/__data/assets/pdf_file/0008/136466/e94888.pdf (accessed August 27, 2014).

Wu, J., Ren, C., Delfino, R.J., Chung, J., Wilhelm, M., and Ritz, B. (2009). Association between local traffic-generated air pollution and preeclampsia and preterm delivery in the south coast air basin of California. *Environmental Health Perspectives*, **117**(11), 1773–1779.

5

PERSONAL EXPOSURE MONITORING AND MODELING

Mark J. Nieuwenhuijsen

5.1 INTRODUCTION

Personal exposure monitoring involves the monitoring of people's personal exposure rather than the environmental media around them, that is, environmental
monitoring. For example, in the case of air pollution, attaching an exposure monitor
or sensor to the person rather than placing a monitor in the area where he or she lives
or works. Personal exposure monitoring is widely accepted and commonly used in
occupational epidemiology (Nieuwenhuijsen 1997), and it is being carried out in
environmental epidemiology with increasing frequency. It could be regarded as
more informative and more representative of people's exposure than environmental
monitoring in environmental epidemiological studies, but its use is often limited by
practical issues. There are not that many environmental epidemiological studies in
which personal exposure measurements have been used as the exposure estimates
(Perera et al. 2006; Kraus et al. 2013; McKenzie et al. 2013; Hampel et al. 2014;
Jedrychowski et al. 2014; Lanzinger et al. 2014; Nyhan et al. 2014; Petersen et al.
2014). It has been used more to validate and/or build models (Nethery et al. 2008a,b;
Montagne et al. 2013, 2014) or to provide a better understanding about where exposure occurs, which can help information epidemiological studies (Jedrychowski et
al. 2006; Lanki et al. 2007; Dons et al. 2011; Johannesson et al. 2011; Minguillón
et al. 2012; Schembari et al. 2012; Dons et al. 2013). New technologies, including
smartphones, other GPS devices, and small sensors, may, however, may make it easier
to use this method, or at least improve existing exposure estimates (Heydenreich &
Wulf 2005; Berghmans et al. 2009; Boogaard et al. 2009; Lane et al. 2010; Mead
et al. 2013; Snyder et al. 2013; Dons et al. 2014; Nieuwenhuijsen et al. 2014). Many
people nowadays have smartphones and with the use of simple Apps they can provide information on location, mobility, physical activity, and even to some extent
environmental exposure levels, which are important features of good exposure
assessment (de Nazelle et al. 2013; Donaire-Gonzales et al. 2013; Nieuwenhuijsen
et al. 2014, 2015). The smartphones, using their GPS, can be used to show objectively
where people spend their time, and therefore which level of exposure they may experience, when overlaid with exposure maps (de Nazelle et al. 2013). Furthermore,
the combination of assessment of personal air pollution concentrations and physical

activity provides the opportunity to estimate the inhaled dose, which may be a better measure than exposure (Buonanno et al. 2013; de Nazelle et al. 2013; Nyhan et al. 2014). For example, de Nazelle et al. (2013) found using modeled nitrogen dioxide (NO_2) data that, on average, time at home, which represented 51% of people's time in a day, and similarly 54% of daily time weighted exposures (Figure 5.1), accounted for 40% of individuals' total inhaled dose. Time at work, 33% of people's daily activity, led to 29% daily time-weighted exposures and 28% of daily inhaled NO_2. In reverse, volunteers only spent 6% of their time in transit, yet this microenvironment contributed to 11% of time-weighted exposures in a day, and 24% of daily inhaled NO_2. Nieuwenhuijsen et al. (2014) showed that using smartphones, apps, and a sensor, the Microaethalometer AE51 traveling routes and black carbon levels along the route could be obtained fairly easily (Figure 5.2).

The small health risks and low exposure levels in environmental epidemiological studies require a refined exposure assessment. Environmental exposure levels tend

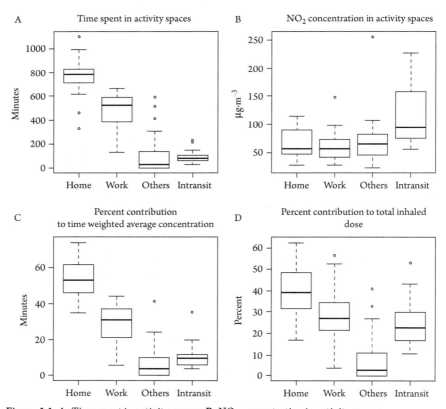

Figure 5.1 A: Time spent in activity spaces. B: NO_2 concentration in activity spaces, derived from fully adjusted model (temporal and microenvironmental factors). C: Percent contribution from different activity spaces to total time-weighted average NO_2 concentration, using concentrations from fully adjusted model (temporal and microenvironmental factors). D: Percent contribution to total NO_2 daily inhaled dose from different activities, using concentrations from fully adjusted model (temporal and microenvironmental factors).

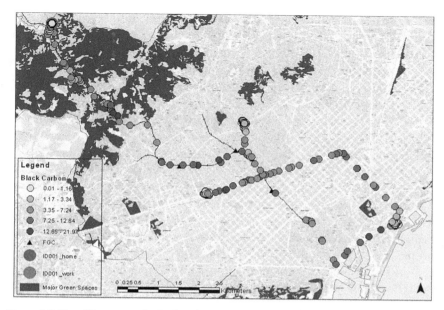

Figure 5.2 Travelling routes obtained using a smartphone app and black carbon levels using a Microaethalometer AE51. The darker the dots the higher the levels of black carbon.

to be much lower than occupational exposure levels and therefore require more sensitive methods of measurement. For example, exposure to particulate matter tends to be measured in milligram per cubic meter in the work place (Nieuwenhuijsen 1997), whereas levels in the general environment tend to be measured in microgram per cubic meter (Janssen 1998). However, environment durations tend to much longer in environmental epidemiology, and susceptible populations, such as pregnant women and their fetuses, children, and the elderly may be affected. They require different sampling durations and strategies.

Exposure to any pollutant is characterized by its nature (e.g., its chemical form or particle size), the concentration, duration, and frequency of contact. Estimates of these characteristics generally can be obtained instrumentally (i.e., using a monitoring device), via questionnaires, through direct observation, or through the use of biomarkers. The emphasis in this chapter is on the measurement of personal exposure with instruments; these provide information mainly on the level of exposure. Information on duration, frequency, and pattern of exposure is generally obtained by questionnaire, observation, or from records and is discussed in chapter 2, although with the increased use of smartphones and other GPS devices and sensors this may be change. Biomonitoring is discussed in chapter 6.

Personal monitoring is generally labor intensive, costly, and difficult to carry out. These factors restrict its use, even though the information obtained generally can be more informative and relevant of people's exposure than other approaches, depending on the circumstances, and increase the scientific value of epidemiological studies. It is usually not possible to carry out personal monitoring on a large number of people. A more efficient use may be to use it to develop and/or validate (statistical) exposure models in a representative sample and/or time period of the population under study (Nethery et al. 2008a,b; Montagne et al. 2013, 2014).

Personal exposure monitoring is perhaps most fully developed in relation to air pollution. Many air pollutants, for example, particulate matter, ozone, CO, and NO_2 in the general environment, have the ability to cause adverse human health effects given a sufficient level of exposure. In this chapter the focus is on personal monitoring of air pollutants, although the same principles could also be applied for personal sampling of noise (Boogaard et al. 2009; Kraus et al. 2013; Nieuwenhuijsen et al. 2014), UV (Heydenreich et al. 2005; McKenzie et al. 2013; Nieuwenhuijsen et al. 2014; Petersen et al. 2014), temperature (Lanzinger et al. 2014, Nieuwenhuijsen et al. 2014), and soil and water contaminants (see chapter 16). However, for the latter, personal factors, such as ingestion rate, obtained by questionnaire (see chapter 2), are combined with environmental levels (see chapter 16) to obtain exposure indices.

Once the decision has been made to use personal monitoring for an epidemiological (including validation) study, a comprehensive sampling strategy needs to be designed and carried out, and the results interpreted. In the process, a number of choices need to be made that will fundamentally affect the way in which the study is carried out, and the value and interpretation of the results. These include whether to adopt a group or individual sampling approach, the number of measurements needed, the duration of monitoring and appropriate averaging time, the type of monitor or method to be used, and how the data will be analyzed, interpreted, and used for the epidemiological study. Crucial to these choices is the fact that, in most circumstances, marked variation occurs in exposure levels, both for the individual and between individuals for any given time. Thus, a single "best estimate" of the average exposure level may not be sufficient; instead, data are needed on levels of variations in exposure. The challenge is to design a strategy that incorporates the variability to the advantage of the epidemiological study in the most efficient way while attempting to avoid potential bias.

Issues regarding the expression of results (e.g., geometric mean [GM] or arithmetic mean [AM]), treatment of data under the detection limit, and quality control are discussed in chapter 1.

5.2 GROUP VERSUS INDIVIDUAL APPROACH

As discussed in chapter 1, two main approaches are available to obtain exposure estimate(s) for a population in an epidemiological study: individual and exposure grouping. In the individual approach, every member of the population is monitored either once or repeatedly, and data are obtained at the individual level. In the group approach, the population is first split into smaller subpopulations or exposure groups based on specific determinants of exposure. In environmental epidemiological studies, exposure groups might be defined, for example, on the basis of distance from an exposure source (e.g., roads or factories). The underlying assumption is that subjects within each exposure group experience similar exposure characteristics, including exposure levels and variation. Subsequently, a representative sample of members from each exposure group is monitored, either once or repeatedly. If the aim is to estimate mean exposure, the average of the exposure measurements is then assigned to all the members in that particular exposure group. (If a sufficient number of samples have been taken from a population, the population could be divided afterward into exposure groups based on the statistical analysis of those samples.) The group approach has rarely been used though in environmental epidemiological studies, and typically measurements are taken on all the subjects in the study (Perera et al. 2006; Kraus et al. 2013; McKenzie et al. 2013; Hampel et al. 2014; Jedrychowski et al. 2014; Lanzinger et al. 2014; Nyhan et al. 2014; Petersen et al. 2014).

Where possible, repeated measurements on individuals should be taken. This enables the estimation of long(er)-term exposure and the within- and between-subject variance in the individual approach and within- and between-subject variance and between-group variance in the group approach (see the following).

5.3 NUMBER OF SUBJECTS AND MEASUREMENTS

The number of subjects to be measured and the number of measurements to be taken on each subject depend on the chosen strategy and the distribution of variability in exposure across the population. In the case of the individual approach, every subject is monitored. Repeated measurements are highly recommended so that the within- and between-subject variance can be estimated, and attenuation in health risk estimates reduced. The number of repeated measurements required can be estimated, and is dependent on the ratio of within- and between-subject variance and the level of attenuation (Liu et al. 1978; chapter 10). In the group approach, the number of measurements depends on the ratio of between-group variance and between- and within-group variance, and the required precision of the estimated mean for each group (Kromhout and Heederik 1995; Kromhout et al. 1996). The number of measurements required for a certain precision can be calculated in various ways, for example,

$$n = \left((t \times CV) / E \right)^2,$$

where n is the number of samples, t is the t-distribution value for the chosen confidence level and $n_0 - 1$ degrees of freedom (e.g., 1.96 for 95% confidence, infinite degrees of freedom), CV is the coefficient of variation (e.g., in geometric standard deviation/ln GM), and E is the chosen level of error (0.1 for 10% variation around the mean). It is important to note that repeated measurements on individuals contribute less to the overall precision of the subgroup mean.

The number of measurements can be increased by sending out (passive) samplers rather than handing them out or by self-monitoring, for example, with NO_2 diffusion tubes, but it may not be possible with other monitors. In this way the number of measurements can be increased, even though the method(s) may not be as reliable. However, the benefits of a larger number of samples may outweigh the loss in reliability.

Whatever the approach, to avoid bias and to fulfill the assumptions of statistical programs, subjects, and measurements should be selected randomly.

5.4 DURATION OF SAMPLING

The duration of the sampling period (or averaging period) depends, among others, on the health outcome of interest in the epidemiological study, the detection limits of the measurement technique, the equipment available, and the level of the pollutant in the environment.

Chronic disease outcomes (e.g., the effects of air pollution on cardiovascular disease) generally require long sampling durations (e.g., days, weeks), and is rarely attempted. Studies of acute disease outcomes (e.g., relationships between air pollution and heart rate variability) may require shorter sampling durations (minutes to less than an hour). Relatively long sampling times may also be necessary for less-sensitive measurement and analysis techniques, for example, use of passive samplers to measure exposure to NO_2, or where low-exposure concentrations are being investigated, such as particulate matter in the general environment, to ensure that enough material is collected for weighing the filters and further laboratory analyses. In the latter case, the duration can be shortened if the flow rate of the sampler is increased, but this may also introduce other problems, such as the increase in weight of the sampler. In general, the variance of the exposure measurements decreases with increasing monitoring time.

5.5 CONTINUOUS OR AVERAGE SAMPLING AND ACTIVE OR PASSIVE SAMPLING

To take personal airborne samples, equipment is needed that is light enough to be carried around without undue inconvenience to the subject and that will not significantly alter his or her usual behavior patterns. The sampler should be placed such that it takes a sample of the inhaled air of the subject, often referred to as the *breathing zone* (within ~30 cm of the nose and mouth). Both active and passive samplers are available for this purpose.

For active sampling, air is drawn by a sampling pump through a collection unit, a sampling head with a filter inside for particulate matter or a Tenax tube for volatile organic compounds (VOCs). The sampling flow rate is dependent on the requirements of the collection unit and may vary from less than 100 ml/min^{-1} for VOC sampling to greater than 4 l/min^{-1} or more for particulate matter sampling.

The exposure concentration in air is determined by dividing the difference in the measured amount of the substance before and after the sampling period (e.g., for particulate matter, the weight on the filter before and after sampling is adjusted for blanks) by the volume of air (in m^3) drawn through the collection unit. The volume of air is the duration of air multiplied by the flow rate. This method provides a concentration over the whole sampling period. For example, in a birth cohort, during the third trimester of pregnancy, pregnant women were asked to wear a small backpack containing a personal monitor during the day-time hours for two consecutive days and to place the monitor near the bed at night. The personal air sampling pumps operated continuously over this period, collecting vapors and particles of less than 2.5 μm in diameter on a precleaned quartz microfiber filter and a precleaned polyurethane foam (PUF) cartridge backup. The samples were analyzed for eight carcinogenic polycyclic aromatic hydrocarbons (PAHs): benz[*a*]anthracene, chrysene, benzo[*b*]fluroanthene, benzo[*k*]fluroanthene, B[a]P, indeno[1,2,3-*cd*]pyrene, disbenz[*a,h*]anthracene, and benzo[*g,h,i*]perylene. The measurements used an exposure index in relation to cognitive function for children at age 3 (Perera et al. 2006).

Passive sampling is based on the principle of diffusion and does not require a sampling pump. It is widely used for gaseous substances, such as NO_2 (Ho Yu et al. 2008; Meng et al. 2012). A problem in sampling environmental pollutants using passive samplers is that the concentration of pollutants present is often low relative to the detection limits of the samplers. This implies the need for relatively long sampling durations and means that the samplers typically provide measures of long-term average concentrations only (e.g., over a period of days or longer). Sometimes there are also problems of accuracy and precision. On the other hand, passive sampling is generally less labor intensive and less costly than active sampling. This provides the possibility of taking more measurements for the same cost and carrying out relatively intense spatial and temporal sampling (e.g., for estimating variance components). Also the longer sampling duration may be an advantage if one needs estimates for longer periods. Recent advances in the design of passive samplers, the application of strict sampling protocols (including repeat measurements at each site), and the use of validation studies comparing passive samplers with more conventional methods, all offer scope to improve the performance of passive sampling. Again this method provides a concentration of the whole sampling period.

Nitrogen dioxide is one of the substances in which personal monitoring has been used in exposure assessment for environmental epidemiological studies (Magnus et al. 1998; Krämer et al. 2000). This is partly due to its potential adverse health effects and its use as a marker for combustion-related (including traffic-related) pollutants. NO_2 is an air pollutant generated mainly by combustion. It occurs both in homes, primarily from gas stoves or heaters, and in outdoor environments, primarily as a result of emission from road vehicles. It is also relatively cheap and easy to monitor, using passive samplers such as the Palmes tube (Palmes et al. 1976) or the

Willems badge (van Reeuwijk et al. 1998). Nitrogen dioxide is absorbed on metal grids, coated with triethanolamine, and then extracted with sulfonic acid and NED A, which produces a colored product that can be analyzed in a photometer.

Krämer et al. (2000) measured outdoor ambient levels of NO_2 and personal exposure to NO_2 with Palmes tubes. They estimated personal exposure to NO_2 with a micro-environment model for an epidemiological study of children. Personal exposure levels to NO_2 (22–27 µg/m^{-3}) were less than half the outdoor ambient levels of NO_2 (44–62 µg/m^{-3}). There was only a weak correlation between personal and outdoor levels ($r = 0.37$), suggesting that outdoor levels were not a good indicator for personal exposure levels. Outdoor levels of NO_2 correlated stronger with the amount of traffic ($r = 0.7$) compared with personal exposure levels, suggesting that personal samples also included sources other than traffic. The correlation between personal exposure to NO_2 with Palmes tubes and estimated personal exposure to NO_2 with a micro-environment model was good ($r = 0.7$). Outdoor NO_2 levels were a stronger predictor of respiratory disease than personal NO_2 levels, perhaps because it was a better marker for traffic-related air pollution. Magnus et al. (1998) measured personal exposure to NO_2 with Palmes diffusion tubes and NO_2 levels in indoor (kitchen, sleeping room, and living room) and outdoor environments for a case–control study of bronchial obstruction in children. Outdoor levels (25.3 µg/m^{-3}) were higher than personal (15.5 µg/m^{-3}) or indoor levels (13.2–14.9 µg/m^{-3}). There was weak correlation between personal and outdoor levels ($r = 0.36$), but stronger correlation between personal and indoor levels (e.g., living room $r = 0.52$, kitchen $r = 0.77$, sleeping room $r = 0.74$). The study found no association between exposure to NO_2 and the development of bronchial obstruction.

More recently there has been a shift to the use of low-cost sensors that work continuously (Snyder et al. 2013; Piedrahita et al. 2014). Snyder et al. (2013) recently reported that there is a change in paradigm in air pollution monitoring, which is being catalyzed by recent advances in multiple areas of electrical engineering that include: 1) microfabrication techniques; 2) microelectro-mechanical systems (MEMSs) that can incorporate microfluidic, optical, and nanotube elements; 3) energy-efficient radios and sensor circuits that have extremely low power consumption; and 4) advanced computing power suitable for handling extremely large databases (e.g., potentially many terabytes, 10^{12} bytes) and user-friendly data visualization. The use of sensors is also greatly increased due to the availability of wireless networks, allowing communications across widely dispersed sensor networks as well as web services (e.g., Xively, https://xively.com/) that allow for information access in near real-time across a broad spectrum of users. The combination of these advancements is helping to drive the development of small, lower-cost, mass-produced sensors. Air pollution sensors can be separated into two main categories, those that measure the concentration of gas phase species and those that measure either particulate matter (PM) mass concentrations or various properties of particles (e.g., scattering or absorption). All sensors systems consist of a few basic elements that include: 1) the sensor element that responds to the species of interest and varies with the pollutant mass in a given volume of sampled air; 2) the transducer that converts the responses to electrical signals; 3) data storage capability or a link to a communication device (e.g., microradio transmitter or cell phone); and 4) a source of power (e.g., battery or energy harvesting). Most commercially available gas sensors are based on two main principles: 1) those that depend on interactions between the sensing material (electrochemical cell or metal oxide semiconductor) and a gas phase component such as nitrogen dioxide (NO_2), ozone (O_3), carbon monoxide (CO), and volatile organic compounds (VOCs); and (2) those that measure absorption of light at visible (e.g., for O_3 and CO_2) or infrared wavelengths (e.g., CO_2), or by chemiluminescence (NO_2). Particulate matter mass can be measured directly by changes in frequency of an oscillating sensor element or indirectly based by light scattering using a proportionality constant that relates the scattered light to a defined (e.g., <2.5 μm) aerodynamic diameter (AD) PM mass concentration. Light scattering and absorption by particles are important particle properties that have direct relationships with visibility and health effects.

Continuous measurements are provided by direct reading instruments, such as the TSI DustTrak ($PM_{2.5}$), TSI P-Trak (ultrafine), and GRIMM monitor for particulate sampling, Microaethalometer AE51 for black carbon, and the Langan CO Enhanced Measurer T15 monitor for CO (Figure 5.3). They can be useful for the study of acute health effects. Magari et al. (2002) measured continuous exposure to $PM_{2.5}$ with a TSI Inc. DustTrak to determine the relation between personal exposure to $PM_{2.5}$ and heart rate variability in 20 relatively young healthy male workers. The arithmetic mean $PM_{2.5}$ concentration over a 24-hour period was 150 μg/m^{-3} (SD = 292 μg/m^{-3}). As expected, smokers had a higher mean $PM_{2.5}$ than nonsmokers, with an arithmetic mean of 216 μg/m^{-3} (SD = 404 μg/m^{-3}) compared with 96 μg/m^{-3}

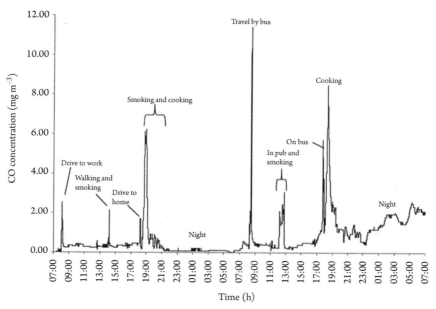

Figure 5.3 Personal carbon monoxide exposure measure using a continuous monitor.

(SD = 158 $\mu g/m^{-3}$) in nonsmokers. The authors used 3-hour $PM_{2.5}$ moving averages and found an association between $PM_{2.5}$ exposure and cardiac autonomic function.

Nyhan et al. (2014) conducted personal PM exposure using personal real-time monitors that were carried at all times by participants. The devices used were Met One Aerocet 531 particle profilers (Met One Instruments, Inc. Grants Pass, OR). The operating principle on which they are based uses laser light scattering technology to count individual particles and calculate the equivalent mass concentration using a proprietary algorithm (Met One Instruments, 2003). Particulate fractions of PM1, PM2.5, PM7, PM10, and TSP (total suspended particles) in ug/m³ within a concentration range of 0 to 1 mg/m³ were measured and logged at 2-minute intervals. Relative humidity (%) and temperature (°C) were measured using a G3120 probe attached to the Aerocet units. A stationary HazDust instrument, which encompasses a low-flow pump and filter (47-mm FRM style) was used for calibrating each of the Aerocet units. Then the study quantitatively assessed the acute relative variation of heart rate variability (HRV) with predicted PM dose in the lungs of commuters. Personal PM exposure, HR, and HRV were monitored in 32 young healthy cyclists, pedestrians, and bus and train passengers. Inhaled and lung deposited PM doses were determined using a numerical model of the human respiratory tract that accounted for varying ventilation rates among subjects and during commutes.

Information from direct reading instruments can be stored in data loggers and downloaded to a computer, where they can be graphed and analyzed, or sent directly to a server. Although direct reading instruments can provide a very informative picture of the variation in exposure over the sampling period, their usage for epidemiological studies is still relatively rare. The instruments are often expensive, they are sometimes not very specific, and accurate calibration is of considerable importance. Also, in case of chronic disease, short-term variations in exposure may not be considered important. More commonly, monitoring is aimed at providing estimates of average concentrations over a measurement period, for example, a day or a few days. Only one concentration value is obtained per measurement period. As noted, time-averaged data of this type are provided by both passive and active monitors.

5.6 SIZE-SELECTIVE SAMPLING

Over the years many epidemiological studies have examined the health effects of airborne particulates. The health hazard from airborne particulates varies with its nature: physical, chemical, toxicological, and/or biological properties. An important property is the aerodynamic diameter, which determines how deeply the particle is likely to penetrate into the respiratory system. Particles have thus been categorized according to the region they are likely to reach in the respiratory system; to measure different size fractions, a personal sampler with different sampling heads is needed. The inhalable particle fraction is the fraction that enters the nose and mouth and has a 50% cut-point diameter of 100 μm. This fraction is often measured in the workplace, but rarely in the general environment (ACGIH 2001). The thoracic fraction is the fraction that enters the thorax and has a 50% cut-point diameter of 10 μm; it is therefore referred to as PM_{10}. The PM_{10} is often measured in the general environment, but rarely in the work place. To measure this fraction, a special PM_{10} sampling head is required; the most frequently used to date is the Harvard Impactor designed by Buckley et al. (1991), which runs at an airflow rate of 4 l/min^{-1}. $PM_{2.5}$, particles with a 50% cut-off diameter of 2.5 μm, which is one of the most important fractions from a health point of view, is the fraction that penetrates deep into the alveolar region. In environmental studies, cyclones are also used to measure this fraction; for example, the GK2.05 cyclone, which runs at 4 l/min$^-$, was designed specifically for the EXPOLIS study (Jantunen et al. 1998). Among the new integrated methods to measure personal and micro-environmental air pollutant concentrations is the multi-pollutant sampler, which was developed to allow personal particulate and gaseous exposures to be measured simultaneously over 24-hour periods (Chang et al. 1999). In its most complete form, the multi-pollutant sampler can be used to measure personal exposures and micro-environmental concentrations of PM_{10}, $PM_{2.5}$, the particle components elemental carbon (EC), organic carbon (OC), sulfate, nitrate, and the elements, and also the gases ozone (O_3), sulfur dioxide (SO_2), and NO_2 simultaneously (see chapter 10 for more details). Finally, ultrafine particulates (UFPs) have a diameter of less than 100 nm and can be measured for example with a TSI CPC 3700 (de Nazelle et al. 2012) or a DiscMini (Fierz et al. 2011).

5.7 FURTHER LABORATORY ANALYSIS

Particulate mass and size are not the only important factors in the development of adverse health effects; the composition of particulates is also important. Therefore, it is useful to analyze particulate samples for their biological and elemental composition (Perera et al. 2006; Johannesson et al. 2011; Minguillón et al. 2012; Montagne et al. 2014a,b). A range of techniques are available for further analysis, including X-ray fluorescence (XRF), inductively coupled plasma-mass spectrometry (ICP-MS), gas chromatography-mass spectrometry (GC-MS), GC-FID, GFAAS, immunoassays, electron scanning microscopy, or reflectance methods. Further information on these techniques can be found in analytical chemistry books.

5.8 RELATIONSHIP BETWEEN AMBIENT AND PERSONAL MEASUREMENTS

In environmental epidemiology, residential air pollution estimates, obtained from stationary ambient air pollution monitors or/and models, are generally used as an exposure index rather than personal exposure measurements. How good a marker are ambient levels for personal exposure? Some of this can be illustrated by results from a study of personal exposure of children and adults in the Netherlands, conducted by Janssen (1998). She took repeated personal measurements of PM_{10} and fine particulates (FPs) (50% cut-point ~3 μm) and compared these with measurements obtained by stationary ambient monitoring.

Table 5.1 shows average levels of personal and outdoor concentrations, and the correlation between personal and outdoor concentrations in Dutch children and adults (after Janssen 1998), and as expected, PM_{10} exposure levels were higher than FP levels (Table 5.1). Children had higher PM_{10} exposure levels than adults, mainly due to high concentrations in classrooms of coarse particles and/or suspension of soil material, caused by the activity of the children. Personal particulate exposure levels were higher than ambient exposure levels, as has often been observed, except perhaps in cases in which the ambient exposure levels are very high (Wallace 1996). Higher personal PM_{10} exposure levels have commonly been attributed to the "personal dust cloud," which is generally not observed with finer particulates (Wallace 1996). The results also showed that personal particulate exposure levels were considerably lower in adults and children not exposed to environmental tobacco smoke (ETS) than for the population as a whole; this confirms that ETS is one of the main sources of indoor air particulate exposure (Wallace 1996).

As Janssen (1998) observed, the correlation was low between personal particulate exposure levels and outdoor fixed-point exposure measurements in the whole population when only one personal and one fixed-point outdoor exposure measurement was used for each subject. The correlation was considerably higher, however, for people not exposed to ETS, especially for FPs. Using repeated measurements of personal and fixed-point outdoor exposure measurements for each subject increased the correlation, in particular for subjects not exposed to ETS and for FPs.

Table 5.1 Average levels of personal and outdoor concentrations, and the correlation between personal and outdoor concentrations in Dutch children and adults

Population	Size fraction	n	Mean personal* ($\mu g/m^{-3}$)	Mean ambient* ($\mu g/m^{-3}$)	Median individual correlation	Cross-sectional correlation**
All subjects						
Adults	PM_{10}	37	62	42	0.5	0.34
Children	PM_{10}	45	105	39	0.63	0.28
Children	FP	13	28	17	0.86	0.41
Non-ETS exposed						
Adults	PM_{10}	23	51	41	0.71	0.50
Children	PM_{10}	25	89	40	0.73	0.49
Children	FP	9	23	18	0.92	0.84

* Mean of individual averages.

** Estimated cross-sectional R, by randomly selecting one measurement per subject.

After Janssen, N. (1998). *Personal exposure to airborne particles. Validity of outdoor concentrations as a measure of exposure in time series studies*. PhD thesis. Wageningen, The Netherlands: Wageningen Agricultural University.

The median of the individual correlation coefficients was 0.9. This suggests that stationary ambient outdoor monitors might be a good indicator of personal exposure to FPs in epidemiological time-series studies that involve linking day-to-day variation in particulate exposure levels to day-to-day variation in health end points. The moderate to high correlation between repeated personal and stationary ambient outdoor measurements can be explained by the exclusion of "fixed" indoor air particulate sources such as smoking and gas cookers, which are likely to change little from day to day compared with outdoor levels. Similar studies have been carried out for gasses such NO_2, and differences have been observed due to the physical and chemical nature of the substance (Magnus et al. 1998; Krämer et al. 2000).

Recently there have been a couple of reviews on the topic. Avery et al. (2010) searched seven electronic reference databases for studies of the within-participant correlation between ambient and personal PM2.5. Eighteen (3%) met inclusion criteria and were abstracted. The studies were published between 1999 and 2008, representing 619 nonsmoking participants aged 6 to 93 years in 17 European and North American cities. Correlation coefficients (median 0.54; range 0.09–0.83) were based on a median of eight ambient-personal PM2.5 pairs per participant (range 5–20) collected over 27 to 547 days. Overall, there was little evidence for publication bias (funnel plot symmetry tests: Begg's log-rank test, $p = 0.9$; Egger's regression asymmetry test, $p = 0.2$). However, strong evidence for heterogeneity was noted (Cochran's Q test for heterogeneity, $p = 0.001$). European locales, eastern longitudes in North America, higher ambient PM2.5 concentrations, higher relative humidity, and lower between-participant variation in r were associated with increased r.

Meng et al. (2012) conducted a quantitative research synthesis to examine factors affecting the strength of the personal-ambient associations across the studies examined with meta-regression. Ambient NO_2 was found to be significantly associated with personal NO_2 exposures, with estimates of 0.42, 0.16, and 0.72 for overall pooled, longitudinal, and daily average correlation coefficients based on random-effects meta-analysis. This conclusion was robust after correction for publication bias with correlation coefficients of 0.37, 0.16, and 0.45. They found that season and some population characteristics, such as pre-existing disease, were significant factors affecting the strength of the personal-ambient associations. They suggested that more meaningful and rigorous comparisons would be possible if greater detail were published on the study design (e.g., local and indoor sources, housing characteristics) and data quality (e.g., detection limits and percent of data above detection limits).

As such there are various advantages and disadvantages of conducting personal and ambient monitoring (Table 5.2) that need to be considered when setting up a campaign for an epidemiological study.

In chapter 12 there is a more detailed discussion of the various issues in personal exposure assessment of particulate matter in the general environment.

Table 5.2 Advantages and disadvantages of conducting personal and ambient

Personal	versus	Ambient/fixed site
Expensive		Cheaper
Small no samples		Covers larger population
Representative of personal exposure		Representative of personal exposure?
Includes various sources		Only site/air

5.9 ANALYSIS OF EXPOSURE VARIABILITY

To better understand the observed exposure levels, it is advisable to get a better understanding of the sources of variability and determinants of exposure. For example, how does the exposure vary from day to day and from subject to subject, and what are the main sources and determinants of exposure? The estimation of variance components, using analysis of variance, and determinants of exposure, using regression techniques, could provide further insight. Although more regularly used in occupational exposure assessment, use in environmental exposure assessment has been limited so far.

5.9.1 Estimation of Variance Components

In most measurement strategies, sampling of both subjects and exposure time is undertaken by measurement of the sample subject over time. A common approach is to predefine exposure strata (i.e., exposure groups, for example, distance from roads) with assumed homogeneous exposure patterns. Stratification criteria are used in environmental studies, such as random sampling that is performed within these strata with subjects chosen at random from all available subjects in each stratum, and sampling periods chosen at random from the total exposure duration of

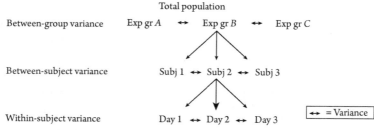

Figure 5.4 Example of variance components in a study population. Between-exposure group variance, exposure variation due to differences in exposure levels between exposure groups. Between-subject variance, exposure variation due to differences in exposure levels between subjects. Within-subject variance, exposure variation due to, for example, day-to-day variability in exposure within subjects. Exp gr, exposure group; Subj, subject.

subjects to be monitored. This measurement strategy is generally affected by three principal sources of variability: between-group variance (Do a priori defined groups really differ?), between-subject variance (Are subjects a priori assigned to a homogeneous exposure group really similar?), and within-subject variance (Do repeated samples on an individual show similar exposure levels?).

These variance components (Figure 5.4) may be estimated by analysis of variance (ANOVA) techniques. Analysis of variance is useful for analyzing the influence of classification variables, known as independent variables, on a continuous response variable, known as the dependent variable. In order to use an ANOVA, three basic assumptions have to be tested:

1. Variables are randomly selected. Non-randomness of sample selection may result in dependency of exposure variables, heterogeneity of variances, or non-normal distributions.
2. Variables and error terms are normally distributed. This is a basic assumption for many statistical techniques, and evaluation of this assumption may reveal outliers or skewed distributions. Occupational and environmental exposure distributions are often lognormally distributed, hence, a logarithmic transformation may be required to obtain a normal distribution. In general, ANOVA is quite robust for non-normality of error terms and only very skewed distributions will have a marked effect.
3. Variables have equal variances. Analysis of variance can tolerate deviations from the equal variance assumption without introducing substantial flaws in the results, particularly when the data are balanced (i.e., equal numbers of observations for every combination of the classification variables). Differences in residual variances within exposure groups up to a factor of 3 to 4 seem acceptable. In environmental measurements, heterogeneity may be introduced by large differences in duration of measurements in the groups monitored.

In ANOVA techniques, the variation in the response variable (e.g., exposure level) is separated into variations due to the classification variables (e.g., subjects and exposure groups) and variation due to random error. The random error includes the measurement error due to the coefficient of variation associated with the measurement technique. Analysis of variance models can be distinguished as random and fixed effect.

A simple one-way ANOVA with random effects is presented in Table 5.3. Variable A has k classes and n is the number of observations per class; say in a survey $k = 3$ and $n = 6$. To find the sum of squares (SS_e) among all 18 samples, the difference between each sample and the overall mean is calculated; these differences are squared and subsequently summed. The sum of squares (SS_a) among exposure groups is calculated likewise by taking the mean difference between each exposure group and the overall mean. The F-statistics is used to test whether the variance of the means of exposure groups is significantly larger than the average variance of observations within the exposure groups. The mean square of error (MS_e) is an

Table 5.3 An ANOVA random-effect model with balanced data

Source	Degrees of freedom	Mean square	F-value	E(MS)
Variable A	$k-1$	$SS_a/(k-1)$	MS_a/MS_e	(SO_4^{2-})
Error	$k(n-1)$	$SS_e/(k(n-1))$		(NO_3^-)
Total	$kn-1$			

unbiased estimate of the residual variance (σ_e^2). The MS of variable A is an unbiased estimate of the variance due to the residual variance in each class (σ_e^2) and the added variance component due to differences among the classes of variable A $(n \times \sigma_a^2)$. In the asbestos survey (σ_e^2) is the within-factory variance and (σ_a^2) is the between-factory variance.

A classical illustration of exposure variability in environmental exposure is based on measurements of exposure to lead and NO_2. For lead on home floors (milligram lead in dust spot sample of $1/m^2$) the within-room variance was substantially lower than the between-room variance ($\lambda = 0.39$). The measurements of personal exposure to NO_2 among mothers and children showed that the within-subject variance was also lower than the between-subject variance (λ of 0.33 and 0.44) (Brunekreef et al. 1987).

Furthermore, Lanki et al. (2007) conducted a study in Amsterdam, the Netherlands, and Helsinki, Finland, during the winter and spring of 1998–1999. In both cities, participants of a larger epidemiological ULTRA study carried a personal measurement system for 24 hours preceding the biweekly clinic visits for determination of exposure to PM2.5 and absorbance. There were 37 non-smoking subjects in Amsterdam and 47 in Helsinki. Personal measurements of PM2.5 were conducted using GK2.05 cyclones (BGI Inc., Waltham, MA), and battery-operated pumps at a flow rate of 4 l/min. Variance components in the data, that is, within-subject and between-subject variation, were calculated using restricted maximum likelihood estimation. In both cities, after exclusion of ETS, the within-subject variation in PM2.5 and absorbance exposures was larger than between-subject variation. In the study, within-subject variation in PM2.5 and absorbance exposures accounted for greater than half of the total variance on days without ETS exposure, which increased between-subject variation. Without ETS, the contribution of within-subject variation to total variance was of the same magnitude for indoor and personal concentrations.

A special case is the nested ANOVA. When measuring subjects repeatedly in different exposure groups, it is obvious that differences may occur between as well as within subjects. Differences within subjects may result in observed differences among exposure groups in which in fact true differences among exposure groups do not exist. The only way to separate the effects of variance between and within subjects is to apply a nested model. In such a model the repeated measurements per

Table 5.4 A nested ANOVA random-effects model with balanced data

Source	Degrees of freedom	Mean square	F-value	E(MS)
Variable A	$k-1$	$SS_a/(k-1)$	MS_a/MS_b	$\sigma^2_e + q\,\sigma^2_b + nq\sigma^2_a$
Variable B (in A)	$k(n-1)$	$SS_b/(k(n-1))$	MS_b/MS_e	$\sigma^2_e + q\sigma^2_b$
Error	$kq(n-1)$	$SS_e/(kq(n-1))$		σ^2_e

A nested ANOVA random-effect model with balanced data variability of exposure and unequal variances across subjects in the exposure groups populations may violate the assumptions of the ANOVA model. Information on the magnitude of the variance components within-subjects, between-subjects, and between-exposure groups can be used to optimize grouping of subjects in epidemiological studies.

subject are nested within each subject and the subjects are nested within each exposure group. Nested effects can be looked upon as an interaction effect (Table 5.4). However, it is difficult to find examples in environmental epidemiology where it has been applied.

5.9.2 Estimation of Important Determinants of Exposure

In the previous section, ANOVA techniques are described that focus on the analysis of factors determining the variability in exposure among individuals. An additional approach is to use linear regression analysis to evaluate the influence of factors on the actual measured personal exposure levels, which may provide a better understanding of where exposure occurs, and which can help epidemiological studies (Jedrychowski et al. 2006; Lanki et al. 2007; Dons et al. 2011, 2013; Johannesson et al. 2011; Minguillón et al. 2012; Schembari et al. 2012). A linear regression model enables the researcher to predict what exposure levels correspond to given values of determinants of exposure. Linear regression analysis with dichotomous variables can be considered as a specific type of ANOVA.

A mathematical expression of a linear regression model is described as:

$$\ln(C_{ij}) = \beta_0 + \beta_1 \, \mathrm{var}_i + \beta_2 \, \mathrm{var}_j,$$

where $\ln(C_{ij})$ is the natural logarithm of exposure concentration (Y), β_0 is the intercept, and β_1 and β_2 are regression coefficients of the independent variables (X). The intercept represents the exposure concentration when the independent variables equal zero. Hence, the intercept may be considered the background exposure level.

The regression coefficients represent the amount of change in the exposure level for each 1-unit change in the independent variables. For any given straight line, this rate of change is always constant. Independent variables may be expressed at a dichotomous level (e.g., presence or absence of local exhaust ventilation, indoor or outdoor activity) or interval level (e.g., hours spent on a specific task, time spent outdoors).

The mathematical expression becomes a statistical model, expressed in the form

$$\ln(C_{ij}) = \beta_0 + \beta_1 \, var_i + \beta_2 \, var_j + E,$$

where E denotes a random variable with mean 0, often called the *error term*. In this statistical model, $\ln(C_{ij})$ is considered a random variable, but in the mathematical expression, $\ln(C_{ij})$ is fixed. The statistical model is used to analyze how well exposure determinants (known, fixed variables X) can predict the exposure level (Y), whereas the mathematical expression is used to assign exposure levels to subjects with unknown exposure levels, based on their time–activity, work, and environmental and work place characteristics. The independent variables are fixed in the statistical model, which is sometimes erroneously associated with the statement that these variables are measured without error. For making statistical inferences the practical implication of the statistical model is that error term E is the only random component on the right-hand side of the equation.

There are five assumptions in order to use linear regression techniques:

1. For any value of the independent value X, Y is a random variable with a mean and variance: in other words, the mean and variance of the random variable Y depend on the value of X. Hence, changes in X are the cause of variations of Y.
2. The Y-values are statistically independent of one other. This assumption may be violated when exposure levels are measured repeatedly on the same subject at different times. For example, if time–activity patterns of a particular subject partly determines his exposure, then it is to be expected that the exposure at one time would be related to the exposure at a later time.
3. The mean value of Y is a linear function of X. This assumption specifies a straight-line function and non-linearity will contribute to the error term.
4. The variance of Y is the same for any X. This assumption of equal variances is quite robust and some differences in variances seem acceptable.
5. For any value of X, Y has a normal distribution. This is a basic assumption, and often a logarithmic transformation is required for work place and environmental measurements. If the normality assumption is not badly violated, the conclusions reached by a regression analysis generally will be reliable and accurate.

Procedures for selecting the best regression equation are based on goodness-of-fit tests, which closely resemble those used in ANOVA techniques. The differences between expected and observed values of Y contribute to the residual variance. The variance in Y, explained by X, is referred to as the *explained variance*, expressed by R^2 in percentage of the total variance. Standard techniques such as residual plots and outlier detection should be used to evaluate the models.

When repeated measurements are available on subjects, mixed effect models are used, with subjects being entered into the model as a random effects and the determinants of interest as a fixed effect.

In the preceding study by Lanki et al. (2007), information on patient and housing characteristics and behavior potentially determining exposure was also collected with questionnaires. Baseline questionnaires filled in by researchers were used to collect information on variables that did not change during the study period (called *permanent determinants* in this study), such as gender, education, and the vicinity of a major street to residence. A self-administered questionnaire, filled in during each 24-hour measurement, was used to obtain information on time-varying determinants, for example, exposure to ETS, time (hours) spent in different microenvironments, and cooking. Statistical analyses were performed using mixed models (PROC MIXED procedure) in SAS statistical software version 8.02 (SAS Institute Inc., Cary, NC). To take into account that several, most likely correlating measurements were conducted on every subject, subject effects were included in the models as random effects (random intercept). Because the repeated measurements were conducted in 2-week intervals, simple compound symmetry was considered a reasonable choice for the covariance structure. Associations of questionnaire variables with PM2.5 and absorbance were first evaluated in models, including only one potential determinant at a time. To evaluate the effects of permanent determinants, subject-specific (individual) averages of PM2.5 and absorbance were included in the models. In the case of time-variant factors, subjects were again treated as random factors. To take into account that confounding factors might cause spurious associations in one-determinant models, multi-determinant models were also constructed. All determinants except the time spent in different microenvironments (outdoors, at home, indoors elsewhere, in a motor vehicle) were treated as binary variables, as there were no strong indications of linear relationships between the determinants and the pollutants in one-determinant models. The "final" model was constructed separately for all measures of exposure by starting from a model including all available determinants, and then dropping the variables one by one based on p-value, until p values of all remaining determinants were less than .1 (backward stepwise elimination). After the selection process, the variables that were found to fulfill the p-value criteria in one city were added in the model of the other one, if not otherwise included. The main determinants of PM2.5 were ETS and cooking, which also affected the levels of absorbance. Other determinants of absorbance were the vicinity of a major street and time spent in traffic. In multi-determinant models, some determinants were associated with the pollutants more clearly in Helsinki than in Amsterdam; for example, the time spent outdoors and opening of windows in the case of absorbance.

5.9.3 Exposure Variability and Implications

The consequences of exposure variability in epidemiological studies have primarily been explored in the context of their effects on the exposure–response relationship. In most research conditions a non-differential misclassification in exposure status (exposed vs. non-exposed) results in an attenuation of the true association between exposure and response (see chapter 10).

When exposure is characterized by a continuous variable, it has been demonstrated that in a study with measurements on all individuals the variance ratio λ (within-subject variance divided by between-subject variance) is directly linked to the attenuation in the observed risk estimate under the classical error model (Liu et al. 1978). Attenuation is expressed by the coefficient of reliability ρ_{xx} that can be approximated by the expression $1/(1 + \lambda)$. Hence, the accuracy of an exposure–response function depends on the degree to which the exposure assessment is successful in providing unbiased estimates of individual exposure levels.

In the alternative grouping approach the attenuation is substantially less than in the individual approach, based on the Berkson error model (see chapter 10), but confidence intervals are wider. Several authors have presented mathematical expressions for estimating group-based attenuation and have evaluated the effect of different grouping strategies on the observed association between exposure and health outcome. In the group approach the aim is to increase the contrast of exposure (ε) between exposure groups, expressed as the ratio between the between-group variance ((σ_{bg}^2)) and the sum of the between- and within-group ((σ_{wg}^2)) variance (i.e., $\varepsilon=(\sigma_{tg}^2)/(\sigma_{bg}^2 +(\sigma_{wg}^2))$), while maintaining reasonably precise exposure estimates of the exposure groups. The precision can be estimated as

$$1/\sqrt{(\sigma_{wg}^2 /k+\sigma_{wg}^2 / kn)}$$

where k is the number of subjects, kn the number of observations in each group, and σ_{wg}^2 the within-subject variance.

Exposure variability may also have implications for the choice of the appropriate measure of exposure, because different measures may be associated with different patterns of exposure variability. A theoretically superior measure of exposure with expected high variability may be less attractive in an epidemiological study than a more proximal measure of exposure with less inherent variability. This point may be illustrated with the applicability of markers of exposure in biological monitoring. Although theoretical arguments may be in favor of biological monitoring, it has to be considered whether markers of exposure can be measured with higher accuracy than environmental agents. Few studies have been published on the utility of markers of exposure in relation to within- and between-subject variability in these markers. Hence, the choice between environmental exposure measurements and measurement of markers of exposure in human material partly depends on the variability in the parameter of interest.

5.9.4 Optimization of Sampling Strategies

In designing an efficient measurement strategy, information is required on the expected variability in exposure among the subjects in the study population. When enough information on exposure variability is available from other studies, statistical equations can assist in the decisions on the most efficient measurement strategy. The appropriate number of measurements depends on the relative accuracy, study size, power, and significance level. Formulae have been presented to calculate the number of subjects in relation to the number of repeated measurements for each subject (White et al. 2008). These formulae combine the classical equations for determining the power of a study with the expressions for evaluating the influence of exposure variability on the precision of the average exposure. The efficiency of increasing the number of repeated measurements or, vice versa, increasing the number of subjects, is partly determined by the variance ratio. In addition, in most epidemiological studies, cost considerations become part of the discussion on the required efficiency of the sampling scheme. For a more detailed discussion on sample size calculations and efficiency of measurement strategies the reader is referred to chapter 10.

5.9.5 Predicting Personal Exposure

Information from the regression models described in the preceding can be used to make prediction models of estimates if information on the determinants of exposure is available. For example, a regression model can be specific in a subpopulation of a study in which measurements are conducted and then applied to the larger population if information on the determinants is available. This approach was adopted in an analysis of factors that influence exposure to nitrogen oxides in the environment (Zipprich et al. 2002). Epidemiological studies that evaluate health effects associated with NO_x commonly rely upon outdoor concentrations of NO_x, NO_2, or residence characteristics as surrogates for personal exposure. In one study, personal exposure over 48 hours and corresponding indoor and outdoor concentrations of NO_x were measured for 48 subjects from 23 households. Demographic, time–activity patterns and household data were collected by questionnaire and used to develop exposure prediction models. In a statistical model, up to 70% of the variation in personal NO_2 and NO_x exposure was explained by two variables (bedroom NO_2 and time spent in other indoor locations; bedroom NO_x, and time spent in the kitchen). These statistical models may reduce the measurement effort considerably in any epidemiological study, because the assessment strategy can largely rely on taking measurements of bedroom exposure to NO_2 and NO_x and on reporting of time–activity patterns in a diary or questionnaire (Zipprich et al. 2002).

5.10 CONCLUSION

Personal monitoring is inevitably labor intensive and expensive. Nevertheless, it is a valuable method because it can dramatically improve exposure assessment in epidemiological studies and thereby add to the scientific credibility of the studies. Intuitively, personal monitoring should provide more accurate exposure estimates than other methods. As has been shown, however, this is highly dependent on the quality and rigor of sampling, the putative agent, and the variability in exposure levels in the study population. Good exposure assessment thus requires careful design of personal monitoring campaigns. Estimates of average exposure levels also provide only one perspective on exposures; equally important are the sources and pathways of exposure and the distribution of variability in exposure levels. In many cases, an understanding of the major determinants of exposure can be as informative as measures of the exposure levels themselves.

REFERENCES

ACGIH. (2001). *Air sampling instruments* (9th ed). ACGIH, Cincinnati.

Avery, C. L., Mills, K. T., Williams, R., McGraw, K. A., Poole, C., Smith, R. L., et al. (2010). Estimating error in using Ambient PM2.5 concentrations as proxies for personal exposures: A review. *Epidemiology*, **21**, 215–223.

Berghmans, P., Bleux, N., Int Panis, L., Mishra, V. K., Torfs, R., and Van Poppel, M. (2009). Exposure assessment of a cyclist to PM10 and ultrafine particles. *Science of the Total Environment*, **407**, 1286–1298.

Boogaard, H., Borgman, F., Kamminga, J., and Hoek, G. (2009). Exposure to ultrafine and fine particles and noise during cycling and driving in 11 Dutch cities. *Atmospheric Environment*, **43**, 4234–4242.

Brunekreef, B., Noy, D., and Clausing P. (1987). Variability of exposure measurements in environmental epidemiology. *American Journal of Epidemiology*, **125**, 892–898.

Buckley, T. J., Waldman, J. M., Freeman, N. C. G., Lioy, P. J., Marple, V. A., and Turner, W. A. (1991). Calibration, intersampler comparison and field application of a new PM-10 personal air sampling impactor. *Aerosol Science and Technology*, **14**, 380–387.

Buonanno, G., Stabile, L., Morawska, L., and Russi, A. (2013) Children exposure assessment to ultrafine particles and black carbon: The role of transport and cooking activities. *Atmospheric Environment*, **79**, 53–58.

Chang, L.-T., Sarnat, J., Wolfson, J. M., Rojas-Bracho, L., Suh, H. H., and Koutrakis, P. (1999). Development of a personal multi-pollutant exposure sampler for particulate matter and criteria Gases. *Pollution Atmosphérique*, **10**, 31–39.

Donaire-Gonzalez, D., de Nazelle, A., Seto, E., Mendez, M., Rodriguez, D., Nieuwenhuijsen, M., and Jerrett, M. (2013). Comparison of physical activity measures using smartphone based CalFit and Actigraph. *Journal Medical Internet Research*, **13**, 15, e111.

Dons, E., Int Panis, L., Van Poppel, M., Theunis, J., and Wets, G. (2012). Personal exposure to Black Carbon in transport microenvironments. *Atmospheric Environment*, **55**, 392–398.

Dons, E., Int Panis, L., Van Poppel, M., Theunis, J., Willems, H., Torfs, R., and Wets, G. (2011). Impact of time–activity patterns on personal exposure to black carbon. *Atmospheric Environment*, **45**, 3594–3602.

Dons, E., Temmerman, P., Van Poppel, M., Bellemans, T., Wets, G., and Int Panis, L. (2013). Street characteristics and traffic factors determining road users' exposure to black carbon. *Science of the Total Environment,* **447,** 72–79.

Dons, E. van Poppel, M., Kochan, B., Wets, G., and Int Panis, L. (2014). Implementation and validation of a modeling framework to assess personal exposure to black carbon. *Environment International,* **62,** 64–71.

Fierz, M., Houle, C., Steigmeier, P., and Burtscher, H. (2011). Design, calibration, and field performance of a miniature diffusion size classifier. *Aerosol Science and Technology,* **45,** 1–10.

Janssen, N. (1998). *Personal exposure to airborne particles. Validity of outdoor concentrations as a measure of exposure in time series studies.* PhD thesis. Wageningen Agricultural University, Wageningen, The Netherlands.

Jantunen, M. J., Hanninen, O., Katsounyanni, K., Knoppel, H., Kuenzli, N., Lebret, E., et al. (1998). Air pollution in European cities: The EXPOLIS study. *Journal of Exposure Analysis and Environmental Epidemiology,* **8,** 495–518.

Jedrychowski, W. A., Perera, F. P., Majewska, R., Camman, D., Spengler, J. D., Mroz, E., et al. (2014). Separate and joint effects of tranplacental and postnatal inhalatory exposure to polycyclic aromatic hydrocarbons: Prospective birth cohort study on wheezing events. *Pediatric Pulmonology,* **49,** 162–172.

Jedrychowski, W. A., Perera, F. P., Pac, A., Jacek, R., Whyatt, R. M., Spengler, J. D., et al. (2006). Variability of total exposure to PM2.5 related to indoor and outdoor pollution sources Krakow study in pregnant women. *Science of the Total Environment,* **366,** 47–54.

Johannesson, S., Rappaport, S. M., and Sallsten, G. (2011). Variability of environmental exposure to fine particles, black smoke, and trace elements among a Swedish population. *Journal of Exposure Science Environmental Epidemiology,* **21,** 506–514.

Hampel, R., Rückerl, R., Yli-Tuomi, T., Breitner, S., Lanki, T., Kraus, U., et al. (2014). Impact of personally measured pollutants on cardiac function. *International Journal of Hygiene and Environmental Health,* **217,** 460–464.

Heydenreich, J., and Wulf, H. C. (2005). Miniature personal electronic UVR dosimeter with erythema response and time-stamped readings in a wristwatch. *Photochemistry and Photobiology,* **81,** 1138–1144.

Ho Yu, C., Morandi, M. T., and Weisel, C. P. (2008). Passive dosimeters for nitrogen dioxide in personal/indoor air sampling: A review. *Journal of Exposure Science and Environmental Epidemiology,* **18,** 441–451.

Kromhout, H., and Heederik, D. (1995). Occupational epidemiology in the rubber industry: Implications of exposure variability. *American Journal of Industrial Medicine,* **27,** 171–185.

Kromhout, H., Tielemans, E., Preller, L., and Heedrik, D. (1996). Estimates of individual dose from current measurements of exposure. *Occupational Hygiene,* **3,** 23–29.

Krämer, U., Koch, T., Ranft, U., Ring, J., and Behrendt, H. (2000). Traffic-related air pollution is associated with atopy in children living in urban areas. *Epidemiology,* **11,** 64–70.

Kraus, U., Schneider, A., Breitner, S., Hampel, R., Rückerl, R., Pitz, M., et al. (2013) Individual daytime noise exposure during routine activities and heart rate variability in adults: A repeated measures study. *Environmental Health Perspectives,* **121,** 607–612.

Lane, N. D., Miluzzo, E., Lu, H., Peebles, D., Choudhury, T., and Campbell, A. T. (2010). A survey of mobile phone sensing. *IEEE Communications Magazine*, **48**, 140–150.

Lanzinger, S., Hampel, R., Breitner, S., Rückerl, R., Kraus, U., Cyrys, J., et al. (2014). Short-term effects of air temperature on blood pressure and pulse pressure in potentially susceptible individuals. *International Journal of Hygiene and Environmental Health*, **217**, 775–784.

Liu, K., Stamler, J. A., Dyer, A., McKeever, J., and McKeever, P. (1978). Statistical methods to assess and minimize the role of intra individual variability in obscuring the relationship between dietary lipids and serum cholesterol. *Journal of Chronic Disease*, **31**, 399–418.

Lanki, T., Ahokas, A., Alm, S., Janssen, N. A., Hoek, G., De Hartog, J. J., et al. (2007). Determinants of personal and indoor PM2.5 and absorbance among elderly subjects with coronary heart disease. *Journal of Exposure Science and Environmental Epidemiology*, **17**, 124–133.

Magari, S. R., Schwartz, J., Williams, P. L., Hauser, R., Smith, T. J., and Christiani, D. C. (2002). The association between personal measurements of environmental exposure to particulates and heart rate variability. *Epidemiology*, **13**, 305–310.

Magnus, P., Nafstad, P., Øie, L., Lødrup Carlsen, K. C., Becher, G., Kongerud, J., et al. (1998). Exposure to nitrogen dioxide and the occurrence of bronchial obstruction in children below 2 years. *International Journal of Epidemiology*, **27**, 995–999.

McKenzie, R., Liley, B., Johnston, P., Scragg, R., Stewart, A., Reeder, A. I., et al. (2013). Small doses from artificial UV sources elucidate the photo-production of vitamin D. *Photochemical and Photobiology Science*, **12**, 1726–1737.

Mead, M. I., Popoola, O. A. M., Stewart, G. B., Landshoff, P., Calleja, M., Hayes, M., et al. (2013). The use of electrochemical sensors for monitoring urban air quality in low-cost, high-density networks. *Atmospheric Environment*, **70**, 186–203.

Meng, Q. Y., Svendsgaard, D., Kotchmar, D. J., and Pinto, J. P. (2012). Associations between personal exposures and ambient concentrations of nitrogen dioxide: A quantitative research synthesis. *Atmospheric Environment*, **57**, 322–329.

Minguillón, M. C., Schembari, A., Triguero-Mas, M., de Nazelle, A., Dadvand, P., Figueras, F., et al. (2012). Source apportionment of indoor, outdoor and personal PM2.5 exposure of pregnant women in Barcelona, Spain. *Atmospheric Environment*, **59**, 426–436.

Montagne, D., Hoek, G., Nieuwenhuijsen, M., Lanki, T., Pennanen, A., Portella, M., et al. (2013). Agreement of land use regression models with personal exposure measurements of particulate matter and nitrogen oxides air pollution. *Environmental Science and Technology*, **47**, 8523–8531.

Montagne, D., Hoek, G., Nieuwenhuijsen, M., Lanki, T., Pennanen, A., Portella, M., et al. (2014). The association of LUR modeled PM2.₅ elemental composition with personal exposure. *Science of the Total Environment*, **493C**, 298–306.

Montagne, D., Hoek, G., Nieuwenhuijsen, M., Lanki, T., Siponen, T., Portella, M., et al. (2014). Temporal associations of ambient PM2.5 elemental concentrations with indoor and personal concentrations. *Atmospheric Environment*, **86**, 203–211.

de Nazelle, A., Fruin, S., Westerdahl, D., Martinez, D., Ripoll, A., Kubesch, N., et al. (2012). A travel mode comparison of commuters' exposures to air pollutants in Barcelona. *Atmospheric Environment*, **59**, 151–159.

de Nazelle, A., Seto, E., Donaire-Gonzalez, D., Mendez, M., Matamala, J., Rodriguez, D, et al. (2013). Improving estimates of air pollution exposure through ubiquitous sensing technologies. *Environmental Pollution*, **176**, 92–99.

Nethery, E., Leckie, S. E., Teschke, K., and Brauer, M. (2008a). From measures to models: An evaluation of air pollution exposure assessment for epidemiological studies of pregnant women. *Occupational and Environmental Medicine,* **65**, 579–586.

Nethery, E., Teschke, K., and Brauer, M. (2008b). Predicting personal exposure of pregnant women to traffic-related air pollutants. *Science of the Total Environment,* **395**, 11–22.

Nieuwenhuijsen, M. J. (1997). Exposure assessment in occupational epidemiology: Measuring present exposures with an example of occupational asthma. *International Archives of Occupational and Environmental Health,* **70**, 295–308.

Nieuwenhuijsen, M. J., Donaire-Gonzalez, D., Foraster, M., Martinez, D., and Cisneros, A. (2014). Using personal sensors to assess the exposome and acute health effect. *International. Journal of Environmental. Research and Public Health,* **11**, 7805–7819.

Nieuwenhuijsen, M. J., Donaire-Gonzales, D., Rivas, I., Cirach, M., Seto, E., Jerrett, M., et al. (2015). Variability and agreement between modeled and personal continuously measured black carbon levels using novel smartphone and sensor technologies. *Environmental Science and Technology,* **49**, 2977–2982.

Nyhan, M., McNabola, A., and Misstear, B. (2014). Comparison of particulate matter dose and acute heart rate variability response in cyclists, pedestrians, bus and train passengers. *Science of the Total Environment,* 468–469, 821–831.

Palmes, E. D., Gunnison, A. F., Dimattio, J., and Tomczyk, C. (1976). Personal sampler for nitrogen dioxide. *American Industrial Hygiene Association Journal,* **37**, 570–577.

Perera, F. P., Rauh, V., Whyatt, R. M., Tsai, W. Y., Tang, D., Diaz, D., et al. (2006). Effect of prenatal exposure to airborne polycyclic aromatic hydrocarbons on neurodevelopment in the first 3 years of life among inner-city children. *Environmental Health Perspectives,* **114**, 1287–1292.

Petersen, B., Wulf, H. C., Triguero-Mas, M., Philipsen, P. A., Thieden, E., Olsen, P., et al. (2014). Sun and ski holidays improve vitamin D status, but are associated with high levels of DNA damage. *Journal of Investigative Dermatology,* **134**, 2806–2813.

Piedrahita, R., Xiang, Y., Masson, N., Ortega, J., Collier, A., Jiang, Y., et al. (2014). The next generation of low-cost personal air quality sensors for quantitative exposure monitoring. *Atmospheric Measurement Techniques Discussion,* 7, 2425–2457.

Schembari, A., Triguero, M., de Nazelle, A., Dadvand, P., Vrijheid, M., Cirach, M., et al. (2012). Personal, indoor and outdoor air pollution levels among pregnant women in a high diesel environment. *Atmospheric Environment,* **64**, 287–295.

Snyder, E. G., Watkins, T. H., Solomon, P. A., Thoma, E. D., Williams, R., Hagler, G. S. W., et al. (2013). The changing paradigm of air pollution monitoring. *Environmental Science and Technology,* **47**, 11369–11377.

van Reeuwijk, H., Fischer, P. H., Harssema, H., Briggs, D. J., Smallbone, K., and Lebret, E. (1998). Field comparison of two NO2 passive samplers to assess spatial variation. *Environmental Monitoring and Assessment,* **50**, 37–51.

Wallace, L. (1996). Indoor particles: A review. *Journal of the Air and Waste Management Association,* **46**, 98–126.

White, E., Armstrong, B. K., and Saracci, R. (2008). *Principles of exposure measurement in epidemiology.* Oxford University Press, Oxford, UK.

Zipprich, J. L., Harris, S. A., Fox, J. C., and Borzelleca, J. F. (2002). An analysis of factors that influence personal exposure to nitrogen oxides in residents of Richmond, Virginia. *Journal of Exposure Analysis and Environmental Epidemiology,* **12**, 273–285.

6

BIOLOGICAL MONITORING

Marie Pedersen, Pierre Droz, and Mark J. Nieuwenhuijsen

6.1 INTRODUCTION

Biological monitoring is mostly used to provide an index of the exposure and/or dose through the analysis of biological samples (NRC 2006). Human biomonitoring is becoming increasingly important in occupational and environmental epidemiological studies (Angerer et al. 2007). Essentially, human biomonitoring assesses whether and to what extent environmental pollutants enter humans through analyses of biological samples such as exhaled breath, urine, breast milk, or blood for a particular chemical of interest and/or its metabolite(s). Human monitoring may also be used to assess early biological effects and/or susceptibility.

Human biomonitoring is widely used to study internal exposures to environmental pollutants throughout population over time. For instance the US National Health and Nutrition Examination Surveys (NHANES) repeatedly determine chemicals in blood and urine from the general population (CDC 2014). In Europe, similar surveys have been/are ongoing (NCR, 2006). These surveys can highlight spatial and temporal trends and when combined with information on potential sources human biomonitoring can be used for preventive action. The European Union–funded projects COPHES/DEMOCOPHES aim to demonstrate that harmonized procedures will enhance the comparability of human biomonitoring surveys (http://www.eu-hbm.info/cophes/human-biomonitoring).

Biomarkers of exposure can be quantified, which is crucial for characterization of exposure, evaluation of potential risk, and policymaking and establishing regulations that are more protective of human health. For example, measurements in humans have been used to assess the efficacy of regulations such as the ban of lead in gasoline, which resulted in a significant decrease in the internal exposure of the general population (Silbergeld 1997).

Human biomonitoring can also help to identify population groups that are at higher risk. For instance, children have higher uptakes of pesticides from diet than adults (Angerer et al. 2007; CDC 2014). In case of phthalates, children have higher uptake and also oxidize a higher amount of the monoesters to toxic metabolites (Wittassek and Angerer 2008).

Human biomonitoring aims to improve the assessment of the exposure and impact on health. Measurement of biomarkers can enable retrospective assessment of exposure, which is useful in cases of accidents and industrial contamination such as in the mid-Ohio Valley in the United States, where the population was exposed to substantial perfluorooctanoic acid (PFOA) because of releases from a chemical plant (Winquist et al. 2013). Hence, integration of biomarkers of exposures in epidemiological studies is useful when the external exposure is difficult to measure. For example, dietary intake of acrylamide, a heat-generated food contaminant, for which the content may vary within similar foods due to difference in food content, cooking temperature, and cooking duration, is very difficult to estimate through food-frequency questionnaires, and measurement of hemoglobin adducts can serve as a biomarker of internal dose in the blood for reactive compounds such as dietary acrylamide (Törnqvist et al. 2002). Moreover, hemoglobin adducts and multiple other biomarkers can be measured in cord blood and used to assess exposure in utero in humans (Barr et al. 2007; Pedersen et al. 2012). Finally, human biomonitoring can contribute to the understanding of mechanisms, toxicokinetics, and effects of environmental pollutants (Wild et al. 2008).

Molecular epidemiology aims to characterize the relations between exposure and disease and to shed light on the "black box" by measuring the multiple biological events involved in environmentally induced disease development (Perera and Weinstein 1982). Following exposure from the external environment, a continuum of biological events may be detected in the human body fluids, cells, or tissues at various stages between the initial exposure and the ultimate health effect (Figure 6.1).

The presence of these measurable events within this continuum can serve as biomarkers in epidemiological studies (NRC 1987). There are several definitions of biomarkers. A biomarker is a characteristic that can be objectively measured and evaluated as an indicator of exposure and/or response to exposure or an intervention. Any chemical, structure, or process that can be measured in the body or its products and influence or predict the incidence or outcome of disease can serve as a biomarker (IARC 1997).

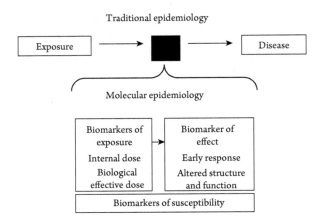

Figure 6.1 Exposure–effect–disease continuum.

Alterations in blood pressure and blood glucose are examples of classical biomarkers. Biomarkers have many valuable applications in medicine for monitoring of human health, disease detection, drug development, clinical trials, and assessment of therapeutic treatment. Biomarkers are unique diagnostic tools for identification of disease or abnormal conditions, diseases prognosis, and response to intervention, but these applications are not discussed in this chapter.

Biomarkers used in epidemiological studies are traditionally classified into those of exposure, effects, and susceptibility, but the distinction between exposure and effects is not always definitive.

A biomarker of exposure is a foreign compound or its metabolite(s), or the product of an interaction between a foreign compound or its metabolites with a cell, DNA, RNA, protein, or lipids. Examples of biomarkers of exposures include internal dose biomarkers such as urinary cotinine, which is often used as an indicator of exposure to tobacco smoke (Benowitz 1999) and biomarkers of effective dose, such as hemoglobin adducts from acrylamide (Törnqvist et al. 2002) or DNA adducts, which are thought to be the initial step of carcinogenicity. Biomarkers of exposure can provide information on chemical exposures in individuals, changes over time, and variability among different populations, and they may provide information on pathways and associated risks.

Biomarkers of effects represent measurable responses that, depending on magnitude, can be recognized as causing an established or potential adverse effect on health or disease. Early effects can be measured in white blood cells as cytogenetic alterations, for example, micronuclei frequency (Fenech 2007). Micronuclei are expressed as small additional nuclei and originate from whole chromosomes and/ or chromosomal fragments, which, during cell division, have not been incorporated in the main nuclei of daughter cells. In healthy adults, higher micronuclei frequency has been associated with cancer risk (Bonassi et al. 2011).

Late biological effect biomarkers refer to biomarkers of altered structure and function of the cell, for example, mutations in tumor suppressor genes, which are the biomarkers most closely related to diseases such as cancer.

Some individuals may be more susceptible due to an inherent or acquired limitation of the body to respond to specific exposures. Genetic polymorphism in genes coding for metabolic activation, detoxification, DNA repair, or biomarkers of nutritional status (e.g., folate) can be measured as indicators of susceptibility (Wild et al. 2008).

Biomarkers vary in the general population in terms of specificity to exposure, persistence, sensitivity, and frequency. The analytical techniques available for detection of internal dose have a high sensitivity and specificity to specific exposures. Effect markers are less exposure-specific, but more closely related to the health outcome.

The promises and limitations of the more recent applications of epigenetic and "omics"-based technologies in epidemiological studies (e.g., genomics), transcriptomics, proteomics, metabolomics, and image-based technologies are described in chapter 14. The "omic"-based techniques are promising tools to identify new biomarkers and elucidate the biological mechanism, especially when applied together with biomarkers with well-described mechanisms such as micronuclei or exposure markers (Fry et al. 2007; van Leeuwen et al. 2008).

Some advantages of measurements of biomarkers in humans compared with external exposure monitoring of airborne substances are:

1. Routes of exposure other than inhalation may exist. This depends on the nature of the exposure and the chemicals to which subjects are exposed. Human biomonitoring provides an integrated measure of exposure through different routes of exposure and takes into account variation in absorption, metabolism, and elimination. Biological monitoring enables estimation of internal exposures though all exposure routes, whereas this would not be possible by ambient air monitoring.
2. Workers often use personal protective equipment. Their efficiency cannot be estimated by air monitoring, but could be with biological monitoring.
3. Physical activity, sex, and body size are known to influence pulmonary ventilation and thus uptake of chemicals. This is not reflected in air monitoring results, but is reflected in biological monitoring results.
4. Exposure may fluctuate widely over time, for example, from day to day. This would require repeated air sampling to estimate the average long-term exposure. This may not be the case for biological monitoring because it could provide information on long-term exposure when the biological half-life is sufficiently long.
5. Individual differences are known to exist among subjects, such as composition of the body ability to absorb, metabolize, eliminate, and repair damage induced by exposure to chemicals. This will have an impact on the level of active species at the site of action, which could be reflected in biological but not air monitoring results.
6. Exposure during specific periods of prenatal development may be critical. Measurement in samples collected at different time points of gestation from pregnant women and their children, for example, maternal blood, maternal urine, placenta, amnion fluid, baby hair, cord blood, and deciduous teeth, can provide valuable information on maternal–placental–fetal toxicokinetics and detail the in utero exposure characterization.

The use of biomarkers in epidemiological studies can, at least partly, overcome these limitations. Measurements of exposure biomarkers in humans can be valuable supplements to the assessment of the external environment because biomarker measures take into account all routes of exposure (i.e., inhalation, dermal, oral, transplacental), variation between individual in terms of exposure and uptake (e.g., the protection afforded by personal protections, influence of physical exercise on uptake, individual differences in the handling of chemicals), and in some situations it reduces the uncertainties produced by day-to-day exposure variability. Measurement of biomarkers of effective dose and early effects reflect individual response to complex exposures in terms of interaction with receptors and ability to repair DNA damage, for example. Bioassays such as the chemically activated lucifer-ase gene expression (CALUX) bioassay have been developed and applied to detect a broad range of exposures with similar toxicity (e.g., dioxin-like activity), assess unknown exposures and potential interactions, and reduce the costs of analyses.

There are a number of challenges and potential disadvantages of human bio-monitoring (Angerer et al. 2007; Wild et al. 2008). Some biomarkers and biologi-cal matrices do not yet have a standardized protocol. Analytical methods can be elaborate and difficult to reproduce. Some methods are expensive. Not all biomark-ers have reliable reference values. Some biomarkers can be difficult to validate, and not all biomarkers can be reliable measured. Validation against other biological and environmental matrices is still necessary for some biomarkers.

If possible the biomarkers applied in the health risk assessment should be sensi-tive, specific, and biologically relevant for the proposed risk and population at risk. Ideally, the method used should be validated as well as practical, inexpensive, and available (IPCS 2001).

Biological material from people (e.g., blood) must only be collected when the added information cannot be obtained from monitoring the external environ-mental or via information from questionnaires or registries (Pedersen et al. 2007). Non-invasive methods for collection of human samples (e.g., placenta, umbilical cord blood, urine, hair, saliva) should be applied whenever possible. Participation must be voluntary, pose no unacceptable discomfort and health risk, and interfere minimally with the study subjects. Sufficient information needed for the interpre-tation of the biomarkers (e.g., smoking status, age, body mass index, health status) should be obtained, and any information relating to an identified or identifiable nat-ural person must be protected. Before collection of human samples the study must be reviewed and approved by the ethical authorities and the data protection agency must be notified. While planning the study, considerations on efficient use of the collected biological material and how to communicate without raising unnecessary fear must be made.

A signed informed consent is a prerequisite for collection of biological samples from humans. The participants must understand that participation is voluntary and that they have the right to withdraw, to know, and not to know the results. The aim of the study, methods, the limitations and perspectives of the study should be clearly explained to the participants and others involved in the study. Care should be taken not to raise unnecessary fear or feelings of guilt, in general, and especially when the study involves workers and/or pregnant women. When biological materials are collected from younger children, the mothers commonly give informed consent on behalf of the children. If the children or caretakers want to withdraw the material donated, it is their right to do so at any time and without giving any reason.

Data interpretation should take into account data on all potential sources of variation, and be carried out with caution because the measured biomarker levels may not necessarily reflect only differences in exposure pattern. Knowledge on variation in response to exposure and baseline levels in the population and how to describe them is needed in health risk assessment, for example, in order to evaluate temporal and spatial trends, and to identify individuals at high risk associated with either highly exposed groups or highly susceptible groups. Communication of the results should be accompanied by expert interpretation, and means of prevention of hazardous exposures should be incorporated as part of the planning in the study design.

The use of biological monitoring should be considered when there are several pathways and routes of exposure and good laboratory methods exist or can be developed.

The issues that need to be considered are the feasibility of the sampling, that is, how easy is it to collect samples, the use of non-invasive methods, biological half-life of the substance of interest, sensitivity and specificity of the method, validation of the methods, and the cost. Some of these may have restricted the use of biological monitoring in occupational and environmental epidemiological studies.

6.2 TYPES OF BIOLOGICAL SAMPLES

A wide range of biological samples can be obtained and analyzed for most chemicals of concern. Blood and urine are the most commonly used matrices (Angerer et al. 2007), but other matrices, such as exhaled breath, hair, nail, fat, deciduous teeth, placenta, amnion fluid, breast milk, feces, sweat, saliva, and semen can also be used (Aw 1995; Table 6.1). Measurements of concentrations of potentially harmful chemicals and/or early biological effects in a critical organ such as the brain, liver, kidney, skeleton, lung, or the developing fetus are rarely possible. Ideally, biological monitoring mirrors the concentration of a hazardous chemical and/or the early biological effect in the critical organ. This may depend on various factors, including external exposure, absorption, distribution, metabolism, and elimination by the body of the chemical.

The choice of biological matrix depends on the study aim, the exposure and effect of interest, the exposure characteristics (e.g., solubility, metabolism, transformation, excretion), feasibility, and how sensitivity, reliability, and invasive is the method used for analysis. Knowledge of the distribution of a substance, the products of its biotransformation within the body, and the time course of these processes is essential when designing a sampling strategy (see chapter 8). It is important to consider the timing of sampling when interpreting data: A blood sample may represent 10 seconds of blood flow; a urine sample may represent 10 hours of collection in the bladder; a hemoglobin adduct reflects accumulated exposures during the past 4 months; a hair sample of 10 cm in length may represent 10 months of hair growth; and a deciduous tooth may reflect accumulated exposure from before birth to the age of teeth shedding. Furthermore, influence by the physiological status of the individual and factors that could result in "noise," such as contamination of laboratory chemicals and equipment or analytical variation, also must be taken into consideration.

Table 6.1 Examples of biological matrix and analytes

Urine	
Parent compounds	Heavy metals, e.g., organic lead, mercury, cadmium, chromium
	Metalloids, e.g., arsenic
	Ketones, e.g., methyl ethyl ketone and methyl isobutyl ketone
	Disinfection by-products, e.g., trichloroacetic acid
	Triclosan
	Bezophenone-3
	Parabens
	Nicotine
Metabolites	Aromatic compounds, e.g., phenol for benzene and phenol, hippuric acid for toluene, methyl hippuric acids for xylenes, mandelic acid for styrene and ethyl benzene, 1-hydroxypyrene for polycyclic aromatic hydrocarbons (PAHs)
	Chlorinated solvents, e.g., trichloroacetic acid for trichloroethylene and 1,1,1-trichloroethane
	Pesticides
	Cotinine for nicotine
	MMA and DMA for inorganic arsenic
	Thiocyanate for tobacco smoke
	Bisphenol A (BPA) monoglucuronide for bisphenol A
	Phthalates
	PFOAs and perfluorooctane sulfonic acids (PFOSs)
Biological effects	Aflatoxin-B1-N7-guanine for mycotoxin
	Malondialdehyde for oxidative stress
	8-Hydroxy2deoxy-guanosine (8-OhdG) for oxidative stress
Blood/serum/plasma	
Parent compounds	Heavy metals, e.g., inorganic lead, mercury, and cadmium
	Aromatic compounds, e.g., toluene
	Chlorinated solvents, e.g., trichloroethylene, perchloroethylene, and 1,1,1-trichloroethane
	Chlorination by-products, e.g., trihalomethanes (THMs)
	Persistent organic pollutants (POPs), e.g., dichlorodiphenyltrichloroethane (DDT), dichlorodiphenyltrichloroethylene (DDE), polychlorinated biphenyls (PCBs), polychlorinsted dibenzo-p-dioxins (PCDDs), dibenzofurans (PCDFs), polybrominated diphenyl ethers (PBDEs)
	BPA
	PFOAs and PFOSs
	Parabens
	Nicotine

(continued)

Table 6.1 Continued

Metabolites	Carboxyhaemaglobin for methylene chloride and carbon monoxide
	Trichloroethanol for trichloroethylene
	Cotinine
	Phthalates
Effective dose	Hemoglobin adducts, e.g., acrylamide, glycidamide
	Albumin adducts
	Dioxin-like, estrogenic and androgenic activity, e.g., CALUX bioassay
Biological effects	DNA adducts, e.g., ^{32}P-postlabeling, HPLC/fluorescence, mass spectrometry, immunological assays
	Genotoxic and cytogenetic damage, e.g., micronucleus assay, comet assay, chromosome aberrations, sister chromatid exchanges

Exhaled breath

Parent compounds	Aromatic compounds, e.g., benzene, toluene, ethyl benzene
	Chlorinated solvents, e.g., trichloroethylene, perchloroethylene, 1,1,1-trichloroethane, and methylene chloride
	Chlorination by-products, e.g., trihalomethanes
	Carbon monoxide for respiratory disturbances
	Nitrogen oxide for asthma
	Alkanes for lipid metabolism
	Alcohol

Hair — *Pesticides, particularly organochlorine pesticides, e.g., hexachlorohexane (HCB), DDT, DDEPOPs, e.g., PCDD/PCDFs, PCBs, PBDEsPAHsPFOAs and PFOSsPhthalates*

Nails

	Metals
	PFOAs and PFOSs

Breast milk

Parent compounds	POPs
	BPA
	Phthalates

Fat — PCBs

Deciduous teeth

Parent compounds	Heavy metals, e.g., organic lead, strontium, manganese
	Nicotine for tobacco smoke
	Organochlorines
	PCBs
	Opiates
	Pharmaceuticals
Metabolites	Cotinine for nicotine

(continued)

Table 6.1 Continued

Saliva	
Parent compounds	Metals, e.g., Ag, Cd, Hg, Mn, Pb
	Perfluoroalkyls
	BPA
	Pesticides
	POPs, e.g., PCBs, PCDDs
Metabolites	Cotinine
	Pesticides
	Phthalates
	Solvents
Placenta	
Parent compounds	Metals
	POPs
	BPA
Metabolites	PAHs
	Phthalates
Biological effects	DNA adducts, e.g., ^{32}P-postlabeling
	Dioxin-like, estrogenic and androgenic activity, e.g., CALUX bioassay

Source: Adapted from Aw 1995; Angerer et al. 2007; Arora and Austin 2013; Alves et al. 2014; CDC, 2014; Michalke et al. 2015.

6.2.1 Urine

A urine sample can be used to determine exposure by detecting the amount of parent compounds present, for example, metals such as lead, mercury, or cadmium. It can also identify the amount of metabolites of specific chemicals, for example, an organic solvent such as benzene (which produces phenol in the urine), toluene (hippuric acid), xylene (methyl hippuric acid), and styrene (mandelic acid). Organophospate pesticides are metabolized to alkylphosphates, which can be detected in the urine. Inorganic arsenic is metabolized in the body by the process of methylation. Inorganic and organic methylated arsenic species can be detected in the urine. This appears to depend upon such things as arsenic burden and individual differences. Phthalates can be measured in urine.

Urine samples are often favored because they are relatively easy to collect compared with blood or other biological samples. Large volumes of urine can be obtained with little discomfort to the study subject. Urine integrates exposure over several hours and may reasonably reflect exposures occurring in the last several days or weeks. Samples are generally collected over a 24-hour period or, for more practical reasons, the first void sample in the morning or at the end of the work shift. Subjects are less likely to decline to cooperate when asked to produce a urine sample rather than blood and it does not require a medically trained person or involve any discomfort. However, urine samples are more prone to external contamination than other biological samples and precautions need to be taken to prevent this.

Several factors should be considered before deciding on using urine samples over other biological samples for biological monitoring; for instance, whether the specific chemical of interest is organic or inorganic, its valency state, and its specificity, as well as the period and duration of exposure. An ideal urinary exposure biomarker would be stable with a relatively long half-life. The metabolite should also be stable during sampling, sample processing, and analysis. If a metabolite is detected, ideally it should be specific to the parent compound of interest.

For metallic mercury, urine is the biological choice for assessing long-term (3- to 4-week) exposure. For recent, acute exposure (1–2 days), blood mercury gives a better indication of exposure. In the case of exposure to inorganic lead, blood lead is preferred over urinary lead because it reflects long-term exposure, the latter being more affected by recent exposure. However, the situation is reversed for exposure to organic lead compounds, with urinary lead being a better index of exposure than blood lead. With exposure to chromium compounds, metabolism results in chromium being excreted in the urine in the trivalent form, regardless of whether exposure and absorption includes hexavalent as well as trivalent forms. Hence, total chromium in the urine will not indicate the relative exposures to different chromium species (Aw 1995). Furthermore, urine sampling may become more complicated where metabolites of some substances are the same as the substance of interest. For example, the chlorination by-product trichloroacetic acid in drinking water is the same as the metabolite of chlorinated solvent such as trichloroethylene, perchloroethylene, and 1,1,1-trichloroethane. Thus when trying to determine the uptake of trichloroacetic acid through ingestion of tap water, exposure to chlorinated solvents should also be estimated and taken into account. Several high-molecular-weight phthalate diesters are also known to have common metabolites. Although analysis of such metabolites is useful to establish phthalate exposure in general, detailed information on the metabolism and excretion kinetics of individual parent phthalates is required to assess their contribution to the measured concentrations of these metabolites.

The concentration of a substance in urine is influenced by a number of factors: the degree of dilution, the kidney function, the body burden of the substance, the metabolic and kinetic pathways, and current and past exposure. Urine is produced continuously by the kidneys as part of a complex process of water and electrolyte control. The kidneys' glomeruli produce an ultrafiltrate (the primary urine) consisting of water, salts, and small molecules at a rate of 125 ml/min^{-1}. A total blood volume of about 300 l is filtered every day. If the glomerular filtration (GFR) is decreased, the capacity for eliminating toxic substances also decreases. In such cases, the concentration of a substance in the urine will become lower, while the body burden increases. This is the case for aluminum, a pollutant that is normally excreted in the urine, but that accumulates in the body of those suffering from severe renal impairment (Berglund et al. 2001). In order to maintain the water balance of the body, water may be reabsorbed. In this process other xenobiotics may be reabsorbed either actively or passively. This is notably the case for lipophilic substances that can cross membranes easily, such as unchanged organic solvents. This reabsorption affects the concentration of substances in urine. To evaluate the concentration of a substance in urine it is often necessary to consider the degree of concentration of the urine. The composition of urine is usually compatible with maintenance of body water and solute content within physiological limits. A short time after consumption of a large volume of fluid, the urine will become diluted, with a low solute content. When water is evaporated, for example, due to perspiration as a result of high environmental temperature or hard physical work, the urine concentration increases. The concentration of a substance can be related to creatinine (a metabolic product of the muscles excreted in the urine in fairly constant quantities) or specific gravity to compensate for the degree of dilution. The excretion rate is higher in males, muscular individuals, and those who eat a lot of meat. Therefore, the substance can be reported in micrograms (or mole) per gram (or mmole) creatinine. Reporting per gram creatinine allows more accurate monitoring of individuals with either very dilute or concentrated urine. The other way to compensate for the degree of dilution is to adjust for a specific gravity. If a urine sample has specific gravity of 1.012, which is fairly diluted urine, and is to be adjusted to represent urine with a more normal specific gravity (1.022), the following calculation can be made:

The concentration in the urine sample $\times$ (1.022 − 1.000)/(1.012 − 1000)

The factor of 1000, which is the specific density of water, must be subtracted from both the numerator and denominator (Berglund et al. 2001). Sometimes the concentration of the substance is not adjusted for and is expressed simply as the measured concentration ($\mu g/l$). This is mainly the case for passively reabsorbed substances, such as solvents. In rare situations, biomarker levels are expressed as rates of excretion (amounts per unit of time) as, for example, mmol/min^{-1}.

6.2.2 Blood

Although long-term diseases are not expected from affected blood cells, it is generally accepted that blood cells can be used as surrogate tissue for biomarker of effect because blood is in steady state with all organs. Blood is a transport medium. After absorption in the gastrointestinal tract or the lungs, substances are transported via the bloodstream to different tissues and organs where they are stored, accumulated, or metabolized. Substances that have been absorbed by tissues will be released and degraded by normal tissue metabolism, transported in the blood, and eventually eliminated from the body. The blood concentration of a substance is influenced by the exposure and concentrations in the tissues (body burden). The relative importance of these two factors varies according to the substance in question and the exposure level (Berglund et al. 2001). A substance in blood is bound to red cells or plasma proteins. For most essential metals, such as iron, copper, and zinc, the body has special transport proteins, such as transferrin, ceruplasmin, and alpha-2-microglobulin. Certain non-essential and toxic substances, metals in particular, bind preferentially to red cells. Cadmium and lead are almost completely bound to red cells. Sometimes it may be necessary to adjust for the hemoglobin concentration or hematocrit when comparing the metal concentration between individuals or groups. The concentration of contaminants in plasma is of particular interest because it constitutes the fraction of the substance in blood that is readily available for transport in and out of tissues. However, for many toxic substances concentrations are so low that they are very difficult to measure. Highly lipophilic compounds (e.g., PCBs, PCDDs, PCDFs, PCBs, PBDEs, and chlorinated pesticides) should be adjusted for cholesterol, triglyceride, or low-density lipid concentration (Berglund et al. 2001). When levels are reported per total blood lipids they become reflective of the total amount of the compound stored in body fat and comparison among studies becomes easier.

Mutagenic and carcinogenic substances bind to macromolecules, especially to proteins. Adducts of reactive chemicals with hemoglobin or serum albumin can be used as biomarkers of internal doses of carcinogens (Törnqvist et al. 2002). Hemoglobin adducts are more commonly monitored because accumulation is still greater than that of serum albumin (Angerer et al. 2007). Moreover, reactive chemicals have to cross a cell membrane, showing that they are sufficiently stable to reach the DNA in the critical organ. Because of these reasons the hemoglobin adducts can be viewed as surrogates of DNA adducts, which are thought to be the initial step of carcinogenicity. Hemoglobin adduct levels in blood enable the estimation of internal exposure as well as biochemical effects. Hemoglobin adducts seem to be better estimates for cancer risk than measuring the genotoxic substances or their metabolites in human body fluids. In advanced laboratories it is possible to routinely determine the adducts of alkylating substances, aromatic amines, and aromatic nitro carbons.

Because cord blood and dried blood spots can be used to investigate environmental exposures in utero, such as heavy metals, persistent organic pollutants (POPs), pesticides, benzene metabolites, acrylamide, perfluorooctanoic acids (PFOAs), and perfluorooctane sulfonates (PFOSs) (Barr et al. 2007; Funk et al. 2008; Pedersen et al. 2012; Stove et al. 2012). Because these matrices reflect in utero exposures better than biomarkers measured in maternal venous blood samples collected during pregnancy, and because they are easier to collect and store, biomarker applications in these matrices are growing. The use of biomarkers in well-characterized samples collected as parts of birth cohorts have great potential (Casas et al. 2013).

DNA can be isolated from the less abundant white blood cells as well as from other matrices, such as placenta or saliva. DNA adducts are markers of exposure to carcinogenic substances, which binds to DNA. They provide an overall measure of exposure, absorption, and metabolic activation of a mixture of DNA adduct-forming compounds, integrated with repair of DNA damage of an individual. There are many different types and methods to detect DNA adducts (Parry and Parry 2012).

Bulky DNA adducts, detected by ^{32}P–post-labeling, are widely accepted as a sensitive biomarker of the biologically effective dose of exposure to genotoxic aromatic compounds, including PAHs and heterocyclic amines, from complex environmental exposures, including those in air, tobacco smoke, and diet, and may be predictive of cancer risk (Phillips and Arlt 2007), whereas ^{32}P–post-labeling due to shortcomings in specificity provides an indicator of total adduct burden. On the other hand, fluorescence detection is limited to fluorescent adducts such as PAHs or aflatoxine. To make a DNA adduct more broadly applicable, development of sensitive, reproducible, high-throughput methods is recommended.

Blood cells can also be evaluated for genotoxic and cytogenetic damage using micronucleus assay (Fenech 2007) or comet assay (single-cell gel electrophoresis), which is increasingly applied in epidemiological studies to measure DNA damage and repair. Principles, applications, and limitations have been summarized by Collins (2004).

Blood samples can be collected to identify parent compounds (or their metabolites) and early effects. Heavy metals such as lead, mercury, and cadmium can be measured in blood. In the United Kingdom, lead blood concentrations are routinely measured for compliance reasons in the work place. For organic solvents such as perchloroethylene and trichloroethylene, the solvents themselves can be identified in blood, whereas for other solvents their metabolites can be detected in blood (e.g., free trichloroethanol for exposure to trichloroethylene). Very low levels of chlorination by-products such as chloroform and chlorodibromomethane can also be detected in blood at apparently lower levels than in exhaled breath (Nieuwenhuijsen et al. 2000; see chapter 16).

The disadvantage of using blood samples for biological monitoring include poorer cooperation because of the discomfort of the procedure, especially if venipuncture is required on a regular basis. Some individuals may faint during venipuncture or even at the thought of the procedure. Facilities have to be in place to deal with this possibility. For those with veins that are not prominent, a degree of skill and experience is required to successfully collect a suitable quantity of blood.

Care must be taken to prevent external contamination of the blood sample, especially when the parent compound is determined. The site of venipuncture has to be adequately cleaned. For determining chromium levels in blood, the use of chromium-free needles have been suggested. For trihalomethanes (THMs), the containers need to be processed to expel compounds that are present in the containers (Aw 1995). Concentrations of chemicals measured in blood samples are expressed in amounts per unit volume, in some cases whole blood is considered and in other situations only plasma is taken into account.

6.2.3 Exhaled Breath

Biological monitoring of exhaled breath involves breathing out into a direct reading instrument or into a sampling bag or other collection device before dispatching the collected sample to a laboratory for analysis. It is preferable to obtain a sample of alveolar breath rather than all the exhaled breath, because it is appears to be the best indicator for blood levels. Special devices have been developed to obtain this fraction (Dyne et al. 1997). The advantages of exhaled breath sampling are that the collection of samples is non-invasive, and repeated samples can be taken within a short period of time. The disadvantages include current lack of agreement on how samples have to be collected, standardization on the type of collection device used, and laboratory methods for analysis. Furthermore, the method may not be as sensitive as blood sampling, which appears to be the case for THMs (see chapter 16). Exhaled breath sampling is suitable for the detection and determination of, for example, benzene, toluene, carbon monoxide, ethyl benzene, n-hexane, carbon tetrachloride, perchloroethylene, trichloroethylene, and trihalomethanes (Aw 1995). Concentrations in exhaled breath are expressed in ppm or mmol/l^{-1}. It should always be mentioned to which fraction of the exhaled breath the data refer: mixed exhaled, alveolar, or end-expired air.

6.2.4 Hair and Nail

Analysis of hair and nail samples has been increasingly successfully used to assess both short- and long-term exposure to arsenic and mercury. The rationale for this is that as nail and hair growth occurs, absorbed arsenic and mercury are incorporated into a portion of the hair and nail. The analysis of hair and nail can provide a measure of exposure over a longer time period, although varying growth rates during the exposure period may need to be taken into account. This may be difficult. Analysis of hair from neonates can enable in utero exposure assessment (Barr et al. 2007).

Although correlation of contamination levels between hair samples and ambient air or internal tissues has been found, external contamination of the hair and nail may give an erroneous indication of the amount absorbed systematically, and certain washing procedures need to be carried out to prevent this. Contamination may occur from consumer products such as the use of hair dye and shampoo, and may affect the subsequent analysis. Procedures to wash and clean the samples before analysis may not adequately remove contaminants absorbed onto the surface of samples. The difference between the concentration of substances measured in head versus pubic hair or in fingernail versus toenail samples may indicate the extent of surface contamination. There are limitations in the interpretation of the results obtained, particularly for individuals rather than groups (Aw 1995).

Analysis of hair is attractive as a non-invasive, cost-effective, and easily applicable biomonitoring tool, but it has some limitations (Schramm 2008). For example, there is a need to standardize the analytical methods; to perform more studies on the kinetic and mechanisms of incorporating organic contaminations into hair and their retention in the hair matrix; to identify the metabolites in hair; to establish reference values for metals and POPs in human hair; to describe possible dose–response relationships; and to better understand hair biology and variations of hair composition by age, sex, race, and so on.

6.2.5 Other Biological Matrices

Analysis of breast milk has been very useful for following time-trend in human exposure to lipophilic chemicals, such as POPs, in particular organochlorine contaminants. Since 1976 the World Health Organization (WHO) has collected and evaluated information on levels of POPs in foods, including human milk (http://www.who.int/foodsafety/areas_work/chemical-risks/pops/en/index1.html). Analyses of milk samples from Swedish women has suggested that the levels of polychlorinated biphenyls (PCBs), polychlorinated dibenzodioxins (PCDDs), and polychlorinated dibenzofurans (PCDFs) declined over time, whereas the temporal trends of polybrominated diphenyl ethers (PBDEs) did not follow any consistent pattern (Lignell et al. 2009). Monitoring breast milk generally has been carried out to estimate the exposure of the child, rather than that of the mother, but the content of lipophilic substances in the milk also represents the body burden of the contaminants in the adipose tissue of the mother. Breast milk is a useful medium because most newborn children obtain all their nutrition from their mother's milk. The concentration of a contaminant is a function of parity, maternal age, weight change, body mass, time of sampling, nutritional status, lactation period, and fat content of the milk (Berglund et al. 2001).

Samples of body fat have been used for determining the extent of exposure to PCBs. Lipophilic substances such as PCBs are not easily biodegradable and therefore persist in the environment and accumulate in adipose tissue. Fat samples may be obtained by needle biopsy or surgical excision. The quantity of fat required for the assay of PCB content is several hundred grams. The amount of PCB determined is in parts per billion or parts per trillion quantities. It is not practical to collect fat samples periodically because it is invasive and thus does not attract many volunteers; therefore, its use is somewhat limited (Aw 1995).

Biological monitoring of semen, teeth, feces, and skeleton has been carried out also, but to a much lesser extent.

6.3 BIOLOGICAL HALF-LIFE

The biological half-life of a substance refers to the time required for clearance of 50% of the substance from the medium. Biological half-lives vary substantially (Table 6.2), and this needs to be taken into account in the sampling strategy. For example, in the case of exposure assessment of chlorination by-products in drinking water, chloroform, generally the main volatile by-product, has a biological half-life of approximately 30 minutes and can be measured in blood and exhaled breath. Trichloroacetic acid, generally the main non-volatile by-product, can be measured in urine and has a half-life of 70 to 120 hours. It is therefore essential that

Table 6.2 Examples of biological indicators and their half-lives

Biological indicator	Approximate $T_{1/2}(h)$
Solvent in breath/blood ES	0.5–2 h
PCB-153 in blood	14 y
Solvents in breath/blood PS	20–70 h
PBDE-147	6 y
DDE in blood	4 y
PFOS in blood	4–5 y
PFOA in blood	3–5 y
Phthalates low molecular weight	3–4 h
Phthalates high molecular weight	24 h
BPA	6 h
Chloroform in breath/blood	0.3–0.5 h
Trichloroacetic acid in urine	50–120 h
Dichloroacetic acid in urine	<2 h
Trichloroethanol in urine	12 h
Mandelic acid in urine	5 h
Phenol in urine	3.5 h
Hippuric acid in urine	1–2 h
Carbon monoxide in breath/blood	5 h
Lead in blood	80 d
Chromium in urine	15–40 h
Cadmium in urine	10–30 y
Mercury in blood	100 h
Hemoglobin adducts	3000[a] h
Albumin adducts	400[a] h

ES, end of work shift sample; PS, prior to work shift sample.

[a] $T_{1/2}$ of hemoglobin/albumin, adducts $T_{1/2}$ may be lower.

Source: Adapted from Droz, P. O., and Wu, M. M. (1991). Biological monitoring strategies. In *Exposure assessment for epidemiology and hazard control* (eds. S. M. Rappaport, and T. J. Smith). Lewis Publishers, Michigan.

chloroform monitoring takes place very quickly after activities associated with chloroform uptake, such as ingestion of, showering and bathing with, and swimming in chlorinated water. Chloroform levels in exhaled breath and blood fall rapidly and the actual uptake may be underestimated the longer the period between exposure and sampling. This, however, is much less of a concern for trichloroacetic acid, for which the main route of uptake is ingestion. A concern for the measurement of trichloroacetic acid is that other chlorinated solvents have trichloroacetic acid as their metabolite. People may be exposed to these kinds of activities repeatedly during the day or during the week and this may be reflected in the biological samples.

Because variability is inherent in biological monitoring, even more so than in personal air sampling, it is important to identify the main categories of variability. Figure 6.2 illustrates the effects of variable exposure. The time profiles of two hypothetical biological indicators, behaving according to a one-compartment kinetic model, are indicated: one with a half-life of 5 hours and the other, 50 hours. As shown in Table 6.2, many indicators have half-lives in this range. In Figure 6.2, there is no variability in exposure at all, and after a certain time (which depends on the half-life), the biological indicator reaches a steady-state level. Sampling after this point would completely define the exposure situation and the health risk if the exposure–response relationship were known. In Figure 6.2, a typical work schedule is taken into account: 8 hours of exposure per day with a 1-hour break, 5 days per week, week after week. In this case the biological sampling becomes a little more complex. The concentration in the biological sample will depend on the sampling time with respect to the work shift for the biological indicator with a half-life of 5 hours, and with respect to the work shift and the day of the week for the biological indicator with a biological half-life of 50 hours. In Figure 6.2, the exposure is not steady any longer; rather, it fluctuates from hour to hour according

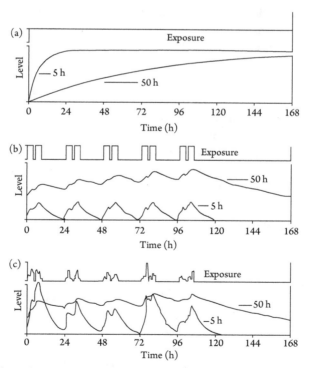

Figure 6.2 Effects of air exposure variability on two biological indicators with half-lives of 5 and 50 hours. Ordinate is an arbitrary scale. Graph (a) constant continuous exposure; (b) constant industrial exposure (8 h/day^{-1}, 1-h break, 5 days/week); (c) fluctuation industrial exposure (1-h air concentrations sampled from a lognormal distribution with $\sigma_g = 2.0$).

to a lognormal distribution (geometric standard deviation of 2.0). The concentration in the biological samples is more variable, especially for the 5-hour biological indicator. This suggests that biological indicators with a short half-life are more sensitive to fluctuations in exposure from day to day and even within 1 day (Droz and Wu 1991). The biological half-life of a substance may differ from person to person, depending on, for example, age, diet, stress, metabolic polymorphism, and disease. These factors may have to be considered when conducting a study. Up to a certain extent variation in biological half-life can be incorporated in a sampling strategy using physiologically based pharmacokinetic (PBPK) modeling (see chapter 8).

6.4 AUTOCORRELATION

Depending on what kind of sampling strategy is chosen, repeated samples may be required (see chapters 1 and 5). Airborne exposures are usually considered as following approximately a lognormal distribution. Although short-term air samples (e.g., 15-min sampling duration) are generally considered to be autocorrelated, there is very little evidence for autocorrelation between 8-hour samples in the work place. Therefore, the latter can be treated as being random. The situation is different for biological indicators, which are themselves autocorrelated due to the finite rates of biological elimination. This can probably be described by using a first-order autoregressive process according to the following model:

$$Y_t = \mu(1 - b_1) + b_1 Y_{t-1} + a_t,$$

where Y_t is the biological indicator on day t, Y_{t-1} is the biological indicator on day $t - 1$, μ is the long-term mean of the biological indicator, b_1 is the first lag autoregressive coefficient, and a_t is a term describing random variation in exposure and individual variability. The autocorrelation coefficient can furthermore be expressed as a function of the half-life $(T_{1/2})$ of the biological indicator:

$$b_1 = e^{-24k} \text{ with } k = 0.693 / T_{1/2}.$$

This is the autocorrelation coefficient of lag 1 (1 day). Coefficients of higher lags can be calculated, for example, for lag σ_e^2.

As could be expected, the longer the half-life of the biological indicator, the larger the autocorrelation coefficient. If $b_1 < 0.10$, it may be assumed that any autocorrelation is negligible, thus one can see that

1. at $T_{1/2}$ smaller than 5 hours, days may be considered as uncorrelated
2. at $T_{1/2}$ between 5 and 50 hours, weeks may be considered as uncorrelated
3. at $T_{1/2}$ between 50 and 200 hours, months may be considered as uncorrelated

A strategy for biological monitoring is easier to establish if the results are unlikely to be autocorrelated. Therefore, the time of sampling should be chosen in order to minimize autocorrelation (p. 176). For biological indicators belonging to case (2), for example, sampling frequency should be restricted to once a week, and for case (3) to once a month. For case (1), sampling can be as frequent as once a day (Droz and Wu 1991).

6.5 DAMPING OF EXPOSURE VARIABILITY

As seen in Figure 6.1, sampling of biological indicators with long half-lives is likely to introduce some damping of the exposure variability. That is, if one compares the distribution of the biological monitoring results with that of, for example, air sampling results, the variance will be lower. For biological indicators with half-lives smaller than 5 hours, this damping effect will be negligible. In this case essentially all the variability of the environmental concentrations is expected to be transmitted to the biological indicators. For indicators with half-lives of 40 hours and greater, less than 50% of the variability will be transmitted. However, for estimating the mean exposure, or the mean target site concentration, biological indicators with long half-lives may be more useful because they are less sensitive to exposure fluctuations (Droz and Wu 1991).

Results from biological monitoring of similarly exposed subjects are subject to intra- and inter-subject variation. Factors that have been taken into account in the interpretation of results include:

1. Those related to the individual: Age, sex, body mass index, genetic differences in the metabolism of the compounds, pregnancy, exercise and physical activity, smoking, medication, consumption of alcohol and dietary factors, and the presence of existing lung, liver, or kidney disease or other illness
2. Those related to exposure: Timing and intensity of exposure in relation to timing of collection of the biological sample, mixed exposures that may affect the metabolism of the compounds absorbed, and route of exposure
3. Those related to the chemical of interest: Half-life, where and how it is metabolized and excreted (Aw 1995)

6.6 VARIABILITY

Exposure variability may also have implications for the choice of the appropriate measure of exposure because different measures may be associated with different patterns of exposure variability. A theoretically superior measure of exposure with expected high variability may be less attractive in an epidemiological study than a more proximal measure of exposure with less inherent variability (see chapter 10). This also governs the applicability of markers of exposure in biological monitoring.

Although theoretical arguments may be in favor of biological monitoring, it has to be considered whether biomarkers of exposure can be measured with higher accuracy and precision than environmental agents. Few studies have been published on the utility of markers of exposure in relation to within- and between-subject variability in these markers. Hence, the choice between environmental exposure measurements and measurement of markers of exposure in human material partly depends on the variability in the parameter of interest.

In general, the measured biomarker levels in epidemiological studies are influenced by several factors in addition to exposure. Intra- and inter-individual variations are caused by factors related to: 1) biological variability between subjects (e.g., genetic susceptibility, age, sex, race, health status, nutritional status); 2) cultural differences (e.g., environment, diet, number of children carried and fed, medication, smoking, alcohol, occupation); and 3) variation in the laboratory techniques applied (e.g., sampling design, time of sampling, spot urine vs. 24-hour urine, protocols, analytical precision of the measurement) (Hansen et al. 2008). The impact of the all these factors of variation on the biomarker levels should be evaluated as part of data interpretation.

The strengths and weaknesses of both measurement approaches were explored in a longitudinal study among boat workers exposed to styrene (Rappaport et al. 1995). The exposure assessment consisted of full-shift personal measurements of styrene exposure per worker carried out over 1 year on seven occasions. Sister chromatid exchanges (SCEs) was used as a marker of exposure. This was measured in lymphocytes from two venous blood samples taken from each worker obtained during the measurement surveys. The correlation between styrene exposure and SCEs was low (11% explained variance). A within- and between-subject variance ratio of 0.33 for styrene exposure was observed and of 2.21 for SCEs. If attenuation of the health risk estimates would be restricted to 10%, three measurements per person would be required for airborne styrene exposure versus 20 measurements per person for SCEs. This latter value would be impossible in epidemiological studies due to the invasive character of the technique and the associated costs. So although intuitively biological monitoring would have been the preferred option for an epidemiological study, detailed analysis showed that this is not the case and that it would be more efficient to obtain air samples. Obviously, this is just one specific example and may not be applicable to all studies or situations.

6.7 MODELS AND DETERMINANTS

Feasibility issues, cost, and time may restrict biological monitoring in epidemiological studies and it is rare that biological samples can be obtained from the entire study population, particularly when it is large. However, biological monitoring could be useful to build dose and/or exposure models in a subpopulation, which subsequently could be applied to a whole population after information is obtained in this population on particular determinants, for example, by questionnaire(see chapter 2). For example, Harris etal. (2002) measured 2,4-dichlorophenoxyacetic acid (2,4 D), 2-(4-chloro-2-methylphenoxy) propionic acid, MCPP (mecoprop), and 3,6-dichloro-*o*-anisic acid (dicamba) in urine (two consecutive 24-h periods) collected from a group of 98 professional turf applicators from 20 companies across southwestern Ontario. The group also filled out questionnaires to acquire information on all known variables that could potentially increase or decrease pesticide exposure to the amount handled to build models for epidemiological studies. They used linear regression to assess the relationship between the concentration of the substances in urine and the questionnaire data. They found that the volume of pesticide (active ingredient) applied was only weakly related to the total dose of 2,4 D absorbed ($R^2 = 0.21$). Two additional factors explained a large proportion of the variation in measured pesticide exposure: the type of spray nozzle used and the use of gloves while spraying. Individuals who used a fan-type nozzle had significantly higher doses than those who used a gun-type nozzle. Glove use was associated with significantly lower doses. Job satisfaction and current smoking influenced the dose but were

Table 6.3 Regression models predicting the log of total dose of mecoprop and 2,4 D in 94 volunteers

Variable	Estimate	SE	p-value	Partial R^2
2,4 D ($R^2 = 0.64$)				
Intercept	−1.09	0.01	0.29	
Log spray	0.96	0.12	0.001	0.44
Nozzle	1.37	0.23	0.001	0.29
Glove wear	−1.50	0.25	0.001	0.29
Satisfaction	−0.39	0.17	0.021	0.06
Smoke	0.51	0.22	0.02	0.06
Mecoprop ($R^2 = 0.67$)				
Intercept	−1.44	0.98	0.14	
Log spray	1.05	0.11	0.001	0.50
Nozzle	1.12	0.22	0.001	0.23
Glove wear	−1.63	0.25	0.001	0.34
Satisfaction	−0.40	0.16	0.02	0.07
Smoke	0.63	0.22	0.005	0.09

Spray: ln (ml product over week + 900); glove wear: if sprayer and not wearing gloves or mixer/loader, then glove wear = 0; if sprayer and wearing gloves, then glove wear = 1; nozzle type: 1 = fan and 0 = gun; job satisfaction: 1, highly satisfied; 2, satisfied; 3, neither satisfied nor unsatisfied; 4, unsatisfied; smoker 1 = yes and 0 = no.

After Harris, S. A., Sass-Kortsak, A. M., Corey, P. N., and Purdham, J. T. (2002). Development of models to predict dose of pesticides in professional turf applicators. *Journal Exposure Analysis and Environmental Epidemiology*, **12**, 130–144.

not highly predictive. In the final multiple regression models, predicting absorbed dose of 2,4 D and mecoprop, approximately 63% to 68% of the variation in doses could be explained by the small number of variables identified (Table 6.3). Biological monitoring in this case was important to be able to determine the true effect of wearing protective equipment such as gloves. This study provided extremely useful information for epidemiological studies, which could focus on obtaining information on these particular variables.

Another example is arsenic, for which uptake is most likely through inhalation and digestion of soil and house dust, including hand to mouth contact, but also through ingestion of contaminated vegetables, fish, and water, as well as smoking. Soil represents an important pathway of exposure, through handling of soil materials (e.g., during play or work), contact with soil-derived dust, and foodstuffs. Exposures to arsenic have attracted particular concern, and several studies have suggested an association between soil arsenic and cancer of the skin, lung, and bladder. This is mainly attributed to the inorganic form of arsenic, although other forms may be as toxic. Inorganic arsenic is reduced by methylation in humans, forming monomethylarsonic acid (MMA) and dimethylarsinic acid (DMA).

Arsenic and its species can be measured in soil and house dust and by biomonitoring in hair, urine, blood, and toenails. Mining and smelting have left certain areas of southwest England with high arsenic levels in soil. There has been considerable concern about these high levels, although it was unclear how much was taken up by the residents. Kavanagh et al. (1998) measured arsenic levels in soil, house dust, and urine of residents in three areas: two exposed areas (Gunnislake and Devon Great Consols) and one unexposed area (Cargreen) (Table 6.4). High levels of arsenic were found in the soil and, to a lesser extent, in house dust. Marked variations were evident, however, between the different areas. Concentrations of As in the soil were

Table 6.4 Arsenic (As) in soil, house dust, and urine in the southwest of England

Ratios between sites	Cargreen	Gunnislake	Devon GC
Soil ($\mu g/g^{-1}$) 1:10:122	37	365	4500
House dust ($\mu g/g^{-1}$) 1:4:24	49	217	1167
Urine ($\mu g/g^{-1}$ creatine)			
Total As 1:2:2	4.7	9.2	10.0
Arsenite (As III)	<LOD	1.7	0.9
Arsenate (As V)	<LOD	0.9	1.3
DMA	4.7	5.6	8.5
MMA	<LOD	0.3	0.7

LOD, below limit of detection; GC, great consols; DMA, dimethylarsinic acid; MMA, monomethylarsonic acid.

Kavanagh, P., Farago, M. E., Thornton, I., Goessler, W., Kuehnelt, D., Schlagenhaufen, C., and Irgolic, K. J. (1998). Urinary arsenic species in Devon and Cornwell residents, UK. *The Analyst*, **123**, 27–30.

up to 122 times greater in areas with high exposure compared to nonexposed areas. For house dust, concentrations were up to 24 times higher. In urine, there was only a twofold difference in arsenic levels between the areas. This suggests that the actual uptake of arsenic from soil and house dust is relatively low. Moreover, biological monitoring needs to be undertaken to obtain good estimates of personal arsenic uptake, since soil or house dust samples cannot be relied upon to provide a reliable dose estimate. The study also suggested that arsenic speciation is very important, for inorganic arsenic levels in the control village were below the detection limit, whereas in the other two areas they were measurable.

6.8 QUALITY CONTROL

Normal quality control procedures apply to the sampling, storage, and laboratory analysis of biological samples (Armstrong et al. 1992; Weber 1996). The measured concentrations are often very low and therefore caution needs to be taken to avoid contamination of the sample by, for example, environmental concentrations and containers and degradation during storage.

REFERENCES

Alves, A., Kucharska, A., Erratico, C., Xu, F., Den Hond, E., Koppen, G., et al. (2014). Human biomonitoring of emerging pollutants through non-invasive matrices: State of the art and future potential. *Analytical and Bioanalytical Chemistry*, **406**, 4063–4088.

Angerer, J., Ewers, U., and Wilhelm, M. (2007). Human biomonitoring: State of the art. *International Journal of Environmental Health*, **210**, 201–228.

Armstrong, B. K., White, E., and Saracci, R. (1992). *Principles of exposure measurement in epidemiology.* Oxford University Press, Oxford, UK.

Arora, M., and Austin, C. (2013). Teeth as a biomarker of past chemical exposure. *Current Opinion in Pediatrics*, **25**, 261–267.

Aw, C. (1995). Biological monitoring. In *Occupational hygiene* (eds. J. M. Harrington, and K. Gardiner, 2nd ed). Blackwell Science, Oxford, UK.

Barr, D. B., Bishop, A., and Needham, L. (2007). Concentrations of xenobiotic chemicals in the maternal-fetal unit. *Reproductive Toxicology*, **23**, 260–266.

Benowitz, N. L. (1999). Biomarkers of environmental tobacco smoke exposure. *Environmental Health Perspectives*, **107**, 349–355.

Berglund, M., Elinder, C.-G., and Jarup, L. (2001). *Human exposure assessment.* World Health Organization, Stockholm, http://www.imm.ki.se.

Bonassi, S., El-Zein, R., Bolognesi, C., and Fenech, M. (2011). Micronuclei frequency in peripheral blood lymphocytes and cancer risk: Evidence from human studies. *Mutagenesis*, **26**, 93–100.

Casas, M., Chevrier, C., Hond, E. D., Fernandez, M. F., Pierik, F., Philippat, C., et al. (2013). Exposure to brominated flame retardants, perfluorinated compounds, phthalates and phenols in European birth cohorts: ENRIECO evaluation, first human biomonitoring results, and recommendations. *International Journal of Environmental Health*, **216**, 230–242.

Centers for Disease Control and Prevention. (2014). http://www.cdc.gov/exposurereport/

Collins, A. R. (2004). The comet assay for DNA damage and repair: Principles, applications and limitations. *Molecular Biotechnology,* **26**, 249–261.

Committee on Biological Markers of the National Research Council (NRC). (1987). Biological markers in environmental health research. *Environmental Health Perspectives,* **74**, 3–9.

Committee on Human Biomonitoring for Environmental Toxicants, National Research Council (NRC). (2006). *Human biomonitoring for environmental chemicals.* National Academies Press, Washington, DC. Available at http://www.nap.edu/catalog/11700.html

Droz, P. O., and Wu, M. M. (1991). Biological monitoring strategies. In *Exposure assessment for epidemiology and hazard control* (eds. S. M. Rappaport, and T. J. Smith). Lewis Publishers, Michigan.

Dyne, D., Cocker, J., and Wilson, H. K. (1997). A novel device for capturing breath samples for solvent analysis. *Science of the Total Environment,* **199**, 83–89.

Fenech, M. (2007). Cytokinesis-block micronucleus cytome assay. *Nature Protocols,* **2**, 1084–1104.

Fry, R. C., Navasumrit, P., Valiathan, C., Svensson, J. P., Hogan, B. J., Luo, M., et al. (2007). Activation of inflammation/NF-kappaB signaling in infants born to arsenic-exposed mothers. *PLoS Genetics,* **3**, e207.

Funk, W. E., Waidyanatha, S., Chaing, S. H., and Rappaport, S. M. (2008). Hemoglobin adducts of benzene oxide in neonatal and adult dried blood spots. *Cancer Epidemiology, Biomarkers and Prevention,* **17**, 1896–1901.

Hansen, A. M., Mathiesen, L., Pedersen, M., and Knudsen, L. E. (2008). Urinary 1-hydroxypyrene (1-HP) in environmental and occupational studies—A review. *International Journal of Environmental Health,* **211**, 471–503.

Harris, S. A., Sass-Kortsak, A. M., Corey, P. N., and Purdham, J. T. (2002). Development of models to predict dose of pesticides in professional turf applicators. *Journal Exposure Analysis and Environmental Epidemiology,* **12**, 130–144.

International Agency on Research in Cancer (IARC). (1997). Application of biomarkers in cancer epidemiology. Workshop report. *IARC Scientific Publications,* **142**, 1–18.

International Programme on Chemical Safety (IPCS), WHO. (2001). Biomarkers in risk assessment: Validity and validation. *Environmental Health Criteria,* **222**, 1–136.

Kavanagh, P., Farago, M. E., Thornton, I., Goessler, W., Kuehnelt, D., Schlagenhaufen, C., and Irgolic, K. J. (1998). Urinary arsenic species in Devon and Cornwell residents, UK. *The Analyst,* **123**, 27–30.

Lignell, S., Aune, M., Darnerud, P. O., Cnattingius, S., and Glynn, A. (2009). Persistent organochlorine and organobromine compounds in mother's milk from Sweden 1996-2006: Compound-specific temporal trends. *Environmental Research,* **109**, 760–767.

Michalke, B., Rossbach, B., Göen, T., Schäferhenrich, A., and Scherer, G. (2015). Saliva as a matrix for human biomonitoring in occupational and environmental medicine. *International Archives of Occupational and Environmental Health,* **88**, 1–44.

Nieuwenhuijsen, M. J., Toledano, M. B., and Elliott, P. (2000). Uptake of chlorination disinfection by-products: A review and a discussion of its implications for epidemiological studies. *Journal Exposure Analysis and Environmental Epidemiology,* **10**, 586–599.

Parry, J. M., and Parry, E. M. (2012). *Genetic toxicology. Principles and methods.* Springer, New York.

Pedersen, M., Merlo, D. F., and Knudsen L. E. (2007). Ethical issues related to biomonitoring studies on children. *International Journal of Environmental Health*, **210**, 479–482.

Pedersen, M., von Stedingk, H., Botsivali, M., Agramunt, S., Alexander, J., Brunborg, G., et al. (2012). Birth weight, head circumference, and prenatal exposure to acrylamide from maternal diet: The European prospective mother-child study (NewGeneris). *Environmental Health Perspectives*, **120**, 1739–1745.

Perera, F. P., and Weinstein, I. B. (1982). Molecular epidemiology and carcinogen-DNA adduct detection: New approaches to studies of human cancer causation. *Journal of Chronic Diseases*, **35**, 581–600.

Phillips, D. H., and Arlt, V. M. (2007). The 32P-postlabeling assay for DNA adducts. *Nature Protocols*, **2**, 2772–2781.

Rappaport, S. M., Symanski, E., Yager, J. W., et al. (1995). The relationship between environmental monitoring and biological markers in exposure assessment. *Environmental Health Perspectives*, **103**, 49–54.

Schramm, K. W. (2008). Hair-biomonitoring of organic pollutants. *Chemosphere*, **72**, 1103–1111.

Silbergeld, E. K. (1997). Preventing lead poisoning in children. *Annual Review of Public Health*, **18**, 187–210.

Stove, C. P., Ingels, A. S., De Kesel, P. M., and Lambert, W. E. (2012). Dried blood spots in toxicology: From the cradle to the grave? *Critical Reviews in Toxicology*, **42**, 230–243.

Törnqvist, M., Fred, M., Haglund, J., Helleberg, H., Paulsson, B., and Rydberg, P. (2002). Protein adducts: Quantitative and qualitative aspects of their formation, analysis and applications. *Journal of Chromatography B*, **778**, 279–308.

van Leeuwen, D. M., Pedersen, M., Hendriksen, P. J., Boorsma, A., van Herwijnen, M. H., Gottschalk, R. W., et al. (2008). Genomic analysis suggests higher susceptibility of children to air pollution. *Carcinogenesis*, **29**, 977–983.

Weber, J. P. (1996). Quality in environmental toxicology measurements. *Therapeutic Drug Monitoring*, **18**, 477–483.

Wild, C. P., Vineis, P., and Garte, S. (2008). *Molecular epidemiology of chronic diseases*. Wiley, New York.

Winquist, A., Lally, C., Shin, H. M., and Steenland, K. (2013). Design, methods, and population for a study of PFOA health effects among highly exposed Mid-Ohio Valley community residents and workers. *Environmental Health Perspectives*, **121**, 893–899.

Wittassek, M., and Angerer, J. (2008). Phthalates: Metabolism and exposure. *International Journal of Andrology*, **31**, 131–138.

7

OCCUPATIONAL EXPOSURE ASSESSMENT IN INDUSTRY- AND POPULATION-BASED EPIDEMIOLOGICAL STUDIES

Melissa C. Friesen, Jérôme Lavoué, Kay Teschke, and Martie van Tongeren

7.1 INTRODUCTION

Epidemiological studies of occupational risk factors are usually either industry- or population-based. Both are often focused on chronic diseases and thus require the reconstruction of exposures over long segments of the subjects' working lives. Industry-based studies are typically defined based on a worker cohort with common exposures to one or a few agents (e.g., cohort study of magnetic fields in the electrical industry), and may evaluate a wide range of health outcomes. Population-based studies are typically defined based on a disease of interest (e.g., a case–control study of lung cancer) or based on a geographic region or population (e.g., the Nordic Occupational Cancer Study, which was enumerated from the national censuses of five Nordic countries; Kjaerheim et al. 2010) and thus represent a wide variety of occupations and industries and multiple agents, each with low prevalence.

This chapter provides an overview of exposure assessment methods commonly used in industry-based (section 7.2) and population-based (section 7.3) studies, and provides recommendations for future directions (section 7.4). Although the approaches, with names such as "job exposure matrices," "self-assessed exposures," "expert assessments," and "measurement-based approaches" suggest that these are distinct methods, the actual methodologies applied in studies vary tremendously and often include elements from several of these approaches. This process is summarized by Stewart et al. (1996), who state, "Historical exposure assessment requires an opportunistic approach, taking advantage of what information is available and developing creative and innovative approaches to exploit that information." (p. 413)

7.2 INDUSTRY-BASED STUDIES

In industry-based studies, the occupational information comes predominantly from the companies involved and often includes extraction of exposure measurements directly pertaining to the work sites and workers in the study (section 7.2.1). In the mid-1990s, half of the 72 industry-based studies published in a selected list of journals used surrogate or expert-based exposure assessment approaches (section 7.2.1); the other half comprised measurement-based approaches (section 7.2.3) (Stewart et al. 1996). Today, there is an even greater inclusion of measurement-based methods and an increasing use of statistical models. A case study is provided in section 7.2.4 to illustrate a state-of-the-art assessment of occupational diesel exhaust for a cohort of miners. The section concludes with recommendations for future exposure assessment efforts (section 7.2.5).

7.2.1 Sources of Exposure Information

The exposure assessment process often begins with a feasibility study that evaluates the quality and type of information available. Company or union employment records may be used to obtain the study subjects' work histories. Because these data are typically related to pay-scale and administrative work units, important exposure-related distinctions in work tasks may not be fully captured. Other data that can be extracted include job descriptions, technological information (i.e., engineering plans, plant layouts, process flow), medical records, and exposure or other measurements. Exposure measurements are collected for a variety of purposes, including testing compliance with regulations and evaluating control measures, and the quality and availability of ancillary information related to the measurements (e.g., sampling location, analytical method, sampling duration, control measures used, reason for sampling) vary. Additional information can also be obtained through interviews and focus groups with long-serving current or retired employees.

Job and/or work area usually form the basis for assigning group-based estimates of exposure intensity that are typically recorded within the structure of a study-specific job exposure matrix (JEM). The JEM incorporates a list of occupations on one axis (often differentiated by department, work area, and/or facility), one or more exposure agents on a second axis, and calendar period on a third axis. The cells provide the occupation-, agent-, and time-specific exposure estimates derived from expert- or measurement-based approaches (i.e., an ordinal, semi-quantitative, or quantitative value). All subjects within an occupation group are assigned the same set of exposure estimates; thus, differences in exposures among workers within the same occupation group, due to variations in specific activities, cannot be captured. A task-based, rather than occupation-based, exposure matrix may be developed when task represents a better proxy of exposure, such as in the construction industry, in which workers with the same occupation perform multiple tasks with variable frequency (Bennett et al. 1996; Benke et al. 2000, 2001; Burstyn 2009; Virji et al. 2009; Dick et al. 2010).

7.2.2 Exposure Surrogates

It has been a long-standing tradition to employ industrial hygienists and other experts to use their expert judgment to estimate exposures to complete the cells of a study-specific JEM. Exposure assessment experts generally understand the main determinants of exposures, they often have direct or indirect experience or knowledge on exposure levels in similar environments, and they have a good overview of the range of jobs and exposure levels that need to be estimated. However, experts may not be able to gain familiarity with all jobs and their environments throughout the time period covered by the study.

In comparisons to measurements, the validity of experts' ratings of exposure intensity has been shown to vary a great deal (Teschke et al. 2002). The agreement is typically higher when experts are provided with at least some exposure data (Hawkins and Evans 1989; Post et al. 1991) or when multiple experts are used (de Cock et al. 1996; Semple et al. 2001; Steinsvag et al. 2007; Friesen et al. 2011). Agents that can be sensed (e.g., noise, wood dust) and broad classes of chemicals that are well known, such as insecticides, cutting fluids, welding fumes, oils, greases, and solvents tend to be estimated more accurately than specific chemical compounds (Teschke et al. 2002). In contrast, little to no improvement has been observed when basic occupation information is supplemented with more detailed information about the job and work practices (de Cock et al. 1996; Stewart et al. 2000). A desktop study found that the agreement with measurements was improved when the expert had greater than 10 years of exposure assessment experience, a higher environmental health science education level, participated in data interpretation training, and access to at least some measurements (Logan et al. 2011). These comparisons usually only evaluate the validity of the ratings for a narrow, recent time period, using measurements collected specifically for the validation study. As a result, they may overestimate validity over a historical study period.

7.2.3 Measurement-Based Approaches

With rare exceptions (e.g., some workers exposed to ionizing radiation), individual exposure measurements are not available for all workers throughout their working life, thus requiring development of group-based estimates (see chapter 5). Measurements available for a subset can be used to calculate an exposure index for each occupational and temporal grouping. Although the arithmetic mean is sensitive to outliers, it remains the most frequently used metric because studies suggest that it better reflects cumulative burden (Seixas et al. 1988; Rappaport 1991). However, the development of the dose metric should be considered in relation to the toxicokinetics and toxicodynamics of the agent of interest (Kriebel and Smith 2010). For example, "peakiness" of noise exposure, that is, the occurrence of short-term very high levels, was identified as potentially contributing to hearing loss in a longitudinal cohort of construction workers (Seixas et al. 2005, 2012).

Statistical modeling of the measurements to identify the determinants of exposure for use in epidemiological studies started to appear in the early 1990s (Burstyn and Teschke 1999; Peretz et al. 2002; Burdorf 2005). The models are used to establish quantitative relationships between exposure levels and potential exposure determinants, such as calendar year, presence, and type of control measures, type of process, or task. The models can then be used to predict exposures wherever the determinants are documented. An early implementation of statistical models was for a cohort mortality study in the sterilization industry (Hornung et al. 1994); year of operation, task, occupational title, product type, presence of exhaust ventilation, aeration, and sterilizer volume explained 80% of the variability in ethylene oxide concentrations in 36 different plants. More recent examples include modeling silica exposure levels in the construction industry (Peters et al. 2011b; Sauvé et al. 2012, 2013; Healy et al. 2014), dust in the silicon carbide industry (Føreland et al. 2013), and trends in inhalation exposure for a wide array of contaminants (Creely et al. 2007).

Burstyn and Teschke (1999) found that early models were simple or multiple linear regression models that assumed independence of the observations (Neter et al. 1996). Now, mixed-effects models, which account for clustering in the data (e.g., within workers or plants) (Peretz et al. 2002), have become the most frequently used approach. Other approaches include:

- Multi-model averaging that considers the relative influence of exposure determinants across a large number of candidate models rather than a single model (Lavoué and Droz 2009)
- Tobit models that analyze censored data, such as measurements below the limit of detection (Sauvé et al. 2013)
- Structural equation models that identify patterns simultaneously for several measurement types (Davis 2012)
- Bayesian models that allow more flexible model structures and that have a probabilistic interpretation (Morton et al. 2010)

There are several challenges in using statistical models to support retrospective exposure assessment. It is critical to consider model selection criteria (i.e., the process of choosing which predictor variables are included in the final model). Extrapolation outside the time range and scope of the exposure models must be done cautiously. Moreover, the representativeness of the measurements to typical exposure scenarios must be considered, such as the purpose of the exposure monitoring, area versus personal measurements, short-term versus full-shift measurements, changes in analytical and sampling methods over time, and the relevance to the expected causative agent. Ideally, validation should be done to examine potential bias in model predictions (Hornung et al. 1994; Burstyn et al. 2002; Friesen et al. 2005); however, obtaining data for validation (especially external data) can be challenging. Alternatively, sensitivity analyses can be conducted to examine the impact of varying the exposure assessment decisions, such as backward extrapolation of time trends (Kromhout et al. 1999). Finally, measurement-based approaches, even with modeling, are rarely able to provide estimates for all missing exposure data. To fill these gaps, researchers have used expert-based approaches that include extrapolation of data to scenarios in which no measurements were available (Birk et al. 2010; Couch et al. 2011; Hewett et al. 2012). They have also used measurement-based approaches that rely on relationships between the agent of interest and other metrics, such as area measurements or a correlated agent (Stewart et al. 2010; Virji et al. 2012).

7.2.4 Case Study: Diesel Exhaust in Miners Study

The measurement-based retrospective exposure assessment study conducted for the Diesel Exhaust in Miners Study (DEMS) represents an innovative and modern approach (Coble et al. 2010; Stewart et al. 2010, 2012; Vermeulen et al. 2010a,b). This study aimed to investigate whether long-term exposure to diesel exhaust, using respirable elemental carbon (REC) as a marker of exposure, was associated with mortality from lung cancer and other causes (Attfield et al. 2012; Silverman et al. 2012). The challenge was to provide historical REC estimates in eight mines in the absence of historical REC measurements. Carbon monoxide (CO) measurements were available back to 1976 and these were modeled to obtain mine-specific time trends, which were applied to a baseline CO-REC side-by-side survey to estimate REC for historical periods that date back to the start of diesel equipment use at each mine (1947–1967). The different steps are described in the following.

7.2.4.1 Collection of Available Historical Data

Measurement data were collected from the companies and other sources, including the US Mine Safety and Health Administration and the older US Mine Enforcement and Safety Administration/Bureau of Mines, along with other work place information to establish a large database on historical measurements of CO and other gases from the mines. In addition, information on the use of diesel engines and levels of ventilation in the mines was established based on company records and interviews with long-serving personnel.

7.2.4.2 Baseline Survey

Personal exposure measurements were carried out for REC, with side-by-side measurements for CO, during a baseline study in seven of the mines. These measurements were used to: 1) develop strategies for assigning workers into similar exposure groups (Coble et al. 2010); 2) assign baseline REC estimates for these groups (Coble et al. 2010); and 3) investigate the relationship between REC and CO levels in the mines (Vermeulen et al. 2010b).

7.2.4.3 Development of Historical Relative Trend Based on Carbon Monoxide Levels

Statistical models for CO levels were developed for each mine using measurement data going back to 1976 and exposure determinants such as the use of diesel engine (as defined by the total horse power provided by the diesel engines adjusted by the amount of time the engines were in use) and the level of mechanical ventilation (Vermeulen et al. 2010a). The model for each mine was used to predict mine-specific annual CO levels going back to the start of diesel use in each mine (1947–1967). Because CO measurements were not available pre-1976, annual estimates for years before 1976 were calculated using the model parameter estimate for the ratio of horsepower to ventilation rate. These estimates were used to derive a relative trend in CO level compared with the baseline level (relative trend = $CO_{year i}/CO_{baseline}$).

7.2.4.4 Historical Extrapolation of Respirable Elemental Carbon

Historical estimates of REC exposure were obtained by using the relative trend in CO levels and applying these to the baseline levels for REC. The relative trends in CO levels were modified based on the percentage of time a worker in a particular job spent in areas that directly received fresh intake air, and the percentage of time a worker spent in areas that received air that had already traveled through some part of the mine.

7.2.4.5 Evaluation of Assessments and Uncertainty

A number of approaches were undertaken to evaluate the exposure assessment method (Stewart et al. 2012). One compared the predicted with measured CO levels from a survey conducted in 1976–1977 that was not used in the model development. The measured and predicted levels were quite similar, with a median difference of just 29%.

7.2.5 Recommendations

In summary, any retrospective exposure assessment is limited by the data available to the researchers. Every attempt should be made to incorporate measurement-based approaches to obtain quantitative exposure estimates. The Diesel Exhaust in Miners Study provides an example of a sophisticated design utilizing measurement data and that used models to fill gaps in historical data. The development of statistical models to identify variables that predict contrast in exposure is preferred over simple stratified means of the available exposure data. Model assumptions must be checked and the application of models outside the scope of measurements must be made cautiously. When measurement-based approaches have gaps, the use of experts to fill those gaps is reasonably supported, especially when their estimates are anchored by exposure estimates and when multiple experts are used. In addition, due to the retrospective nature of the assessment it is difficult to validate estimates. However, the many areas of uncertainty in the exposure assessment process can be evaluated via uncertainty analyses of the epidemiological results.

7.3 POPULATION-BASED STUDIES

In population-based studies, subjects are not selected based on occupation. As a result, occupational exposures often need to be estimated for a very large number of different jobs and industries. The occupational information predominantly comes from the study participants (section 7.3.1) because it is usually impractical to collect available data from all relevant work places. Thus, exposure assessment nearly always relies on surrogate or expert-based methods (sections 7.3.2–7.3.5). However, the use of measurements that have been collected from similar jobs or work places to refine surrogate-based approaches has been increasing. Depending on the information available and the exposure prevalence, exposure metrics can be qualitative (exposed/not exposed), ordinal, semi-quantitative, or quantitative intensity estimates. In addition, estimates of probability or prevalence and frequency of exposures, as well as confidence in the assignment, are often generated. These additional data can be used in the development of exposure indices (i.e., cumulative exposure) or can be used in sensitivity analyses. This section concludes with recommendations for future exposure assessment efforts (section 7.3.6).

7.3.1 Sources of Exposure Information

In population-based studies, occupational information is predominantly obtained from administrative databases (e.g., medical records, registry data, death certificates) or through questionnaires or interviews with study participants or their proxies. Administrative data sources generally include only limited occupational information, such as job title and employer or industry. The scope of the occupational component of interviews can vary substantially, from the current or longest held job to a detailed lifetime work history capturing all jobs ever held and their start and stop years. The occupational component may include a section in which the participant identifies, from a checklist of agents, what he or she was exposed to, and may include generic open-ended questions about tasks, tools, and equipment used, and chemicals and materials handled. In addition, supplemental exposure-oriented job- and industry-specific questions may be asked of subsets of subjects (Gerin et al. 1985; Stewart et al. 1998). For instance, a participant who reported that she worked as a welder may be asked additional welding-specific questions. Increasing the scope increases the time burden on the participant but improves the ability to identify between-subject differences in exposure. However, collecting detailed occupational information may not be feasible for participants diagnosed with a serious and life-threatening disease. One may obtain occupational information from a proxy respondent, such as the subject's spouse or child; it will usually be less detailed, although reasonably reliable (Kaerlev et al. 2003; Villanueva and Garcia 2006; Tagiyeva et al. 2011). Information about occupations is usually quite accurate—both that from employment records and from self-reported employment histories (Kromhout and Vermeulen 2001; Teschke et al. 2002).

Open-ended responses on occupation and industry must be classified based on standardized coding systems, which may be used as an exposure proxy (section 7.3.2) or as the basis for other exposure assessment methods (sections 7.3.4 and 7.3.5). This coding has typically been done manually, sometimes (and prefer-ably) by two or more independent coders who then resolve discordant assignments. Occupation and industry classification systems differ between countries and also change over time; thus, pooling studies can be time intensive to re-code into a com-mon system (Kogevinas 2003; 't Mannetje and Kromhout 2003). Re-coding efforts can be facilitated by the use of cross-walks between systems (van Tongeren et al. 2013) and have been found to result in similar exposure estimates to manual cod-ing when a JEM is applied to the resulting codes (Koeman et al. 2013). However, when multiple matches are identified, manual resolution may be needed to assign the most appropriate code. Recent efforts to automate coding using computer algo-rithms have observed moderate to excellent agreement between the manual and automated assignments (Patel et al. 2012; Burstyn et al. 2014). Freely available web tools have also been developed to aid in classifying jobs (e.g., http://www.cdc.gov/niosh/topics/coding/overview.html; www.caps-canada.ca).

A source of direct exposure data in population studies is biological specimens (e.g., urine, blood, hair) that can be analyzed for chemical agents and/or their metab-olites. Biological measures of exposures represent varying time windows of previ-ous exposure, depending on the half-life of the agent in the body (see chapter 6). Biological measures of long half-life agents (e.g., cadmium) may represent expo-sures years or even decades ago, but many chemicals (e.g., organic solvents) have much shorter half-lives, so measures would represent more recent exposure. An additional challenge is that exposure measures from post-disease or treatment bio-specimens may be not be comparable to pre-morbid measures (e.g., cancer can be a wasting disease, potentially altering contaminant concentrations in adipose tissue samples taken after diagnosis).

7.3.2 Occupation and Industry as an Exposure Proxy

Job and industry groupings are commonly used as surrogate metrics of exposure in epidemiological analyses. Careful consideration of exposures that may be common to occupations or industries shown to be at elevated risk can be a useful initial step toward the identification of risk from certain exposures. This is illustrated by the International Agency for Research on Cancer's assessment of several occupational risk factors as "carcinogenic to humans" (Group 1) based on occupation or indus-try as surrogates of exposure, including chimney sweeping (soot), painters, work in aluminum production, and work in the rubber-manufacturing industry (Baan et al. 2009). The main problem is that specific agents cannot be clearly identified as risk factors and thus it is difficult to identify target agents for prevention efforts. For example, carpenters are exposed to wood dust, but they also have potential exposure to solvents, formaldehyde-based resins, paints and varnishes, and bioaerosols from their own work, and many other agents, such as metal fumes and insulation materials, from other trades with whom they may work closely. In addition, although finishing carpenters may be highly exposed to wood dust, framing carpenters working in construction outdoors likely have much lower exposure. Therefore, an elevated risk in a job can only be interpreted as suggestive of risk for specific agents. In addition, if only some individuals in a job are exposed to a particular agent, its effect may be masked if no elevation in risk is observed in the heterogeneously exposed job group.

7.3.3 Self-Assessment of Occupational Exposures

Many studies have asked participants to self-assess occupational exposure using checklists. The reliability and validity of the self-reported information has been well studied and found to be highly variable between studies and between agents (Teschke et al. 2002; Donnay et al. 2011; Svendsen and Hilt 2011; Hardt et al. 2014). Agents that are easily sensed (e.g., odiferous chemicals, visible dusts, perceptible vibrations) are more likely to be recognized by subjects and reported. Using familiar terminology to subjects promotes more accurate reporting (e.g., asking about varsol exposure, rather than its component hydrocarbons). Subjects involved in choosing chemicals for work place use (e.g., farmers buying pesticides) are more likely to remember exposures than those without this level of control or knowledge. Prompting recall with a list of specific agents of interest (i.e., querying whether a subject was exposed to any "dusts, fumes, gases, or vapors") results in higher sensitivities than open-ended questioning, without an equivalent loss in specificity. Subjects who are provided with relative or objective benchmarks against which to judge their potential for exposures do so better than those considering their own exposure in isolation.

The use of self-assessments based on checklists as a primary exposure metric in epidemiological analyses is hampered by the potential for recall bias (Fonn et al. 1993; Hardt et al. 2014). It is generally accepted that any exposure assessment must be done blind to disease status, and this is clearly not feasible for self-assessment of exposure. Reporting differences can also occur based on gender, age, time since exposure, and socio-demographic characteristics (Gustafson 1998; Kennedy and Koehoorn 2003; Parks et al. 2004; Hooftman et al. 2005; Quinn et al. 2007; Sembajwe et al. 2010; Eng et al. 2011; Locke et al. 2014). Given these challenges, using the results of exposure checklists directly in epidemiological analyses is rarely recommended, especially when exposure is reported post-diagnosis for a subset of subjects. However, these exposure checklists, when supplemented by other occupational information about potential exposure determinants, can provide a useful starting point for expert-based assessments (section 7.3.5).

7.3.4 Job Exposure Matrices

Starting in the 1980s, "generic" (as opposed to industry-specific) JEMs began to be developed to efficiently apply expert exposure decisions in population-based case–control studies. These generic JEMs defined the "occupation" axis as the range of jobs and industries that might be observed in the general population based on one of the standardized occupation classification systems (section 7.3.1). The generic JEM could then be easily linked to the subjects' coded jobs. Thus, the JEM would allow subjects who have different jobs but similar exposures to be identified, to help in identifying the particular agents responsible for elevated risks.

The earliest generic JEM provided a dichotomous exposure status ("exposed" vs. "not exposed") for 376 known and suspected carcinogens for 500 combinations of occupations and industries coded using standard US classifications (Hoar et al. 1980). A 2001 review identified 19 early generic JEMs (Kromhout and Vermeulen 2001). Most provided an ordinal or semi-quantitative exposure intensity metric (i.e., low, medium, high exposure). A few included the probability of exposure (Steineck et al. 1989), proportion of the working time exposed (Imbernon et al. 1991), or a time axis to account for temporal trends (Ferrario et al. 1988). Two especially notable generic JEMs were developed in Finland (FINJEM, ~100 agents) and in France (Matgéné, 22 agents). These JEMs provided quantitative exposure estimates and, where possible, incorporated measurements with which to anchor exposure intensity estimates (Kauppinen et al. 1998; Pukkala et al. 2005; Févotte et al. 2011; Kauppinen et al. 2014). An additional useful feature in Matgéné is that it is available in multiple occupation and industry coding systems. In addition to chemical agents, JEMs have been developed for risk factors such as electromagnetic fields (Bowman et al. 2007; Turner et al. 2014), electric shocks (Vergara et al. 2012; Huss et al. 2013), low back pain (Solovieva et al. 2012), noise (Choi et al. 2012; Sjöström et al. 2013), physical and psychosocial stressors (Rijs et al., 2014), endocrine-disrupting agents (Brouwers et al. 2009), and shiftwork (Fernandez et al. 2014).

Generic JEMs have several limitations. They cannot account for variability in exposures that occur within a job, which may cause exposure misclassification. The exposure indices may distinguish between different aspects of exposure (i.e., probability, intensity, frequency) and, for simplicity, users may wish to aggregate the indices. For instance, many users of FINJEM use an index that multiplies the probability and intensity (Pukkala et al. 2005). However, this aggregation was found to cause bias in unexpected directions in some circumstances because truly unexposed people within an occupation with any non-null probability will be considered exposed, whereas truly exposed people will get their exposure estimates diminished by the multiplication with probability (Burstyn et al. 2012).

Several challenges occur when attempting to transport a JEM across jurisdictions to other study settings. First, cross-walks have to be created between the standard classifications systems used, potentially requiring time-consuming transcription procedures and manual resolution (van Tongeren et al. 2013). Second, differences in the industrial profile or in enforcement and the nature of health and safety regulations can greatly affect regional occupational exposure estimates. Several studies have evaluated the transportability of FINJEM to other Scandinavian countries (Kauppinen et al. 2009), Australia (Benke, Fritschi, and Aldred 2001), and Canada (Lavoué et al. 2012). Although extrapolation was possible for some agents, this may not be the case for all agents and countries and, thus each should be evaluated on a case-by-case basis. To account for regional differences, several teams have constructed region-specific JEMs by adapting FINJEM to better reflect occupational exposures in other Scandinavian countries (Kauppinen et al. 2009), Spain (García et al. 2013), New Zealand ('t Mannetje et al. 2011), and internationally (van Tongeren et al. 2013). These adaptations were performed using expert judgment and required the development of cross-walks between the Finnish and other occupational classification systems.

Other recent adaptions include the systematic use of measurements to calibrate JEMs to a concentration scale. Recent examples include the development of a silica JEM for the SYNERGY study (Peters et al. 2011b), benzene and lead JEMs for a large prospective cohort of Shanghai women (Friesen et al. 2012; Koh et al. 2014), and an electromagnetic field JEM for the INTEROCC study (Turner et al. 2014). Three of these studies modified Wild's (2002) statistical framework to systematically combine expert judgment and exposure measurements (Peters et al. 2011b; Friesen et al. 2012; Koh et al. 2014). In these studies, all occupations in the study were linked to a JEM with ordinal expert ratings. The JEM rating and measurements were combined in a mixed-effects statistical model framework in which the JEM rating and calendar year (to account for temporal trends) were incorporated as fixed effects and occupation, industry, and/or geographical region were incorporated as random effects. This structure implies that exposure for an occupation/industry/region will be calculated as a weighted average of the measurements from all occupations/industry/regions that had the same rating estimate and the occupation/industry/region-specific estimate, with the weights varying based on the amount of data and their variability. This approach provided greater contrast among individuals in the final exposure estimates than could be obtained by using only the expert JEM ratings.

Generic JEMs have been compared predominantly with expert-based methods (section 7.3.5), due to the lack of gold standards, thus focusing on the agreement between estimates rather than their validity. Teschke et al. (2002) found generally low to fair agreement across studies, with JEMs generally showing lower sensitivity but higher specificity than expert-based approaches. In more recent comparisons, higher agreement was achieved for specific agents, but not for all agents (Lavoué et al. 2012; Offermans et al. 2012). Despite these limitations, Pukkala et al. (2005) were able to detect known associations between exposure to silica based on FINJEM estimates and lung cancer. Similarly, Peters (2012) found similar risk estimates for silica exposure when using an expert-based JEM and expert assessments in SYNERGY, a multicenter study of lung cancer.

7.3.5 Expert Assessment: Job-by-Job
Assessment and Decision Rules

In population-based studies, expert judgment is frequently used to assign exposure estimates to the agents of interest. Although very similar to the expert judgment process used in industry-based studies (section 7.2.2), there are three key differences. First, the task requires assigning exposure to the wide range of occupations and industries that appear in subjects' occupational histories rather than only jobs within a single industry. Second, the information on which the experts make their assignments comes directly from study subjects rather than employers. Without detailed reports from subjects, experts cannot be aware of specific worksite characteristics. The experts often supplement their existing knowledge of an exposure by reviewing the published literature to identify which occupations and industries may have the exposure of interest, identify determinants of exposure, and anchor their estimates of exposure intensity (Bakke et al. 2007; Park et al. 2009; Pronk et al. 2009). Third, expert assignments occur most often at the subject-level, rather than occupational group-level; that is, one or more experts review the subject-specific information captured in the lifetime work histories, exposure checklists, and job- and industry-specific questionnaires for each job one at a time. Because the typical participant reports six to eight jobs over his or her lifetime, and a case–control study may contain several thousand individuals, individual assessments can be very time consuming and costly.

One concern is the lack of consistency in the assessments carried out by experts assessing similar exposures within and among studies. On average, the agreement between experts is moderate, but can vary widely from poor to excellent depending on the agent (Teschke et al. 2002; 't Mannetje et al. 2003; Correa et al. 2006; Steinsvag et al. 2007; Friesen et al. 2011; Rocheleau et al. 2011; Brouwer et al. 2014; Chen et al. 2014). Unfortunately, good agreement does not imply good validity; however, assessing the validity of expert ratings in population-based study designs is difficult because of the lack of gold standards with which to compare the expert estimates. Only three studies thus far have provided a limited evaluation of the validity of experts' ratings for population-based studies (Benke et al. 1997; Tielemans et al. 1999; Fritschi et al. 2003). These studies have found variable sensitivities and specificities, but obtained reasonable discrimination between high and low exposures with the use of job- and industry-specific questionnaires.

Job-by-job expert review has been criticized as a "black box" assessment (Kromhout 2002; Teschke et al. 2002) because the rationale for the exposure decisions is rarely defined and may vary among experts. Additionally, there is no mechanism to apply the decision rules used by the expert to other studies, making expert assessment much less efficient than the use of JEMs. In response, methodological research into approaches to improve the transparency of the decisions by developing and reporting decision rules that link questionnaire responses to exposure decisions has been growing. Such decision rules have resulted in similar exposure estimates to a job-by-job review (Behrens et al. 2012; Pronk et al. 2012;

Friesen et al. 2013; Carey et al. 2014; Peters et al. 2014). A web-based software application (www.occideas.org) has been developed to facilitate the application of decision rules for newly initiated studies (Fritschi et al. 2009). Decision rules can also be extracted from previously made expert assignments using machine learning approaches (Black et al. 2004; Wheeler et al. 2013). For example, Wheeler et al. (2013) extracted the underlying decision rules used in a job-by-job expert assessment of occupational diesel exhaust exposure using classification and regression tree models. The decision rules could be described using a series of *if . . . then . . .* conditions that could then be reviewed and modified by other experts. The resulting predictions had excellent agreement with the expert's assignments. The model outputs also estimated the probability that the assignment was correct; this measure of uncertainty could be used to prioritize jobs for expert review.

Expert-based assessment is increasingly using measurement data to identify determinants of exposure that can be used to develop exposure intensity estimates. Several studies have extracted published or publicly available measurements and their ancillary data into databases to aid these efforts. Such data have been used to develop statistical models to identify factors that predicted contrast in exposure concentrations; the results were used to predict exposure for the exposure scenarios reported by the study participants. For example, a model to estimate historical trichloroethylene exposure included predictors based on industrial hygiene principles, such as mechanism of exposure release into the air, proximity to emission source, and presence of local and general exhaust ventilation (Hein et al. 2010). To apply the model in a case–control study of brain cancer, an expert inferred values for each variable based on participants' responses to task-based questions (Neta et al. 2012). In another example, a model to estimate historical metalworking fluid concentrations incorporated surrogates of exposure that could be more directly extracted from the occupational questions, including type of industry, type of metalworking fluid, and type of operation (grinding vs. other) (Friesen et al. 2014). The resulting quantitative estimates were evaluated in a case–control study of bladder cancer. The exposure–response relationship for straight metalworking fluids was consistent with the findings from an industry cohort study, with both studies showing a twofold increased risk in the highest exposure category (Friesen et al. 2009; Colt et al. 2014). Most published measurement data are reported as summary measures (e.g., arithmetic and geometric means). Methods to analyze the data that account for both the number of measurements and the variability of measurements have used simulation of the individual measurements from the summary measures (Lavoue et al. 2007) or mixed-effects meta-regression models to analyze the summary measures (Koh et al. 2014).

7.3.6 Recommendations

In population-based studies, ideally the exposure assessment will be based on as detailed occupational information as possible to be able to capture subject-specific differences in exposure. Exposures in the population are often low in prevalence, so exposure assessments used in epidemiological analyses should be designed to maximize specificity (Kromhout and Vermeulen 2001). This means that subjects whose exposure status is uncertain should be classified into an uncertain category, such as "possible," so that the exposed and unexposed groups are not diluted with misclassified subjects (Dosemeci and Stewart 1996). Exposure intensity estimates should be anchored by exposure measurements, preferably using statistical models to identify temporal trends and predictors of contrasts in exposure. Limited resources and scarcity of data support use of a mixture of approaches in a study and a focus of resources on subjects and jobs with high likelihood of exposure. For instance, a generic JEM may be used to prioritize jobs in which it is necessary to use expert judgment. The expert-based assessments should be made by teams of experts who transparently report the rationales for the exposure decisions. For studies in which the collection of occupational information is limited, there is a "new generation" of generic JEMs—that incorporate exposure measurements, that flag occupations in which exposure may be highly heterogeneous for additional review, and that consider regional differences between the study population and the population for which the JEM was designed. They continue to show promise and will continue to play a major role in multi-center studies that cover large populations and for which other assessment approaches are too costly or not available. However, null findings in population-based studies should be considered cautiously because of the potential for non-differential exposure misclassification that may mask exposure–disease associations. Because no gold standard exists, sensitivity analyses should be conducted to evaluate the robustness of exposure–disease associations to exposure assessment decisions.

7.4 CONCLUSION

This chapter provided an overview of methods for assessing exposure in epidemiological studies that investigate exposure–disease relationships. There is a long and rich history of such studies, which have generated a wealth of data that have been used to design and implement policies to reduce exposures and improve workers' health. Industry-based studies are often cohort studies, although nested case–control analyses are often carried out within such cohorts so that more detailed data on exposure and confounding factors can be collected. Population-based studies are generally case–control studies, although in recent years large population-based cohort studies have been initiated. They are designed to have high power to detect exposure–response associations for a wide range of agents. In such large-scale studies, individual case-by-case assessments are cost prohibitive, and thus a combination of approaches that incorporate JEMs and decision rules are needed. In addition, these studies are beginning to adopt exposome approaches, whereby a large array of potential exposures are assessed using -omics technology in biological specimens. Such large-scale studies are now possible due to the reduction of the cost in -omics analyses, enabling analyses of large numbers of biological samples. A difficulty for studies of chronic diseases with long latency is that the results of such -omics assessments usually reflect more recent exposure rather than exposures that occurred years earlier. A challenge for large-scale occupational epidemiological studies is to adapt current methodologies or develop new methods that allow for high-throughput assessment of exposure.

REFERENCES

Attfield, M. D., Schleiff, P. L., Lubin, J. H., Blair, A., Stewart, P. A., Vermeulen, R., et al. (2012). The Diesel Exhaust in Miners Study: A cohort mortality study with emphasis on lung cancer. *Journal of the National Cancer Institute,* **104**, 869–883.

Baan, R., Grosse, Y., Straif, K., Secretan, B., El Ghissassi, F., Bouvard, V., et al. (2009). Special report: Policy a review of human carcinogens-part F: Chemical agents and related occupations. *Lancet, Oncology,* **10**, 1143–1144.

Bakke, B., Stewart, P. A., and Waters, M. A. (2007). Uses of and exposure to trichloroethylene in US industry: A systematic literature review. *Journal of Occupational and Environmental Hygiene,* **4**, 375–390.

Behrens, T., Mester, B., and Fritschi, L. (2012). Sharing the knowledge gained from occupational cohort studies: A call for action. *Occupational and Environmental Medicine,* **69**, 444–448.

Benke, G., Fritschi, L., and Aldred, G. (2001). Comparison of occupational exposure using three different methods: Hygiene panel, job exposure matrix (JEM), and self reports. *Applied Occupational and Environmental Hygiene,* **16**, 84–91.

Benke, G., Sim, M., Forbes, A., and Salzberg, M. (1997). Retrospective assessment of occupational exposure to chemicals in community-eased studies: Validity and repeatability of industrial hygiene panel ratings. *International Journal of Epidemiology,* **26**, 635–642.

Benke, G, Sim, M., Fritschi, L., and Aldred, G. (2000). Beyond the job exposure matrix (JEM): The task exposure matrix (TEM). *Annals of Occupational Hygiene,* **44**, 475–482.

Benke, G., Sim, M., Fritschi, L., and Aldred, G. (2001). A task exposure database for use in the alumina and primary aluminium industry. *Applied Occupational and Environmental Hygiene,* **16**, 149–153.

Bennett, J. S., Feigley, C. E., Underhill, D. W., Drane, W., Payne, T. A., Stewart, P. A., et al. (1996). Estimating the contribution of individual work tasks to room concentration: Method applied to embalming. *American Industrial Hygiene Association Journal,* **57**, 599–609.

Birk, T., Guldner, K., Mundt, K. A., Dahmann, D., Adams, R. C., and Parsons, W. (2010). Quantitative crystalline silica exposure assessment for a historical cohort epidemiologic study in the German porcelain industry. *Journal of Occupational and Environmental Hygiene,* **7**, 516–528.

Black, J., Benke, G., Smith, K., and Fritsch, L. (2004). Artificial neural networks and job-specific modules to assess occupational exposure. *Annals of Occupational Hygiene,* **48**, 595–600.

Bowman, J. D., Touchstone, J. A., and Yost, M. G. (2007). A population-based job exposure matrix for power-frequency magnetic fields. *Journal of Occupational and Environmental Hygiene,* **4**, 715–728.

Brouwer, M., Huss, A., Vermeulen, R., Nijssen, P., de Snoo, G., and Kromhout, H. (2014). Expert assessment of historical crop specific pesticide use in The Netherlands. *Occupational and Environmental Medicine*, **71**, 717–722.

Brouwers, M. M., van Tongeren, M., Hirst, A. A., Bretveld, R. W., and Roeleveld, N. (2009). Occupational exposure to potential endocrine disruptors: Further development of a job exposure matrix. *Occupational and Environmental Medicine*, **66**, 607–614.

Burdorf, A. (2005). Identification of determinants of exposure: Consequences for measurement and control strategies. *Occupational and Environmental Medicine*, **62**, 344–350.

Burstyn, I. (2009). Measurement error and model specification in determining how duration of tasks affects level of occupational exposure. *Annals of Occupational Hygiene*, **53**, 265–270.

Burstyn, I., Boffetta, P., Burr, G. A., Cenni, A., Knecht, U., Sciarra, G., et al. (2002). Validity of empirical models of exposure in asphalt paving. *Occupational and Environmental Medicine*, **59**, 620–624.

Burstyn, I., Lavoué, J., and Van Tongeren, M. (2012). Aggregation of exposure level and probability into a single metric in job-exposure matrices creates bias. *Annals of Occupational Hygiene*, **56**, 1038–1050.

Burstyn, I., Slutsky, A., Lee, D. G., Singer, A. B., An, Y., and Michael, Y. L. (2014). Beyond crosswalks: Reliability of exposure assessment following automated coding of free-text job descriptions for occupational epidemiology. *Annals of Occupational Hygiene*, **58**, 482–492.

Burstyn, I., and Teschke, K. (1999). Studying the determinants of exposure: A review of methods. *American Industrial Hygiene Association Journal*, **60**, 57–72.

Carey, R. N., Driscoll, T. R., Peters, S., Glass, D. C., Reid, A., Benke, G., et al. (2014). Estimated prevalence of exposure to occupational carcinogens in Australia (2011-2012). *Occupational and Environmental Medicine*, **71**, 55–62.

Chen, Y. C., Coble, J. B., Deziel, N. C., Ji, B. T., Xue, S., Lu, W., and Friesen, M. C. (2014). Reliability and validity of expert assessment based on airborne and urinary measures of nickel and chromium exposure in the electroplating industry. *Journal of Exposure Science and Environmental Epidemiology*, **24**, 622–628.

Choi, Y.-H., Hu, H., Tak, S., Mukherjee, B., and Park, S. K. (2012). Occupational noise exposure assessment using o*net and its application to a study of hearing loss in the US general population. *Occupational and Environmental Medicine*, **69**, 176–183.

Coble, J. B., Stewart, P. A., Vermeulen, R., Yereb, D., Stanevich, R., Blair, A., et al. (2010). The Diesel Exhaust in Miners Study: II. Exposure monitoring surveys and development of exposure groups. *Annals of Occupational Hygiene*, **54**, 747–761.

Colt, J. S., Friesen, M. C., Stewart, P. A., Park, D.-U., Johnson, A., et al. (2014). A case-control study of occupational exposure to metalworking fluids and bladder cancer risk among men. *Occupational and Environmental Medicine*, **71**, 667–674.

Correa, A., Min, Y. I., Stewart, P. A., Lees, P. S. J., Breysse, P., Dosemeci, M., et al. (2006). Inter-rater agreement of assessed prenatal maternal occupational exposures to lead. *Birth Defects Research Part A-Clinical and Molecular Teratology*, **76**, 811–824.

Couch, J. R., Petersen, M., Rice, C., and Schubauer-Berigan, M. K. (2011). Development of retrospective quantitative and qualitative job-exposure matrices for exposures at a beryllium processing facility. *Occupational and Environmental Medicine*, **68**, 361–365.

Creely, K. S., Cowie, H., Van Tongeren, M., Kromhout, H., Tickner, J., and Cherrie, J. W. (2007). Trends in inhalation exposure—a review of the data in the published scientific literature. *Annals of Occupational Hygiene*, **51**, 665–678.

Davis, M. E. (2012). Structural equation models in occupational health: An application to exposure modelling. *Occupational and Environmental Medicine*, **69**, 184–190.

de Cock, J., Kromhout, H., Heederik, D., and Burema, J. (1996). Experts' subjective assessment of pesticide exposure in fruit growing. *Scandinavian Journal of Work Environment and Health*, **22**, 425–432.

Dick, F. D., Semple, S. E., van Tongeren, M., Miller, B. G., Ritchie, P., Sherriff, D., et al. (2010). Development of a task-exposure matrix (TEM) for pesticide use (TEMPEST). *Annals of Occupational Hygiene*, **54**, 443–452.

Donnay, C., Denis, M. A., Magis, R., Fevotte, J., Massin, N., Dumas, O., et al. (2011). Under-estimation of self-reported occupational exposure by questionnaire in hospital workers. *Occupational and Environmental Medicine*, **68**, 611–617.

Dosemeci, M., and Stewart, P. A. (1996). Recommendations for reducing the effects of exposure misclassification on relative risk estimates. *Occupational Hygiene*, **3**, 169–176.

Eng, A., 't Mannetje, A., McLean, D., Ellison-Loschmann, L., Cheng, S., and Pearce, N. (2011). Gender differences in occupational exposure patterns. *Occupational and Environmental Medicine*, **68**, 888–894.

Fernandez, R. C., Peters, S., Carey, R. N., Davies, M. J., and Fritschi, L. (2014). Assessment of exposure to shiftwork mechanisms in the general population: The development of a new job-exposure matrix. *Occupational and Environmental Medicine*, **71**, 723–729.

Ferrario, F., Continenza, D., Pisani, P., et al. (1988). Description of a job-exposure matrix for sixteen agents which are or maybe related to respiratory cancer. In *Progress in occupational epidemiology*. (eds. C. Hogstedt, and C. Reuterwall). 379–382. Elsevier, Amsterdam.

Févotte, J., Dananché, B., Delabre, L., Ducamp, S., Garras, L., Houot, M., et al. (2011). Matgéné: A program to develop job-exposure matrices in the general population in France. *Annals of Occupational Hygiene*, **55**, 865–878.

Fonn, S., Groeneveld, H. T., Debeer, M., and Becklake, M. R. (1993). Relationship of respiratory health status to grain dust in a Witwatersrand grain mill: Comparison of workers' exposure assessments with industrial hyigene survey findings. *American Journal of Industrial Medicine*, **24**, 401–411.

Føreland, S., Bakke, B., Vermeulen, R., Bye, E., and Eduard, W. (2013). Determinants of exposure to dust and dust constituents in the Norwegian silicon carbide industry. *Annals of Occupational Hygiene*, **57**, 417–431.

Friesen, M. C., Coble, J. B., Katki, H. A., Ji, B. T., Xue, S. Z., Lu, W., et al. (2011). Validity and reliability of exposure assessors' ratings of exposure intensity by type of occupational questionnaire and type of rater. *Annals of Occupational Hygiene*, **55**, 601–611.

Friesen, M. C., Coble, J. B., Lu, W., Shu, X. O., Ji, B. T., Xue, S. Z., et al. (2012). Combining a job-exposure matrix with exposure measurements to assess occupational exposure to benzene in a population cohort in Shanghai, China. *Annals of Occupational Hygiene*, **56**, 80–91.

Friesen, M. C., Costello, S., and Eisen, E. A. (2009). Quantitative exposure to metalworking fluids and bladder cancer incidence in an autoworkers cohort. *American Journal of Epidemiology*, **169**, 1471–1478.

Friesen, M. C., Davies, H. W., Teschke, K., Marion, S., and Demers, P. A. (2005). Predicting historical dust and wood dust exposure in sawmills: Model development and validation. *Journal of Occupational and Environmental Hygiene*, 2, 650–658.

Friesen, M. C., Park, D. U., Colt, J. S., Baris, D., Schwenn, M., Karagas, M. R., et al. (2014). Developing estimates of frequency and intensity of exposure to three types of metalworking fluids in a population-based case-control study of bladder cancer. *American Journal of Industrial Medicine*, 57, 915–927.

Friesen, M. C., Pronk, A., Wheeler, D. C., Chen, Y. C., Locke, S. J., Zaebst, D. D., et al. (2013). Comparison of algorithm-based estimates of occupational diesel exhaust exposure to those of multiple independent raters in a population-based case-control study. *Annals of Occupational Hygiene*, 57, 470–481.

Fritschi, L., Friesen, M. C., Glass, D., Benke, G., Girschik, J., and Sadkowsky, T. (2009). OccIDEAS: Retrospective occupational exposure assessment in community-based studies made easier. *Journal of Environmental and Public Health*, 2009, 957023.

Fritschi, L., Nadon, L., Benke, G., Lakhani, R., Latreille, B., Parent, M. E., and Siemiatycki, J. (2003). Validation of expert assessment of occupational exposures. *American Journal of Industrial Medicine*, 43, 519–522.

García, A. M., González-Galarzo, M. C., Kauppinen, T., Delclos, G. L., and Benavides, F. G. (2013). A job-exposure matrix for research and surveillance of occupational health and safety in Spanish workers: Matemesp. *American Journal of Industrial Medicine*, 56, 1226–1238.

Gerin, M., Siemiatycki, J., Kemper, H., and Begin, D. (1985). Obtaining occupational exposure histories in epidemiologic case-control studies. *Journal of Occupational and Environmental Medicine*, 27, 420–426.

Gustafson, P. E. (1998). Gender differences in risk perception: Theoretical and methodological perspectives. *Risk Analysis*, 18, 805–811.

Hardt, J. S., Vermeulen, R., Peters, S., Kromhout, H., McLaughlin, J. R., and Demers, P. A. (2014). A comparison of exposure assessment approaches: Lung cancer and occupational asbestos exposure in a population-based case-control study. *Occupational and Environmental Medicine*, 71, 282–288.

Hawkins, N. C., and Evans, J. S. (1989). Subjective estimation of toluene exposures: A calibration study of industrial hygienists. *Applied Industrial Hygiene*, 4, 61–68.

Healy, C. B., Coggins, M. A., Van Tongeren, M., MacCalman, L., and McGowan, P. (2014). Determinants of respirable crystalline silica exposure among stoneworkers involved in stone restoration work. *Annals of Occupational Hygiene*, 58, 6–18.

Hein, M. J., Waters, M. A., Ruder, A. M., Stenzel, M. R., Blair, A., and Stewart, P. A. (2010). Statistical modeling of occupational chlorinated solvent exposures for case-control studies using a literature-based database. *Annals of Occupational Hygiene*, 54, 459–472.

Hewett, P., Morey, S. Z., Holen, B. M., Logan, P. W., and Olsen, G. W. (2012). Cohort mortality study of roofing granule mine and mill workers. Part I: Estimation of historical crystalline silica exposures. *Journal of Occupational and Environmental Hygiene*, 9, 199–210.

Hoar, S. K., Morrison, A. S., Cole, P., and Silverman, D. T. (1980). An occupation and exposure linkage system for the study of occupational carcinogenesis. *Journal of Occupational and Environmental Medicine*, 22, 722–726.

Hooftman, W. E., van der Beek, A. J., Bongers, P. M., and van Mechelen, W. (2005). Gender differences in self-reported physical and psychosocial exposures in jobs with both female and male workers. *Journal of Occupational and Environmental Medicine*, 47, 244–252.

Hornung, R. W., Greife, A. L., Stayner, L. T., Steenland, N. K., Herrick, R. F., Elliott, L. J., et al. (1994). Statistical model for prediction of retrospective exposure to ethylene oxide in an occupational mortality study. *American Journal of Industrial Medicine*, **25**, 825–836.

Huss, A., Vermeulen, R., Bowman, J. D., Kheifets, L., and Kromhout, H. (2013). Electric shocks at work in Europe: Development of a job exposure matrix. *Occupational and Environmental Medicine*, **70**, 261–267.

Imbernon, E., Goldberg, M., Bonenfant, S., Chevalier, A., Guénel, P., Vatré, R., et al. (1991). Occupational respiratory cancer and exposure to asbestos. A case control study in a cohort of worker in the electricity and gas industry. *American Journal of Industrial Medicine*, **28**, 339–352.

Kaerlev, L., Lynge, E., Sabroe, S., and Olsen, J. (2003). Reliability of data from next-of-kin: Results from a case-control study of occupational and lifestyle risk factors for cancer. *American Journal of Industrial Medicine*, **44**, 298–303.

Kauppinen, T., Heikkilä, P., Plato, N., Woldbaek, T., Lenvik, K., Hansen, J., et al. (2009). Construction of job-exposure matrices for the Nordic Occupational Cancer Study (NOCCA). *Acta Oncologica*, **48**, 791–800.

Kauppinen, T., Toikkanen, J., and Pukkala, E. (1998). From cross-tabulations to multipurpose exposure information system: A new job-exposure matrix. *American Journal of Industrial Medicine*, **33**, 409–417.

Kauppinen, T., Uuksulainen, S., Saalo, A., Mäkinen, I., and Pukkala, E. (2014). Use of the Finnish information system on occupational exposure (FINJEM) in epidemiologic, surveillance, and other applications. *Annals of Occupational Hygiene*, **58**, 380–396.

Kennedy, S. M., and Koehoorn, M. (2003). Exposure assessment in epidemiology: Does gender matter? *American Journal of Industrial Medicine*, **44**, 576–583.

Kjaerheim, K., Martinsen, J. I., Lynge, E., Gunnarsdottir, H. K., Sparen, P., Tryggvadottir, L., et al. (2010). Effects of occupation on risks of avoidable cancers in the Nordic countries. *European Journal of Cancer*, **46**, 2545–2554.

Koeman, T., Offermans, N. S. M., Christopher-De Vries, Y., Slottje, P., Van Den Brandt, P. A., Goldbohm, R. A., et al. (2013). JEMs and incompatible occupational coding systems: Effect of manual and automatic recoding of job codes on exposure assignment. *Annals of Occupational Hygiene*, **57**, 107–114.

Kogevinas, M. (2003). Commentary: Standardized coding of occupational data in epidemiological studies. *International Journal of Epidemiology*, **32**, 428–429.

Koh, D. H., Nam, J. M., Graubard, B. I., Chen, Y. C., Locke, S. J., and Friesen, M. C. (2014). Evaluating temporal trends from occupational lead exposure data reported in the published literature using meta-regression. *Annals of Occupational Hygiene*, Epub 5 Sep 2014. pii: meu061.

Kriebel, D., and Smith, T. J. (2010). *A biologic approach to environmental assessment and epidemiology*. Oxford University Press, New York.

Kromhout, H. (2002). Commentary. *Occupational and Environmental Medicine*, **59**, 594–594.

Kromhout, H., Loomis, D. P., and Kleckner, R. C. (1999). Uncertainty in the relation between exposure to magnetic fields and brain cancer due to assessment and assignment of exposure and analytical methods in dose-response modeling. *Annals of the New York Academy of Science*, **895**, 141–155.

Kromhout, H., and Vermeulen, R. (2001). Application of job-exposure matrices in studies of the general population: Some clues to their performance. *European Respiratory Review*, **11**, 80.

Lavoue, J., Begin, D., Beaudry, C., and Gerin, M. (2007). Monte carlo simulation to reconstruct formaldehyde exposure levels from summary parameters reported in the literature. *Annals of Occupational Hygiene*, **51**, 161–172.

Lavoué, J., and Droz, P. O. (2009). Multimodel inference and multimodel averaging in empirical modeling of occupational exposure levels. *Annals of Occupational Hygiene*, **53**, 173–180.

Lavoué, J., Pintos, J., Van Tongeren, M., Kincl, L., Richardson, L., Kauppinen, T., et al. (2012). Comparison of exposure estimates in the Finnish job-exposure matrix FINJEM with a JEM derived from expert assessments performed in Montreal. *Occupational and Environmental Medicine*, **69**, 465–471.

Locke, S. J., Colt, J. S., Stewart, P. A., Armenti, K. R., Baris, D., Blair, A., et al. (2014). Identifying gender differences in reported occupational information from three US population-based case-control studies. *Occupational and Environmental Medicine*, **71**, 855–864.

Logan, P. W., Ramachandran, G., Mulhausen, J. R., Banerjee, S., and Hewett, P. (2011). Desktop study of occupational exposure judgments: Do education and experience influence accuracy? *Journal of Occupational and Environmental Hygiene*, **8**, 746–758.

Morton, J., Cotton, R., Cocker, J., and Warren, N. D. (2010). Trends in blood lead levels in UK workers, 1995-2007. *Occupational and Environmental Medicine*, **67**, 590–595.

Neta, G., Stewart, P. A., Rajaraman, P., Hein, M. J., Waters, M. A., Purdue, M. P., et al. (2012). Occupational exposure to chlorinated solvents and risks of glioma and meningioma in adults. *Occupational and Environmental Medicine*, **69**, 793–801.

Neter, J., Kutner, M., Nachtsheim, C. J., and Wasserman, W. (1996). *Applied linear statistical models* (4th ed.). WCB McGraw-Hill/Irwin, New York.

Offermans, N. S. M., Vermeulen, R., Burdorf, A., Peters, S., Goldbohm, R. A., Koeman, T., et al. (2012). Comparison of expert and job-exposure matrix-based retrospective exposure assessment of occupational carcinogens in The Netherlands Cohort Study. *Occupational and Environmental Medicine*, **69**, 745–751.

Park, D., Stewart, P. A., and Coble, J. B. (2009). A comprehensive review of the literature on exposure to metalworking fluids. *Journal of Occupational and Environmental Hygiene*, **6**, 530–541.

Parks, C. G., Cooper, G. S., Nylander-French, L. A., Hoppin, J. A., Sanderson, W. T., and Dement, J. M. (2004). Comparing questionnaire-based methods to assess occupational silica exposure. *Epidemiology*, **15**, 433–441.

Patel, M. D., Rose, K. M., Owens, C. R., Bang, H., and Kaufman, J. S. (2012). Performance of automated and manual coding systems for occupational data: A case study of historical records. *American Journal of Industrial Medicine*, **55**, 228–231.

Peretz, C., Goren, A., Smid, T., and Kromhout, H. (2002). Application of mixed-effects models for exposure assessment. *Annals of Occupational Hygiene*, **46**, 69–77.

Peters, S. M. (2012). Qunatitative exposure assessment in community-based studies: The case for respirable crystalline silica and lung cancer. In *Quantitative exposure assessment in community-based studies* (pp. 101–114). Thesis Utrecht University.

Peters, S., Glass, D. C., Milne, E., and Fritschi, L. (2014). Rule-based exposure assessment versus case-by-case expert assessment using the same information in a community-based study. *Occupational and Environmental Medicine*, **71**, 215–219.

Peters, S., Vermeulen, R., Cassidy, A., t'Mannetje, A., van Tongeren, M., Boffetta, P., et al. (2011a). Comparison of exposure assessment methods for occupational carcinogens in a multi-centre lung cancer case-control study. *Occupational and Environmental Medicine*, **68**, 148–153.

Peters, S., Vermeulen, R., Portengen, L., Olsson, A., Kendzia, B., Vincent, R., et al. (2011b). Modelling of occupational respirable crystalline silica exposure for quantitative exposure assessment in community-based case-control studies. *Journal of Environmental Monitoring*, **13**, 3262–3268.

Post, W., Kromhout, H., Heederik, D., Noy, D., and Duijzentkunst, R. S. (1991). Semiquantitative estimates of exposure to methylene chloride and styrene: The influence of quantitative exposure data. *Applied Occupational and Environmental Hygiene*, **6**, 197–204.

Pronk, A., Coble, J., and Stewart, P. A. (2009). Occupational exposure to diesel engine exhaust: A literature review. *Journal of Exposure Science and Environmental Epidemiology*, **19**, 443–457.

Pronk, A., Stewart, P. A. Coble, J., Katki, H. A., Wheeler, D. C., Colt, J. S., et al. (2012). Comparison of two expert-based assessments of diesel exhaust exposure in a case-control study: Programmable decision rules versus expert review of individual jobs. *Occupational and Environmental Medicine*, **69**, 752–758.

Pukkala, E., Guo, J., Kyyrönen, P., Lindbohm, M.-L., Sallmén, M., and Kauppinen, T. (2005). National job-exposure matrix in analyses of census-based estimates of occupational cancer risk. *Scandinavian Journal of Work, Environment and Health*, **31**, 97–107.

Quinn, M. M., Sembajwe, G., Stoddard, A. M., Kriebel, D., Krieger, N., Sorensen, G., et al. (2007). Social disparities in the burden of occupational exposures: Results of a cross-sectional study. *American Journal of Industrial Medicine*, **50**, 861–875.

Rappaport, S. M. (1991). Assessment of long-term exposures to toxic substances in air. *Annals of Occupational Hygiene*, **35**, 61–121.

Rijs, K. J., van der Pas, S., Geuskens, G. A., Cozijnsen, R., Koppes, L. L., van der Beek, A. J., and Deeg, D. J. (2014). Development and validation of a physical and psychosocial job-exposure matrix in older and retired workers. *Annals of Occupational Hygiene*, **58**, 152–170.

Rocheleau, C. M., Lawson, C. C., Waters, M. A., Hein, M. J., Stewart, P. A., Correa, A., et al. (2011). Inter-rater reliability of assessed prenatal maternal occupational exposures to solvents, polycyclic aromatic hydrocarbons, and heavy metals. *Birth Defects Research Part A—Clinical and Molecular Teratology*, **91**, 350–350.

Sauvé, J.-F., Beaudry, C., Bégin, D., Dion, C., Gérin, M., and Lavoué, J. (2012). Statistical modeling of crystalline silica exposure by trade in the construction industry using a database compiled from the literature. *Journal of Environmental Monitoring*, **14**, 2512–2520.

Sauvé, J.-F., Beaudry, C., Bégin, D., Dion, C., Gérin, M., and Lavoué, J. (2013). Silica exposure during construction activities: Statistical modeling of task-based measurements from the literature. *Annals of Occupational Hygiene*, **57**, 432–443.

Seixas, N., Neitzel, R., Sheppard, L., and Goldman, B. (2005). Alternative metrics for noise exposure among construction workers. *Annals of Occupational Hygiene*, **49**, 493–502.

Seixas, N. S., Neitzel, R., Stover, B., Sheppard, L., Feeney, P., Mills, D., et al. (2012). 10-year prospective study of noise exposure and hearing damage among construction workers. *Occupational and Environmental Medicine*, **69**, 643–650.

Seixas, N. S., Robin, T. G., and Moulton, L. H. (1988). The use of geometric and arithmetic mean exposures in occupational epidemiology. *American Journal of Industrial Medicine*, **14**, 465–477.

Sembajwe, G., Quinn, M., Kriebel, D., Stoddard, A., Krieger, N., and Barbeau, E. (2010). The influence of sociodemographic characteristics on agreement between self-reports and expert exposure assessments. *American Journal of Industrial Medicine*, **53**, 1019–1031.

Semple, S. E., Proud, L. A., Tannahill, S. N., Tindall, M. E., and Cherrie, J. W. (2001). A training exercise in subjectively estimating inhalation exposures. *Scandinavian Journal of Work Environment and Health*, **27**, 395–401.

Silverman, D. T., Samanic, C. M., Lubin, J. H., Blair, A. E., Stewart, P. A., Vermeulen, R., et al. (2012). The Diesel Exhaust in Miners Study: A nested case-control study of lung cancer and diesel exhaust. *Journal of the National Cancer Institute*, **104**, 855–868.

Sjöström, M., Lewné, M., Alderling, M., Willix, P., Berg, P., Gustavsson, P., et al. (2013). A job-exposure matrix for occupational noise: Development and validation. *Annals of Occupational Hygiene*, **57**, 774–783.

Solovieva, S., Pehkonen, I., Kausto, J., Miranda, H., Shiri, R., Kauppinen, T., et al. (2012). Development and validation of a job exposure matrix for physical risk factors in low back pain. *PloS One*, **7**, e48680.

Steineck, G., Plato, N., and Alfredsson, L. (1989). Industry-related urothelial carcinogens: Application of a job exposure matrix to census data. *American Journal of Industrial Medicine*, **16**, 209–224.

Steinsvag, K., Bratveit, M., Moen, B. E., and Kromhout, H. (2007). Inter-rater agreement in the assessment of exposure to carcinogens in the offshore petroleum industry. *Occupational and Environmental Medicine*, **64**, 582–588.

Stewart, P. A., Carel, R., Schairer, C., and Blair, A. (2000). Comparison of industrial hygienists' exposure evaluations for an epidemiologic study. *Scandinavian Journal of Work, Environment and Health*, **26**, 44–51.

Stewart, P. A., Coble, J. B., Vermeulen, R., Schleiff, P., Blair, A., Lubin, J., et al. (2010). The Diesel Exhaust in Miners Study: I. Overview of the exposure assessment process. *Annals of Occupational Hygiene*, **54**, 728–746.

Stewart, P. A., Lees, P. S., and Francis, M. (1996). Quantification of historical exposures in occupational cohort studies. *Scandinavian Journal of Work, Environment and Health*, **22**, 405–414.

Stewart, P. A., Stewart, W. F., Siemiatycki, J., Heineman, E. F., and Dosemeci, M. (1998). Questionnaires for collecting detailed occupational information for community-based case control studies. *American Industrial Hygiene Association Journal*, **59**, 39–44.

Stewart, P. A., Vermeulen, R., Coble, J. B., Blair, A., Schleiff, P., Lubin, J. H., et al. (2012). The Diesel Exhaust in Miners Study: V. Evaluation of the exposure assessment methods. *Annals of Occupational Hygiene*, **56**, 389–400.

Svendsen, K., and Hilt, B. (2011). The agreement between workers and within workers in regard to occupational exposure to mercury in dental practice assessed from a questionnaire and an interview. *Journal of Occupational Medicine and Toxicology*, **6**, 8.

Tagiyeva, N., Semple, S., Devereux, G., Sherriff, A., Henderson, J., Elias, P., et al. (2011). Reconstructing past occupational exposures: How reliable are women's reports of their partner's occupation? *Occupational and Environmental Medicine*, **68**, 452–456.

Teschke, K., Olshan, A. F., Daniels, J. L., De Roos, A. J., Parks, C. G., Schulz, M., et al. (2002). Occupational exposure assessment in case-control studies: Opportunities for improvement. *Occupational and Environmental Medicine*, **59**, 575–593; discussion 594.

Tielemans, E., Heederik, D., Burdorf, A., Vermeulen, R., Veulemans, H., Kromhout, H., et al. (1999). Assessment of occupational exposures in a general population: Comparison of different methods. *Occupational and Environmental Medicine*, **56**, 145–151.

't Mannetje, A., Fevotte, J., Fletcher, T., Brennan, P., Legoza, J., Szeremi, M., et al. (2003). Assessing exposure misclassification by expert assessment in multicenter occupational studies. *Epidemiology*, **14**, 585–592.

't Mannetje, A., and Kromhout, H. (2003). The use of occupation and industry classifications in general population studies. *International Journal of Epidemiology*, **32**, 419–428.

't Mannetje, A., McLean, D. J., Eng, A. J., Kromhout, H., Kauppinen, T., Fevotte, J., et al. (2011). Developing a general population job-exposure matrix in the absence of sufficient exposure monitoring data. *Annals of Occupational Hygiene*, **55**, 879–885.

Turner, M. C., Benke, G., Bowman, J. D., Figuerola, J., Fleming, S., Hours, M., et al. (2014). Occupational exposure to extremely low-frequency magnetic fields and brain tumor risks in the INTEROCC study. *Cancer Epidemiology, Biomarkers and Prevention*, **23**, 1863–1872.

van Tongeren, M., Kincl, L., Richardson, L., Benke, G., Figuerola, J., Kauppinen, T., et al. (2013). Assessing occupational exposure to chemicals in an international epidemiological study of brain tumours. *Annals of Occupational Hygiene*, **57**, 610–626.

Vergara, X. P., Kheifets, L., Silva, M., Bracken, T. D., and Yost, M. (2012). New electric-shock job exposure matrix. *American Journal of Industrial Medicine*, **55**, 232–240.

Vermeulen, R., Coble, J. B., Lubin, J. H., Portengen, L., Blair, A., Attfield, M. D., et al. (2010a), The Diesel Exhaust in Miners Study: IV. Estimating historical exposures to diesel exhaust in underground non-metal mining facilities. *Annals of Occupational Hygiene*, **54**, 774–788.

Vermeulen, R., Coble, J. B., Yereb, D., Lubin, J. H., Blair, A., Portengen, L., et al. (2010b). The Diesel Exhaust in Miners Study: III. Interrelations between respirable elemental carbon and gaseous and particulate components of diesel exhaust derived from area sampling in underground non-metal mining facilities. *Annals of Occupational Hygiene*, **54**, 762–773.

Villanueva, V., and Garcia, A. M. (2006). Validity and reliability of surrogate informatin for controls in a case-control study on Alzheimer's disease. *Journal of Alzheimer's Disease*, **10**, 409–416.

Virji, M. A., Woskie, S. R., Waters, M., Brueck, S., Stancescu, D., Gore, R., et al. (2009). Agreement between task-based estimates of the full-shift noise exposure and the full-shift noise dosimetry. *Annals of Occupational Hygiene*, **53**, 201–214.

Virji, M. A., Park, J. Y., Stefaniak, A. B., Stanton, M. L., Day, G. A., Kent, M. S., et al. (2012). Sensitization and chronic beryllium disease at a primary manufacturing facility, part 1: Historical exposure reconstruction. *Scandinavian Journal of Work, Environment and Health*, **38**, 247–258.

Wheeler, D. C., Burstyn, I., Vermeulen, R., Yu, K., Shortreed, S. M., Pronk, A., et al. (2013). Inside the black box: Starting to uncover the underlying decision rules used in a one-by-one expert assessment of occupational exposure in case-control studies. *Occupational and Environmental Medicine*, **70**, 203–210.

Wild, P. (2002). Combining expert ratings and exposure measurements: A random effect paradigm. *Annals of Occupational Hygiene*, **46**, 479–487.

8

PHARMACOKINETIC MODELING IN EPIDEMIOLOGY

Marc-André Verner

8.1 INTRODUCTION

The assessment of exposure to chemicals in epidemiology is most frequently performed based on biomarkers of exposure (i.e., levels measured in biological specimens) or environmental measurements in media that are relevant to exposure (e.g., air, water, food, dust). Although these measurements provide insights into human exposure, they have multiple limitations that may bias exposure–outcome associations and lead to false negatives or false positives in observational studies. Issues with using biomarker or environmental levels to assess exposure include:

- Measured environmental levels may not provide an accurate or precise estimate of the internal exposure.
- Measuring levels during etiologically relevant periods may be impractical or available levels may not be representative of exposure when the chemical insult occurred.
- Biological levels can be influenced by physiological processes that are also related to the health outcome of interest (confounding).
- Biological levels can be modulated by the health outcome itself (reverse causality).

In epidemiological studies, it is sometimes impossible or impractical to collect biological or environmental samples that are representative of exposure during windows of vulnerability. For example, studies of health outcomes observed in adults or the elderly may not be able to measure exposure during early life windows, unless they undertake a longitudinal birth cohort and follow subjects until they develop the disease. Even in the setting of longitudinal birth cohorts, it may be unfeasible to obtain serial biological samples during periods of rapid changes in physiology (e.g., growth) and exposure (e.g., lactational exposure, dust ingestion) because of the costs and the burden on study participants. In these cases, researchers may have to rely on one or a few samples that were drawn at a time that is more convenient than toxicologically relevant. These studies could benefit from tools like pharmacokinetic models to estimate exposure retrospectively or prospectively in study subjects and better characterize exposure during critical windows of vulnerability.

Another shortcoming of using biomarker or environmental levels as a measure of exposure in epidemiological studies is the possibility that inter-individual variability in physiological processes influences the association between measured levels and the health outcome of interest. For a given external dose, the resulting levels in biological specimens can vary from one individual to another depending on variability in pharmacokinetic processes like distribution in the body, biotransformation rates, and excretion rates and routes. Likewise, the same biomarker levels at a given time in different individuals do not necessarily imply equal exposure. In certain cases, the physiological parameters that are influencing internal levels are also associated with the health outcome and, consequently, confound the association. It is possible to reduce confounding by statistically controlling for the influence of physiological parameters that are easily measured in epidemiological studies (e.g., body mass index). However, it may be impossible to control for other parameters that are harder to measure (e.g., glomerular filtration rate, temporal changes in the volume of body lipids). Where confounding by unmeasured physiological processes exists, it is paramount to adequately quantify the influence of these physiological processes to avoid underestimating or overestimating the strength of the epidemiological association. In certain cases, the health outcome itself could influence the biological levels of chemicals and give the impression of a causal association between the exposure and the outcome (i.e., reverse causality). In these cases, pharmacokinetic models could be used to characterize the impact of physiological variability on biomarker levels and their association with health outcomes.

In this chapter, we discuss how pharmacokinetic modeling, and especially physiologically based pharmacokinetic modeling, can be used to better interpret measured biomarker or environmental levels, generate exposure estimates, and characterize the influence of physiological processes on epidemiological associations. Some examples of applications are also presented.

8.2 WHAT IS PHYSIOLOGICALLY BASED PHARMACOKINETIC MODELING?

Physiologically based pharmacokinetic (PBPK) modeling is the mathematical representation of the physiological, biochemical, and physicochemical processes that govern the absorption, distribution, metabolism, and excretion of a chemical in the body. The first step in developing a PBPK model is to conceptually represent the physiological characteristics of the organism of interest while accounting for the pathways of uptake and the disposition of the chemical under study. Tissues that are involved in the pharmacokinetics of the chemical are represented as compartments, assembled into a network of compartments connected by blood circulation. Then, the movement of chemicals in and out of the different compartments is described mathematically with a set of mass balance differential equations that are based on organism- and chemical-specific parameters

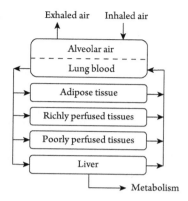

Figure 8.1 Conceptual representation of a PBPK model for a lipophilic volatile organic compound.

(e.g., blood perfusion rates, metabolism rate, tissue:blood partition coefficients). In other words, an absorbed dose of a chemical will be gradually distributed across the various organs of the body, depending on its affinity for these tissues. Once the model is completed, simulations can be performed for different exposure scenarios and resulting tissue or blood concentrations can be validated against experimental data.

Say we want to develop a model for occupational exposure by inhalation to a volatile organic compound that is lipophilic and metabolized by the liver. We first need to make sure relevant tissues and processes involved in the uptake and disposition of that compound are represented in the PBPK model. In this example, the model would have to include the gas exchange in the lungs (absorption), the adipose tissue (distribution), and the liver (metabolism). The chemical is also likely to distribute to other tissues, but they may not be individually as important as the adipose tissue and the liver for the pharmacokinetics of that compound. Physiologically based pharmicokinetic modelers often lump these remaining tissues into one or multiple compartments based on shared pharmacokinetic properties, like the richly perfused and poorly perfused tissues. The PBPK model could therefore include five compartments (Figure 8.1): a gas exchange compartment, the adipose tissue, the liver, the richly perfused tissues, and the poorly perfused tissues. Arrows in this model represent the movement of the chemical in and out of compartments, through blood circulation, inhalation, or metabolism. The rate at which the chemical will enter the body, distribute to the different compartments, and be metabolized is calculated based on parameters like the ventilation rate, blood:air and tissue:blood partition coefficients, blood perfusion rates, the volume of the different compartments, and metabolic constants.

The uptake by inhalation can be modeled by assuming instantaneous equilibrium among alveolar air, venous blood, and arterial blood. Because the chemical concentration in the alveoli is assumed to be in equilibrium, the net balance of chemical in lung blood (inputs-outputs) is 0 (Eq. 8.1):

$$Q_{pulmonary} \times C_{inhaled} - Q_{pulmonary} \times C_{exhaled} + Q_{cardiac} \times C_{venous} - Q_{cardiac} \times C_{arterial} = 0 \qquad \text{(Eq. 8.1)}$$

where $Q_{pulmonary}$ is the pulmonary ventilation, $C_{inhaled}$ is the inhaled air concentration, $C_{exhaled}$ is the exhaled air concentration, $Q_{cardiac}$ is the cardiac output, C_{venous} is the venous blood concentration, and $C_{arterial}$ is the arterial blood concentration. $C_{exhaled}$ is calculated from the arterial blood concentration and the blood:air partition coefficient ($P_{blood:air}$):

$$C_{exhaled} = \frac{C_{arterial}}{P_{blood:air}} \qquad \text{(Eq. 8.2)}$$

By rearranging the equation, the concentration in arterial blood can be calculated as follows:

$$C_{arterial} = \frac{Q_{pulmonary} \times C_{inhaled} + Q_{cardiac} \times C_{venous}}{Q_{cardiac} + (Q_{pulmonary} / P_{blood:air})} \qquad \text{(Eq. 8.3)}$$

The rate of entry in the different compartments can be calculated by multiplying the arterial blood concentration by the tissue-specific blood perfusion rate (Q_{tissue}). Likewise, the rate at which the chemical will leave the compartment is characterized by the tissue venous blood concentration and the blood perfusion rate. The mass balance differential equation for compartments where there is no metabolism is calculated as follows (Eq. 8.4):

$$\frac{dAmount_{tissue}}{dt} = Q_{tissue} \times C_{arterial} - Q_{tissue} \times C_{venous\ from\ tissue} \qquad \text{(Eq. 8.4)}$$

where the venous blood concentration is (Eq. 8.5):

$$C_{venous\ from\ tissue} = \frac{C_{tissue}}{P_{tissue:blood}} \qquad \text{(Eq. 8.5)}$$

and concentration in the tissue is (Eq. 8.6):

$$C_{tissue} = \frac{Amount_{tissue}}{Volume_{tissue}} \qquad \text{(Eq. 8.6)}$$

In metabolizing tissues, an additional expression is included in the mass balance differential equation to describe the rate of metabolism. The rate of saturable metabolism can be calculated using a Michaelis-Menten equation (Eq. 8.7):

$$\frac{dAmount_{metabolized}}{dt} = \frac{Vmax \times C_{venous\,from\,liver}}{Km + C_{venous\,from\,liver}} \tag{Eq. 8.7}$$

where Vmax is the maximum metabolism rate and Km is the affinity constant or, in other words, the concentration at which the metabolism rate is half the Vmax. In a PBPK model in which metabolism occurs in the liver, the liver compartment mass balance differential equation is (Eq. 8.8):

$$\frac{dAmount_{liver}}{dt} = Q_{liver} \times C_{arterial} - Q_{liver} \times C_{venous\,from\,liver} - \frac{Vmax \times C_{venous\,from\,liver}}{Km + C_{venous\,from\,liver}} \tag{Eq. 8.8}$$

The concentration in venous blood coming out of the different compartments and returning to the lungs is calculated from the compartment-specific venous blood concentration and the perfusion rates (Eq. 8.9):

$$C_{venous} = \frac{\sum\left(C_{venous\,from\,tissue} \times Q_{tissue}\right)}{\sum Q_{tissue}} \tag{Eq. 8.9}$$

The different parameters used in the model can be found in the literature, measured using *in vitro* or *in vivo* models, or estimated using predictive models. Information on organ volume and blood perfusion rates is available from different sources. Algorithms have been developed to estimate organ volumes based on body weight alone (Young et al. 2009) or a combination of different parameters like age, body weight, and body height (Haddad et al. 2006). Blood perfusion rates in the different organs are usually expressed as a fraction of the cardiac output, which can be estimated based on age, body weight, gender, and energy expenditure (Brochu et al. 2012). Ventilation rates are also available in the literature (Brochu et al. 2012). Tissue:blood and blood:air partition coefficients are often available in the literature for well-studied chemicals. When modeling a chemical for which partition coefficients have not been measured, quantitative-structure activity relationship (QSAR) models and predictive algorithms can be used to estimate these parameters (Peyret et al. 2010). Metabolic constants can be scaled from animal data, *in vitro* biotransformation assays using human tissues (e.g., microsomes, hepatocytes), or estimated using QSAR regression models.

The PBPK model example given here is relatively simple. More compartments and processes may need to be included when developing a PBPK model for chemicals that have more complex pharmacokinetics (e.g., slow diffusion into tissues, multiple routes of exposure or excretion) or when simulating exposures during different stages of life (e.g., life-course models, models of pregnancy and lactation). For a more detailed description of model development and mass-balance differential equations, please refer to Krishnan and Andersen (2001).

8.3 PHYSIOLOGICALLY BASED PHARMICOKINETIC MODEL SIMULATION

Once a PBPK model is developed, simulations can be performed for different expo-sure scenarios or physiological inputs. Depending on how the model parameters are calculated (e.g., compartment volumes, ventilation rate), model inputs could include age, body weight, and physical exertion. Exposure could be defined in terms of the chemical's concentration in the air and the periods of exposure. As an exam-ple, the venous blood level profile of a worker who is 30 years of age, weighs 70 kg, works an 8-hour shift (with a 1-hour break for lunch), and is exposed to an average 20 ppm of styrene by inhalation was simulated using the PBPK model described in Jonsson and Johanson (2002) (Figure 8.2).

Physiologically based pharmicokinetic models can output a variety of dose metrics. As shown in Figure 8.2, the model can provide a complete concentration time-course in blood or a given tissue. In addition, the maximum concentration (Cmax) in blood or tissues can be identified. Where the overall exposure is of inter-est, the blood/tissue concentration can be integrated over a certain period: This measure is called the area under the concentration versus time curve (AUC).

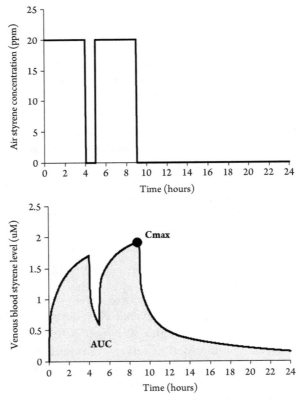

Figure 8.2 Simulated occupational exposure to styrene (20 ppm) during an 8-hour work shift.

When measured biological levels are available, simulated levels can be compared with experimental data to validate the PBPK model. Data from controlled exposure experiments are preferred for model validation because exposure is precisely measured, many physiological measurements can be obtained (e.g., body weight, ventilation), and serial biological specimens can be collected. However, conducting controlled exposures may not be possible for certain chemicals, such as carcinogens or environmental chemicals with long half-lives. In these cases, biomonitoring data from occupational or environmental epidemiological studies could be used to assess model accuracy and precision.

Physiologically based pharmicokinetic modeling also allows evaluating inter-individual variability in biological levels by incorporating variability into physiological parameters (Bois et al. 2010). Instead of running a simulation with a specific set of model parameter values for a single individual (like in the preceding example), model simulations can be performed iteratively using a Monte Carlo procedure to simulate exposure for individuals of a population. At each iteration, values for the different model parameters (e.g., partition coefficients, metabolic constants) are sampled from probabilistic distributions and fed into the model to perform a simulation. Subsequently, results from iterative model simulations can be compiled to derive a distribution of biological levels in a population.

8.4 APPLICATIONS OF PHYSIOLOGICALLY BASED PHARMICOKINETIC MODELING IN EPIDEMIOLOGY

8.4.1 Estimating Internal Exposure

Physiologically based pharmicokinetic and simple pharmacokinetic models are drawing increasing attention in epidemiology for prospective or retrospective exposure assessment or for cumulative exposure estimation. Here we present some examples of studies in which modeled exposure estimates have been used in environmental epidemiology.

Certain chemicals are transferred from the mother to the infant through breast-feeding. The period during which infants are breastfed is a critical period of development for different systems, including the brain and the immune system. However, collecting infants' blood during periods of potentially heighted vulnerability can be challenging for any number of reasons (e.g., ethics, costs, logistics). Physiologically based pharmicokinetic models of human lactation can be used to estimate children's levels during and after breastfeeding. In a longitudinal birth cohort study of Inuits, infants' monthly polychlorinated biphenyl (PCB) levels were estimated using the PBPK model presented in Verner et al. (2009), which was validated against plasma levels measured in 6-month-olds from the same cohort ($n = 105$); the Spearman's rank correlation coefficient between measured and simulated 2,2',4,4',5,5'-hexachlorobiphenyl (PCB-153) levels was 0.89. Estimated levels for each postnatal month of life were subsequently used to evaluate the association between infants' levels and behavior at 11 months of age. Whereas measured prenatal levels were associated with infants' inattention, only estimated postnatal levels (especially around the fourth month) were associated with increased activity. The use of PBPK modeling in this study allowed the identification of a postnatal window of vulnerability without having to collect serial blood samples from infants. The same PBPK model was also used in a longitudinal birth cohort study of children from multiple cities in Spain (Gascon et al. 2013). In this study, measured prenatal levels and estimated postnatal levels of three persistent organic pollutants (PCB-153, hexachlorobenzene [HCB], p,p'-dichlorodiphenyldichlroethylene [p,p'-DDE]) were used to evaluate their association with cognitive and psychomotor development at 14 months of age as measured using the Bayley Scales of Infant Development (BDSID). A significant association was only observed with measured prenatal PCB-153 levels and psychomotor development.

It has been suggested that the breast tissue is especially sensitive to environmental stressors during puberty and early adulthood (Tokunaga et al. 1994). Yet, most epidemiological studies of breast cancer and environmental contaminants used levels measured at the time of diagnosis or a few years before to assess exposure (Lopez-Cervantes et al. 2004). To back-extrapolate early life levels of persistent organic pollutants from levels measured later in life, a life-course PBPK model was developed (Verner et al. 2008). This model accounts for changes in body weight, height, pregnancies, and breastfeeding to simulate subject-specific lifetime exposure profiles. In the context of a breast cancer study, subject-specific information on physiology, breastfeeding, and blood levels could be used in the PBPK model to back-extrapolate early life levels of persistent organic pollutants to subsequently evaluate their association with outcomes that occur later in life. However, the precision and accuracy of the PBPK model have yet to be tested against repeated measurements in women.

Although not a PBPK model per se, a one-compartment pharmacokinetic model developed by Shin et al. (2011b) coupled with a model for individual exposure (Shin et al. 2011a) was used to predict serum concentrations of perfluorooctanoic acid (PFOA) in residents from eastern Ohio and western West Virginia. Predicted serum PFOA levels were correlated with measured serum PFOA levels (Spearman's rank correlation coefficient = 0.67) when including all study participants (n = 45,276) who did not report working for the DuPont company. The correlation was stronger when restricting analyses to study participants who provided information on water consumption and stayed in the same residence and worked at the same place for the 5 years before blood sampling (n = 1074; Spearman's rank correlation coefficient = 0.82). Estimated PFOA levels at different ages (e.g., at birth, from 0 to 10 years) were used in epidemiological studies of kidney function (Watkins et al. 2013), cancer (Barry et al. 2013; Vieira et al. 2013), pregnancy outcome (Savitz et al. 2012a,b), and ulcerative colitis (Steenland et al. 2013).

Whereas characterizing internal exposure is a crucial step in epidemiological studies, estimating external exposure from biomarker levels can also be of interest to translate epidemiological findings into human risk assessment and policymaking. This process, called "reverse dosimetry," can be achieved using PBPK modeling

(Clewell et al. 2008). For example, PBPK models can be used to perform Monte Carlo simulations for a given external exposure level (e.g., concentration of a chemical in the air, food, water) to generate a distribution of blood levels. Simulated blood levels can subsequently be expressed as exposure conversion factors by dividing the external exposure level by the simulated blood level (external level/blood level). The probability distribution of external exposure levels can be reconstructed by multiplying an observed biomarker level by the distribution of simulated exposure conversion factors. A more detailed description of this approach can be found in Tan et al. (2006), who reconstructed chloroform exposure from measured blood levels.

8.4.2 Optimal Sampling Time

It is not always clear how many biological samples need to be collected or when they should be collected to adequately classify study subjects' exposure in epidemiological studies. The right sampling schedule depends on several parameters, including chemical-specific properties (e.g., half-life), exposure route (e.g., oral, dermal, inhalation), exposure pattern (e.g., three times daily, continuous exposure), within- and between-person variability in exposure, and the toxicologically relevant exposure metric (e.g., maximum blood level, cumulative exposure). Pharmacokinetic models can be used to evaluate blood or tissue level profiles for different exposure scenarios and, in turn, help determine sampling times when biomarker levels are most representative of the exposure metric of interest.

As an example, a PBPK model was employed to identify the best time to sample blood or exhaled air to obtain the most accurate estimate of overall exposure to styrene in the workplace (Verner et al. 2012). The model was used to perform Monte Carlo simulations for different physiological parameters and different patterns of exposure and workload. The exposure metric of interest was the 24-hour area under the blood level versus time curve. Subsequently, regression analyses were carried out to identify the time when blood or exhaled air levels were most representative of the 24-hour area under the curve, that is, the time when levels were most strongly associated with the 24-hour area under the curve (highest R^2). Results suggested that blood and exhaled air samples should be taken at the end of the work shift or shortly thereafter.

Epidemiological studies on chemicals with relatively short half-lives like bisphenol A and pyrethroids often rely on spot urine samples to assess exposure in study subjects. Unfortunately, the variability in measured levels may be mostly attributable to within-person variability rather than between-person variability, hence impeding the identification of associations between exposure and health outcomes. Pharmacokinetic models, such as the one presented in Aylward et al. (2012), could be used to simulate exposures in the population and determine how many samples are necessary to reach an acceptable level of resolution in exposure estimates and when samples are most representative of exposure. The Aylward et al. (2012) model incorporates input on half-life and variation in exposure over time, and thus can be used for a wide variety of agents with short half-lives.

8.4.3 Confounding

In epidemiological studies, some physiological parameters can influence both biological levels of contaminants and the outcome, creating the impression that there is no association when there is one, or that there is an association where there isn't. Pharmacokinetic models are increasingly being used to evaluate the impact of such parameters on epidemiological associations.

Many epidemiological studies reported an association between prenatal exposure to polychlorinated biphenyls (PCBs) and reduced birth weight (Govarts et al. 2012). However, most of these studies did not statistically adjust for gestational weight gain. Women with a high gestational weight gain usually have a corresponding increase in the volume of the adipose tissue in which lipophilic persistent organic pollutants are stored, hence diluting the body burden, and they usually deliver heavier babies. As a result, women with high gestational weight gain tend to have lower PCB levels and deliver heavier babies, whereas women with low gestational weight gain tend to have higher levels and deliver smaller babies. To evaluate the influence of gestational weight gain on the association between prenatal PCB exposure and birth weight, a pharmacokinetic model of women's lifetime exposure, gestation, and lactation (Verner et al. 2013) was used to simulate a population through an iterative Monte Carlo procedure; for each simulated woman, physiological model inputs (e.g., pre-pregnancy body weight, gestational weight gain) and exposure were sampled from distributions, and fat gain during pregnancy and birth weight were predicted based on sampled gestational weight gain using linear regression models. Simulated PCB levels in maternal blood during pregnancy or cord blood at delivery were associated with simulated birth weight, although the association was weaker than the one observed in the meta-analysis of 12 European studies by Govarts et al. (2012). These results suggested that a portion of the association between prenatal PCBs and birth weight was attributable to confounding by gestational weight gain. Indeed, following the publication of the simulation study, Govarts et al. (2014) reanalyzed their data adjusting for gestational weight gain in seven cohorts where this information was collected and observed a 48% reduction in the effect estimate.

Physiologically based pharmacokinetic models are expected to play an increasing role in understanding the influence of pharmacokinetic processes on the association between exposure biomarkers and health outcomes. By comparing results from observational studies to those obtained in simulated populations, epidemiologists will be able to better identify and quantify confounding by physiological processes.

8.4.4 Reverse Causality

Some health outcomes can have an influence on the pharmacokinetics of chemicals. For example, weight loss in cancer patients could increase biological levels of lipophilic contaminants because of the decrease in the volume of distribution (i.e., smaller fat volume) (Chevrier et al. 2000). In a case–control study, this would result in cancer patients having higher biological levels than controls and give the impression that these contaminants increase the risk of developing cancer. Another example in which reverse causality is suspected is the epidemiological association between blood lead levels and chronic renal failure. Reduced glomerular filtration rate in chronic renal failure patients can delay urinary lead excretion, which results in higher blood lead levels in study cases than in controls (Evans and Elinder 2011). Where issues of reverse causality are difficult to circumvent with statistical methods or study design, pharmacokinetic models could be used to quantify the impact of health outcomes on biological levels.

In a study of children and adolescents from a population highly exposed to PFOA, Watkins et al. (2013) evaluated the association between exposure to perfluoroalkyl substances (PFAS) and kidney function as indicated by estimated glomerular filtration rate. They used two different metrics to characterize exposure: measured concurrent serum PFAS levels (including PFOA), and predicted concurrent and historical serum PFOA concentrations using a validated environmental, exposure, and pharmacokinetic model based on individual residential histories (Shin et al. 2011b). When using measured concurrent serum levels, they observed an association between PFAS levels and reduced glomerular filtration rate. On the other hand, neither predicted concurrent or historical levels were associated with glomerular filtration rate. Because PFAS are excreted through the kidneys, and reduced kidney function may slow excretion, these results led authors to hypothesize that reduced glomerular filtration rate probably caused the increased measured concurrent serum PFAS levels rather than the other way around.

Similarly, concerns have been raised about the direction of many associations observed in epidemiological studies, such as the association between DDE and body mass index (Wolff et al. 2007) and the association between PCBs and diabetes (Longnecker 2006). The use of PBPK modeling may be able to shed light on the influence of pharmacokinetic variability on measured biological levels and reduce uncertainty when interpreting observed epidemiological associations.

8.5 CONCLUSION

Pharmacokinetic modeling shows potential for improving exposure assessment in epidemiological studies. As discussed in this chapter, these models allow estimating exposure prospectively or retrospectively when collecting biological specimens during etiologically relevant periods is not possible. In addition, the impact of physiological processes on biomarker levels can be estimated from model simulations, thus leading to a better understanding of confounding and direction of epidemiological associations. The low costs associated with performing simulations and the increasing availability of validated PBPK models in the literature should stimulate the use of modeling for study design and analyses in epidemiology.

REFERENCES

Aylward, L. L., Kirman, C. R., Adgate, J. L., McKenzie, L. M., and Hays, S. M. (2012). Interpreting variability in population biomonitoring data: Role of elimination kinetics. *Journal of Exposure Science and Environmental Epidemiology*, **22**(4), 398–408.

Barry, V., Winquist, A., and Steenland, K. (2013). Perfluorooctanoic acid (PFOA) exposures and incident cancers among adults living near a chemical plant. *Environmental Health Perspectives*, **121**(11-12), 1313–1318.

Bois, F. Y., Jamei, M., and Clewell, H. J. (2010). PBPK modelling of inter-individual variability in the pharmacokinetics of environmental chemicals. *Toxicology*, **278**(3), 256–267.

Brochu, P., Brodeur, J., and Krishnan, K. (2012). Derivation of cardiac output and alveolar ventilation rate based on energy expenditure measurements in healthy males and females. *Journal of Applied Toxicology*, **32**(8), 564–580.

Chevrier, J., Dewailly, E., Ayotte, P., Mauriege, P., Despres, J. P., and Tremblay, A. (2000). Body weight loss increases plasma and adipose tissue concentrations of potentially toxic pollutants in obese individuals. *International Journal of Obesity and Related Metabolic Disorders*, **24**(10), 1272–1278.

Clewell, H. J., Tan, Y. M., Campbell, J. L., and Andersen, M. E. (2008). Quantitative interpretation of human biomonitoring data. *Toxicology and Applied Pharmacology*, **231**(1), 122–133.

Evans, M., and Elinder, C. G. (2011). Chronic renal failure from lead: Myth or evidence-based fact? *Kidney International*, **79**(3), 272–279.

Gascon, M., Verner, M. A., Guxens, M., Grimalt, J. O., Forns, J., Ibarluzea, J., et al. (2013). Evaluating the neurotoxic effects of lactational exposure to persistent organic pollutants (POPs) in Spanish children. *Neurotoxicology*, **34**, 9–15.

Govarts, E., Casas, M., Schoeters, G., Eggesbo, M., Valvi, D., Nieuwenhuijsen, M., et al. (2014). Prenatal PCB-153 exposure and decreased birth weight: The role of gestational weight gain. *Environmental Health Perspectives*, **122**(4), A89.

Govarts, E., Nieuwenhuijsen, M., Schoeters, G., Ballester, F., Bloemen, K., de Boer, M., et al. (2012). Birth weight and prenatal exposure to polychlorinated biphenyls (PCBs) and dichlorodiphenyldichloroethylene (DDE): A meta-analysis within 12 European Birth Cohorts. *Environmental Health Perspectives*, **120**(2), 162–170.

Haddad, S., Tardif, G. C., and Tardif, R. (2006). Development of physiologically based toxicokinetic models for improving the human indoor exposure assessment to water contaminants: Trichloroethylene and trihalomethanes. *Journal of Toxicology and Environmental Health, Part A*, **69**(23), 2095–2136.

Jonsson, F., and Johanson, G. (2002). Physiologically based modeling of the inhalation kinetics of styrene in humans using a bayesian population approach. *Toxicology and Applied Pharmacology*, **179**(1), 35–49.

Krishnan, K., and Andersen, M. E. (2001). Physiologically based pharmacokinetic modeling in toxicology. In *Principles and methods of toxicology* (4th ed.) (ed. A. Wallace Hayes). Taylor & Francis, Philadelphia.

Longnecker, M. P. (2006). Pharmacokinetic variability and the miracle of modern analytical chemistry. *Epidemiology*, **17**(4), 350–351.

Lopez-Cervantes, M., Torres-Sanchez, L., Tobias, A., and Lopez-Carrillo, L. (2004). Dichlorodiphenyldichloroethane burden and breast cancer risk: A meta-analysis of the epidemiologic evidence. *Environmental Health Perspectives*, **112**(2), 207–214.

Peyret, T., Poulin, P., and Krishnan, K. (2010). A unified algorithm for predicting partition coefficients for PBPK modeling of drugs and environmental chemicals. *Toxicology and Applied Pharmacology,* **249**(3), 197–207.

Savitz, D. A., Stein, C. R., Bartell, S. M., Elston, B., Gong, J., Shin, H. M., et al. (2012a). Perfluorooctanoic acid exposure and pregnancy outcome in a highly exposed community. *Epidemiology,* **23**(3), 386–392.

Savitz, D. A., Stein, C. R., Elston, B., Wellenius, G. A., Bartell, S. M., Shin, H. M., et al. (2012b). Relationship of perfluorooctanoic acid exposure to pregnancy outcome based on birth records in the mid-Ohio Valley. *Environmental Health Perspectives,* **120**(8), 1201–1207.

Shin, H. M., Vieira, V. M., Ryan, P. B., Detwiler, R., Sanders, B., Steenland, K., et al. (2011a). Environmental fate and transport modeling for perfluorooctanoic acid emitted from the Washington Works Facility in West Virginia. *Environmental Science & Technology,* **45**(4), 1435–1442.

Shin, H. M., Vieira, V. M., Ryan, P. B., Steenland, K., and Bartell, S. M. (2011b). Retrospective exposure estimation and predicted versus observed serum perfluorooctanoic acid concentrations for participants in the C8 Health Project. *Environmental Health Perspectives,* **119**(12), 1760–1765.

Steenland, K., Zhao, L., Winquist, A., and Parks, C. (2013). Ulcerative colitis and perfluorooctanoic acid (PFOA) in a highly exposed population of community residents and workers in the mid-Ohio valley. *Environmental Health Perspectives,* **121**(8), 900–905.

Tan, Y. M., Liao, K. H., Conolly, R. B., Blount, B. C., Mason, A. M., and Clewell, H. J. (2006). Use of a physiologically based pharmacokinetic model to identify exposures consistent with human biomonitoring data for chloroform. *Journal of Toxicology and Environmental Health, Part A,* **69**(18), 1727–1756.

Tokunaga, M., Land, C. E., Tokuoka, S., Nishimori, I., Soda, M., and Akiba, S. (1994). Incidence of female breast cancer among atomic bomb survivors, 1950-1985. *Radiation Research,* **138**(2), 209–223.

Verner, M. A., Ayotte, P., Muckle, G., Charbonneau, M., and Haddad, S. (2009). A physiologically based pharmacokinetic model for the assessment of infant exposure to persistent organic pollutants in epidemiologic studies. *Environmental Health Perspectives,* **117**(3), 481–487.

Verner, M. A., Charbonneau, M., Lopez-Carrillo, L., and Haddad, S. (2008). Physiologically based pharmacokinetic modeling of persistent organic pollutants for lifetime exposure assessment: A new tool in breast cancer epidemiologic studies. *Environmental Health Perspectives,* **116**(7), 886–892.

Verner, M. A., McDougall, R., and Johanson, G. (2012). Using population physiologically based pharmacokinetic modeling to determine optimal sampling times and to interpret biological exposure markers: The example of occupational exposure to styrene. *Toxicology Letters,* **213**(2), 299–304.

Vieira, V. M., Hoffman, K., Shin, H. M., Weinberg, J. M., Webster, T. F., Fletcher, T. (2013). Perfluorooctanoic acid exposure and cancer outcomes in a contaminated community: A geographic analysis. *Environmental Health Perspectives,* **121**(3), 318–323.

Watkins, D. J., Josson, J., Elston, B., Bartell, S. M., Shin, H. M., Vieira, V. M., et al. (2013). Exposure to perfluoroalkyl acids and markers of kidney function among children and adolescents living near a chemical plant. *Environmental Health Perspectives,* **121**(5), 625–630.

Wolff, M. S., Anderson, H. A., Britton, J. A., and Rothman, N. (2007). Pharmacokinetic variability and modern epidemiology—the example of dichlorodiphenyltrichloroethane, body mass index, and birth cohort. *Cancer Epidemiology, Biomarkers & Prevention*, **16**(10), 1925–1930.

Young, J. F., Luecke, R. H., Pearce, B. A., Lee, T., Ahn, H., Baek, S., et al. (2009). Human organ/tissue growth algorithms that include obese individuals and black/white population organ weight similarities from autopsy data. *Journal of Toxicology and Environmental Health, Part A*, **72**(8), 527–540.

9

DERMAL AND INADVERTENT INGESTION EXPOSURE ASSESSMENT

Sean Semple and John W. Cherrie

9.1 INTRODUCTION

Most epidemiological studies examining the relationship between exposure to hazardous substances and adverse health outcomes have focused on inhalation exposure. Although this is appropriate for many substances, and particularly for those materials having direct effects on the lung, failure to consider the importance of exposure and uptake of material deposited on the skin may lead to over or under-estimation of the risk. The skin is regarded as the largest organ of the body and plays an important role in protecting us from physical, biological, and chemical insults from our surrounding environment. With a surface area of approximately 2 m², the skin also provides an important route for many chemicals to enter the body. Many lipophillic chemicals can pass through the unbroken skin, whereas others can exert important health effects locally, for example, by causing irritation or sensitization of the skin.

Dermal exposure occurs in many settings, both in the workplace environment and in wider non-workplace settings such as home and leisure activities. Dermal contact with chemicals may be a result of immersion of hands and forearms in solutions such as degreasants, or may arise from the handling of objects or surfaces that have a thin covering layer of the contaminant. Dermal exposure can also arise from splashes or accidental spills directly onto the body or clothing, or may occur when spraying operations produce fine aerosols that are then deposited on the body. Non-occupational exposures may follow similar routes and may additionally include scenarios such as whole-body immersion (bathing), showering, washing, and direct intentional application of consumer products. Examples include consumer dermal exposure to disinfection by-products such as trihalomethanes present in the public water supply (see chapter 16) and application of cosmetics and sunscreens to our skin.

Solvents, pesticides, and trihalomethanes are some of the largest chemical groups for which dermal exposure and uptake has required assessment in any consideration of health effects. Xylene, toluene, benzene, and carbon tetrachloride are, or have been, among the most commonly used solvents and are used either as thinners, degreasants, additives to prevent icing, or as ingredients in protective coatings.

Trihalomethanes are formed during the chlorination of water and uptake occurs during showering, bathing, and swimming.

Particles do not pass though undamaged skin, although they may dissolve in sweat and the constituent substances may then permeate through the *stratum corneum* barrier (e.g., metal ions) (Stefaniak et al. 2014). Pesticides, which may be used in agriculture, in public spaces such as parks or golf courses, and in home or garden uses, are generally non-volatile and as a result dermal exposure can often be the primary exposure route with the uptake fraction received from inhalation being low (Wolfe et al. 1967). Pesticide compounds, such as lindane, paraquat, and carbaryl are, or have been, used extensively worldwide. In less-developed countries poor control and failure to use protective equipment during application and crop re-entry activities produces many pesticide poisoning deaths each year. In countries in which professional use of pesticides is not carefully controlled, there is a strong chance that pesticide residues are taken into the home on clothing or as contamination on the body (Thompson et al. 2014).

A wide variety of other materials such as mercury, tetraethyl lead additives in petrol, acrylates used in dentistry, or the nitroglycols used in explosives manufacture, are all hazardous substances that may be absorbed through the skin. There are a number of reviews of chemicals that pose dermal hazards (e.g., Grandjean 1990; Semple 2004).

Dermal exposure assessment is still a relatively immature science with only limited understanding of the exposure process and what biologically relevant exposure metrics should be used for measurement. The importance of the dermal route in chemical risk assessment and hence in epidemiology can be traced to work carried out by Durham and Wolfe (1962). Since then interest in dermal exposure and uptake has been pioneered by researchers investigating occupational exposure to pesticides (e.g., Davis et al. 1983; Brouwer et al. 1992). Pesticide exposure continues to be a major area of interest for dermal exposure research.

As part of the occupational exposure limit framework in many countries, chemicals that could contribute substantially to total body burden by uptake via the unbroken skin and cause serious systemic health effects may be assigned a skin notation; for example, the American Conference of Governmental Industrial Hygienists apply the "skin" note to over 200 substances (ACGIH 2012).

The relative importance of the dermal exposure route may have increased due to developments in control technology and improved hygiene measures, leading to substantial reductions in inhalation exposures over time. It has been argued that with decreasing airborne concentrations across many workplaces and environments, the relative proportion of total body uptake attributable to dermal exposure may have increased. There is, however, a counter argument that control of the airborne fraction will consequentially reduce the degree of surface contamination and hence dermal exposure levels, as demonstrated by Vermeulen et al. (2000) in a study of changes in dermal and inhalation exposure levels in the rubber industry.

Some chemicals, such as those in personal care products, are deliberately applied to the skin. Estimation of the amount of exposure in these circumstances is, at least in principal, more easily undertaken because the concentration of the substance of interest can be quantified in the product, plus the frequency and extent of use can be measured (e.g., Koniecki et al. 2011). However, there are few studies that actually quantify these data in user populations.

One of the main problems in developing dermal exposure assessment strategies has been the lack of a biologically relevant exposure metric. Just as with inhalation exposure, it is often unknown whether it is the cumulative amount of material absorbed, the average quantity over a certain reference period, or exposure peaks that produce ill-health effects. Further, sampling methods have developed in an unstandardized manner and often without thought to how the fraction sampled relates either to exposure or to uptake. For example, when measuring the quantity of material on the skin at the end of a work shift we may simply be sampling the fraction that has not already been absorbed, or lost to the environment, over the exposure period, therefore gaining little insight into the mass uptake and hence the dermal contribution. Scientific progress in this area continues to be slow.

The relationship between exposure and uptake is a complex one for the dermal pathway. Many studies focus on the quantity of material deposited on the workers' skin as the factor regulating dermal uptake. Although it is true that dermal absorption cannot physically exceed the mass of material deposited on the skin, it is the concentration of the substance that drives the diffusive process (Cherrie and Robertson 1995). The mass uptake of a chemical through the skin is not necessarily a constant proportion of the mass deposited on the skin, and in fact just measuring the mass of a contaminant on the skin may give very misleading information about the possible risks from skin exposure (Frasch et al. 2014).

Often dermal exposure is viewed purely in terms of the percutaneous uptake of chemicals. It is important, however, to remember that three types of chemical–skin interactions exist, and an understanding of these is vital to properly characterize the dermal exposure. First, the chemical may pass through the skin and contribute to the systemic load, thereby producing systemic health effects on target organs such as the liver, kidneys, and brain. Alternatively, the chemical can induce local effects ranging from irritation to burns and degradation of the barrier properties of the skin. Last, the chemical can evoke allergic skin reactions through complex immune-system responses that can subsequently trigger dermatitis or other allergic disease. There may often be interactions between these modes of action. For example, a chemical can irritate the skin surface thus leading to significant increases in percutaneous penetration of that, or other, chemicals. However, in each case the chemical must diffuse through the outer layers of the skin before any adverse health outcome is possible.

Finally, contamination on the hands is generally closely linked to inadvertent ingestion of hazardous substances through hand to mouth contacts. For some time it has been recognized that children may habitually place objects and their fingers in their mouth, but there is good evidence that to a lesser extent this is also the case for adults (Cherrie et al. 2006). It seems likely that this exposure pathway will add to the overall exposure arising from skin contamination.

9.2 UNDERSTANDING SKIN–CHEMICAL INTERACTIONS

Skin is made up of an outer layer, the stratum corneum or epidermis, a water-resistant layer of dead keratinocytes, and an inner layer termed the dermis. The dermis is composed of living cells and also the microstructure of the skin, including blood vessels, nerves, hair follicles, and sweat glands.

When chemicals deposit onto the thin liquid layer on the outer surface of the skin, a concentration gradient is generated across the "membrane" of the skin. Assuming that the concentration of the material within the body is less than that on the epidermal surface, a diffusive mass transfer will be set up with the rate of diffusion regulated by the chemical and physical properties of the material and skin. This passive movement from outer skin to the dermis and hence to blood capillaries is governed by Fick's Law, which states that at steady state, the rate of diffusion across a barrier will be directly proportional to the concentration gradient across that barrier.

The transfer of material across the skin can be characterized by two factors. The lag time is the time it takes from application on the skin surface until the material enters the receptor medium or blood supply. The duration of the lag time can range from minutes for chemicals such as the phenoxycarboxylic herbicides 2,4 D and MCPA, to many hours for materials such as the polycyclic aromatic hydrocarbon chrysene. After the lag time is complete we have steady-state conditions with linear increments in the quantity of material passing through the skin with time, provided there is sufficient contaminant to sustain diffusion. The steady-state diffusion flux (J) is measured in units of mass per unit area per time period ($mg/cm^2/hr$) and is directly proportional to the concentration gradient (C) across the skin membrane. For a given concentration gradient, the rate of flux is regulated by the permeability constant (K_p) measured in units of cm/h. Knowledge of K_p for a chemical is thus essential to be able to predict or estimate the quantity or fraction of a material deposited on the skin that will be absorbed into the body. Many methods of assessing dermal uptake rely on experimental determinations of absorbed fraction, in which the dermal absorbed dose is compared to the applied mass. Recent work has suggested that this commonly employed "infinite dose" approach may be suitable for chemicals with poor absorption characteristics but may overestimate uptake for materials that are more rapidly absorbed through the skin (Frasch et al. 2014).

Bowman and Maibach (2000) examined some of the factors that influence the flux of contaminant material across the skin. The region of the skin has been shown to have a large effect on the penetration of a given chemical. Differences of as much as 50-fold may be found between highly permeable areas such as scrotal skin when compared with less permeable tissue from the legs and abdomen. Occlusion, where applied material is covered to prevent evaporation from the surface of the skin, has also been shown to increase the quantity of absorbed material by up to five times. Gordon et al. (1998) demonstrated that human volunteers bathing in water containing chloroform, the main trihalomethane, absorbed some 30 times more chloroform at temperatures of 40°C when compared with 30°C. This is likely to be due to increased blood flow to the surface of the skin at higher temperatures. Recent work has additionally shown that just 30 seconds of topical application of heat can dramatically increase the uptake of pharmaceuticals (Oliveira et al. 2014). Experiments have also shown that irritated skin can have dermal uptake levels an order of magnitude greater than in nonirritated skin, and work by Fartasch and colleagues (2012) showed that skin that has been regularly occluded or involved in wet-handling tasks suffers from poorer barrier function when an irritant material is then applied. Box 9.1 lists a number of important factors that influence the uptake of chemicals through the skin.

Various groups (e.g., Sartorelli et al. 1998; Wilkinson and Williams 2001) have used simple diffusion cells to calculate the rate of flux across the skin for a variety of solvents, polycyclic aromatic hydrocarbons, organophosphorus insecticides, and phenoxy-carboxylic herbicides. Interlaboratory studies have shown that flux rates determined in this way are reasonably robust, with human variability in skin likely to be responsible for most of the differences found (van de Sandt et al. 2004). Patel and Cronin (2001) showed that the permeability of compounds may be modeled using quantitative structure–activity relationship techniques. This method employs correlation techniques to identify physicochemical properties such as the octanol/water partition coefficient (K_{ow}), the molecular weight, and the water solubility of the material that may be closely related to the permeability. Recent work (Riviere & Brooks 2011) has shown that such models are closely associated with the skin type used to generate the base data.

Bunge and Ley (2002) have suggested that in some circumstances solids may penetrate the skin more easily than aqueous solutions, but the material must generally first enter a solution phase by mixing with the sweat and sebum layer on the

---

Box 9.1 Factors Influencing the Uptake of Chemicals Through the Skin

Concentration

Duration

Surface area

Skin thickness

Skin location

Skin condition

Humidity

Temperature

Vehicle effects

Presence of sweat

Particle size (particularly when particles are in the nano-size range)

Molecular weight

Permeability co-efficient

skin. Kezic et al. (2002) have demonstrated that in some circumstances more dilute solvents may find it easier to transfer across the skin than concentrated solutions. This illustrates that our current understanding that diffusion across the skin is directly proportional to the concentration of material is a simplification, and the reality may be more complex. There is still a long way to go in fully understanding the thermodynamic activity of the diffusion process of many mixtures of chemicals through skin. Differences in the experimental setup, application methods, and measurement techniques make it difficult to compare findings across groups working in the field of percutaneous penetration, and there is a need for a standardized experimental protocol that will allow the identification of vehicle, anatomical location, and other physical effects, on the rate of flux across the skin.

The absorption of nanoparticles through the skin and the possible adverse health effects that this may produce are currently subject to considerable debate. Watkinson and colleagues (2013) examined sunblock preparations and suggested that intact nanoparticles do not penetrate the stratum corneum. A recent literature review concluded "that absorption of nanoparticles through the skin is possible although occurs to a very low degree and that the level of penetration, depending on chemistry and experimental conditions, may be greater than for larger particles" (Poland et al. 2013).

9.3 MEASURING DERMAL EXPOSURE

9.3.1 What to Measure

There are four key elements that are important in measuring dermal exposure: exposure intensity, surface area exposed, duration, and frequency of exposure. Exposure intensity is most often measured as a mass of material deposited over a given area. However, as described earlier, the parameter driving diffusion and hence uptake is the concentration of the material on the skin surface, and so any true measure of exposure intensity should be expressed in terms of skin surface concentration. Unfortunately no accepted sampling methods to measure concentration exist and instead the mass per unit area is often used as a surrogate. The suitability of mass as a surrogate for concentration differs in different exposure scenarios, especially between the "finite dose" situations experienced in many environmental measurements and the "infinite dose" exposure events often characteristic of occupational settings. Mass may also be an unsuitable surrogate in situations in which the concentration of the contaminant changes during the measurement period, as for example, occurs when pesticides are diluted before use. Measurement of the dermal exposure intensity is often divided into "potential exposure," the amount of material that is deposited on an individual's clothing and gloves; and "actual exposure," the amount of material that comes into contact with the skin.

The second element necessary to characterize dermal exposure is the surface area exposed. This can be assessed by direct visualization techniques (see later). The surface area exposed is likely to be subject to high degrees of day-to-day, between-subject, and anatomical variation. Wassenius et al. (1998) carried out a study to examine the variability of skin exposure of machine operators exposed to cutting fluids. Using video recording of work tasks and data on fluid evaporation times, this paper describes how workers' hands were wet for anything from 0% to 100% of the job time. Tasks with short cycle times were more likely to have a higher degree of relative wet time but overall the degree of skin exposure was shown to be highly variable and independent of machine type or task process. A study of dermal exposure during spray painting (Lansink et al. 1997) demonstrated that paint over-spray is not uniformly deposited over the body. More than 50% of the total mass of dermal exposure was to the lower legs and less than 3% to the hands. The study also found that only approximately 10% of the worker's coverall surface was covered with paint. The high degree of variation in terms of anatomical location and the amount of surface area covered will play an important role in determining the degree of systemic uptake of the chemical.

The last important parameter required is a measure of the duration and frequency of the exposure event. The duration of contact may be of little importance if the material remains on the skin or clothing for a much longer period thereafter. In these situations the time until removal (e.g., by washing, evaporation, or uptake) may be the controlling factor. However, the duration and frequency of contact may play a larger role, particularly when the rate of evaporation or uptake is high. It is important that the type and frequency of sampling are chosen to reflect these factors.

Dermal exposure assessment can be achieved by either direct physical measurement of deposited material, indirect methods such as visualization and bio-monitoring, or by modeling using statistical or deterministic procedures. All have advantages and disadvantages in terms of accuracy, practical considerations, expense, and what they actually tell us about dermal exposure. None of the methods are suitable for all chemical types and exposure scenarios and many suffer from a lack of standardized methodologies. Direct measurement can be further divided into surrogate skin methods, for example, based on patches of adsorbent material, and removal techniques in which the residual contaminant on the skin is generally washed or wiped from the skin surface.

9.3.2 Surrogate Skin Techniques

Surrogate skin includes whole-body suits and absorbent patch sampling. By using suits or patches attached to the outside of the body, both techniques aim to sample the total amount of the substance that would be deposited on the skin or clothing. This is often described as potential dermal exposure. Whole-body suits cover the entire body surface and may be augmented with a hat or hood for the head and gloves for the hands. They can be analyzed in terms of body part to identify those anatomical regions receiving greatest exposure. Patches are worn at various representative locations on the body, with the mass collected on each patch being extrapolated depending on the patch size relative to the size of the body area being sampled. Sampling protocols, such as the World Health Organization method (WHO 1982) and the Organisation for Economic Co-operation and Development guidelines (OECD 1997) for patch sampling, vary in terms of the number of patches, their location, size, and sampling material. Even the size of each anatomical region represented by similarly placed patches differs between protocols.

One of the primary weaknesses of patch sampling is the potential introduction of large errors when the exposure is non-uniform. If a patch for a given body area is subject to a splash or spill, the method will overestimate the potential dermal exposure for that body area. The converse is also true when proportionally less is deposited on the patch compared with the surrounding area. Work by Tannahill et al. (1996) compared exposure measurements made by whole-body sampling with those from patch sampling. In general there was a linear relationship between the two methods, although the authors note that the accuracy of the patch method increased with increasing numbers of patches. In summary, when exposure is likely to be non-uniform the use and interpretation of patch sampling should be undertaken with caution.

Other difficulties with patch sampling include patch overloading and problems with detachment in highly active work situations or confined environments. Careful consideration of the quantity of chemical likely to be deposited and the absorption capabilities of the patch material should take place prior to sampling. Close observation of subjects may be required to replace patches that appear overloaded or become detached during sampling.

The use of whole-body suits, typically lightweight cotton overalls, is often used to sample potential dermal exposure among spray painters and pesticide applicators, and has been used to collect dermal exposure data across a wide variety of exposure scenarios (van Hemmen 2002). Other investigators have also used similar suits worn by children and toddlers to investigate exposure to pesticide residues in nurseries (Cohen Hubal et al. 2000).

The "reservoir" effects of clothing may also introduce errors with surrogate skin measurements. Chemicals may soak into overalls or clothing and then slowly transfer to the patch or whole-body suit over time. Direct dermal exposure may occur for only a short period of the working day, but contaminated or wet clothing is often worn by workers for the remainder of the shift. In such situations interior patches or suits removed after the dermal exposure event would be likely to underestimate the true exposure.

Two other aspects of surrogate skin sampling are likely to introduce error into the exposure assessment process. First, absorbent materials such as cotton will not behave in the same manner as skin. Fluid applied to the skin will take one of three routes. It may run off the skin, as is the case with the majority of a liquid deposited after a splash, spill, or immersion event. Alternatively, the liquid may evaporate from the warm skin surface into the surrounding air, or it may be absorbed into the stratum corneum by diffusive processes. Cotton and other similar sampling materials are more likely to absorb fluids than real skin and also the fluid is less likely to evaporate due to lower surface temperatures. Hence surrogate skin methods are likely to overestimate the amount of a chemical available for uptake through the skin. Second, and in common with most dermal measurement techniques, surrogate skin sampling measures the mass of the contaminant instead of the concentration. Although mass is a useful measure and is often used as a surrogate of concentration, the mass of material deposited on the skin in occupational settings is likely to far exceed the mass uptake.

9.3.3 Removal Techniques

Removal techniques can be divided into wiping, washing, or tape stripping. All of these methods aim to collect the quantity of the material present on the surface of the skin or, in the case of tape stripping, bound to the outer layer of the stratum corneum. Wiping may be carried out dry, or with absorbent material soaked in water, alcohol, or any other appropriate solvent. Wipes are usually used on the hands but may be employed to measure any area of the skin. Templates are commonly used to ensure that only a predetermined skin area is wiped. No standardized protocol exists describing the number of wipes or the amount of force that should be applied when collecting wipe samples and it is thus difficult to compare results obtained across studies. However, these techniques are often used because of their apparent simplicity; for example, Kim et al. (2013) used hand washing as part of an assessment of the assessment of health risks from exposure to chlorpyrifos and dichlorvos in children at childcare facilities.

Hand-washing methods follow similar principles with the hand being placed in a sealed bag containing a volume of water or other solvent and vigorous shaking used to remove the chemical from the surface of the skin. Brouwer et al. (2000) found that six different wipe sampling strategies, each with a variety of skin loadings, were shown to have sampling efficiencies ranging from 41% to 104% with standard deviations between 6% and 28%, indicating high degrees of variability. Similar variation in sampling efficiencies were evident for hand-wash sampling studies with four methods across 10 pesticides at a range of skin loadings, giving mean wash efficiencies from 23% to 96%.

Tape stripping removes the outermost layer or layers of the stratum corneum of the skin with the aim of quantifying compounds present in the skin. This has been used extensively for the assessment of exposure to a range of chemicals (e.g., Nylander-French 2000; Kammer et al. 2011), including acrylates, jet fuel, polycyclic aromatic hydrocarbons, and epoxy components. These methods are clearly more invasive than surrogate skin and other removal techniques and suffer from error introduced by the lack of a method to standardize measurements to the quantity of stratum corneum cells removed, although work by Boeniger and Nylander-French (2002) aims to overcome this problem. Stripping does, however, give an indication of the amount of a substance that has already been absorbed into the skin, something that both wipe and washing methods will fail to record.

9.3.4 Visualization Methods

Deposition of material onto the clothing and skin can also be assessed using direct visualization techniques. Fluorescent tracers can be added to the bulk solution of the liquid under study and the deposition of this fluid may then be visualized using ultraviolet light. This method was initially developed by Fenske et al. (1986) and later developed by Roff in 1994 to produce a dodecahedral illumination system (fluorescent interactive video exposure system—FIVES). Later, a similar video imaging technique to assess dermal exposure (VITAE) was employed by Bierman et al. (1998) to measure the exposure of agricultural workers to pesticides. By calibrating image analysis software to fluorescent intensity based on the mass per unit area, these systems are able to quantify total-body exposure at the point of image acquisition, and to also measure the skin surface area exposed, although this is often not reported. However, the system requires careful calibration and the quantity of tracer added to the bulk solution must also be closely regulated to ensure that interpretable images are produced. Issues such as timing of "sampling" to prevent saturation of the image are similar to those relevant to surrogate skin sampling. Practical difficulties also exist in terms of expense, time to carry out the measurement, the acceptability of adding fluorescent tracers to the material being applied, and binding of the tracer to the skin preventing the same worker being measured on consecutive days.

9.3.5 Biomonitoring

Biomonitoring of blood, breath, or urine for the target substance or a metabolite (see chapter 6) may also be employed to measure the passage of chemicals through the skin and therefore, indirectly, the degree of dermal exposure (e.g., for trihalomethane uptake). For biomonitoring to be effective the pharmacokinetics of the material must be well understood and exposure from other routes such as inhalation or ingestion should be negligible (see chapter 8). For this reason biomonitoring remains a research tool rather than a methodology used in the field of dermal exposure assessment, although it is routinely used to assess total exposure. Chamber experiments in which workers' skin is exposed to liquids (Kezic et al. 2001) or high concentrations of vapor (Brooke et al. 1998) while they are supplied with uncontaminated air to breathe, allow the measurement of the uptake of chemicals through the skin.

A recent example of the use of biological monitoring in investigating the contribution of dermal exposure to ethylene oxide during an accidental release was reported by Boogaard et al. (2014). They showed that under very high concentrations of ethylene oxide (>1000 ppm), workers wearing breathing apparatus were adequately protected from inhalation exposure risks (the inhalation occupational exposure limit for ethylene oxide is 0.5 ppm, averaged over 8 hours). However, dermal uptake, as estimated from pharmacokinetic models and from biological monitoring of workers exposed during an incident, showed that in such circumstances dermal uptake may become the leading exposure route and may result in unacceptable exposure.

9.3.6 Modeling

Measuring techniques are becoming increasingly sophisticated and standardized, and advances in this field will allow greater collection of dermal exposure data across a range of industries, processes, and environmental conditions. Although this is good news for future epidemiological studies that wish to incorporate the influence of dermal exposure on the risk of health effects, the situation for retrospective studies is not so positive. Few good-quality measurements of dermal exposure exist, and those that have been gathered have produced exposure metrics of questionable value.

As a result, modeling dermal exposure has been the focus of considerable work. The estimation and assessment of substance exposure (EASE) system developed by the UK HSE and a similar technique by the US EPA (Mulhausen and Damiano 1998) are generic models primarily used for risk assessment purposes. These procedures model likely exposure levels from information on process type and chemical used, but categorize exposure into broad ranges and so are of limited use. Initial validation work by Hughson and Cherrie (2001) has demonstrated that EASE tends to overestimate dermal exposures by up to two orders of magnitude. Additionally, from an epidemiological standpoint, it is of little value to evaluate the mass or volume of a substance that is deposited on the worker without progressing to determine the quantity absorbed into the systemic circulation. Only by estimating both deposition and uptake through the skin can we provide a "biologically relevant" assessment of the hazard that is likely to be related to any systemic ill-health effect.

The UK HSE used a database of dermal exposure measurements to produce an empirical model and indicative distributions for a range of tasks from the pesticide and biocide application sector (Phillips and Garrod 2000). This work created a basic job-exposure matrix with four levels of potential dermal exposure and three types of profiles, to reflect the degree of variability across different tasks. Deterministic modeling has also been developed. Again, these models tend to be process specific. Brouwer et al. (2001) examined the parameters controlling the deposition of paint spray aerosol onto painters' skin and clothing. The model produced a good correlation between estimated and measured exposures.

The development of the conceptual model by Schneider et al. (1999) has provided a structured framework to characterize and analyse exposure scenarios by dividing them into a range of sources, compartments, and transport processes. This model has been further developed (Gorman Ng et al. 2012) to take account of the interaction between dermal and ingestion exposure routes as illustrated in Figure 9.1. In summary, the model focuses on sources that may emit into the work environment via four pathways, which link the source of exposure from the process or activity being undertaken to the person. Sources emit a mass of contaminant material to a number of compartments: the air compartment; surfaces in the environment; the outside or inside of the worker's clothing; or to the worker's skin (Hands and Arms Layer). From there it may transfer to the peri-oral area around the nose and mouth or directly to the oral cavity where ingestion may take place. Each compartment can exchange contaminant substances with other compartments.

Emission (E) to air may be by evaporation, spraying, grinding, or some other activity. Emission to the other compartments can occur by splashing, spilling, spraying, or other mechanisms. Compartments may be defined by the mass and concentration of contaminant, the area of the compartment covered by the material, or in the case of the air compartment, its volume. The contaminant may "flow" in or out of each compartment, giving rise to increases or decreases in mass therein. For example, material may be *lost* (L) from the surface contamination layer to the air, to the outer or inner clothing layer, or the skin contamination layer. In addition, there may be *deposition* (Dp) from the air to surfaces, or *transfer* (T) from the surface contamination layer to the skin contamination layer or the outer clothing layer. Additionally, contaminant in the oral cavity may be *swallowed* (Sw) and ingested.

Transfer or removal from surfaces to the skin contamination layer may be mediated by contact between the worker's body and the surface. The direction of the contaminant transfer will depend on whether there is more available contamination on the skin or the surface, the wetness of the hand, the properties of the surface, and many other factors.

In the conceptual model, clothing is recognized as an important protective measure for people handling hazardous substances. It is described by two compartments with a barrier layer that restricts the passage of substances to the skin. A substance can either permeate from the outer clothing layer (a diffusion process) or penetrate (bulk flow) to the inner layer, or bypass the clothing and be transferred directly to the skin contamination layer.

In each compartment there are two other processes that may operate: *decontamination* (D) and *redistribution* (Rd). Decontamination, for example, by washing hands, results in the loss of some of the contaminant from the system. Redistribution is the process of modifying the pattern of contamination within a compartment, for example, by transferring some contaminant from one area of the body to another, perhaps by touching the face with dirty hands. Redistribution does not change the mass in a compartment but may alter the area covered or the contaminant concentration.

Other generic models for the estimation of dermal exposure include DREAM for occupational exposure and CONSEXPO for consumer product exposure events. DREAM (van-Wendel-de-Joode et al. 2003) is a new method for semi-quantitative dermal exposure assessment that may prove useful in epidemiology. The detailed questionnaire characterizes tasks and produces estimates of dermal exposure levels using the conceptual model as a framework and has

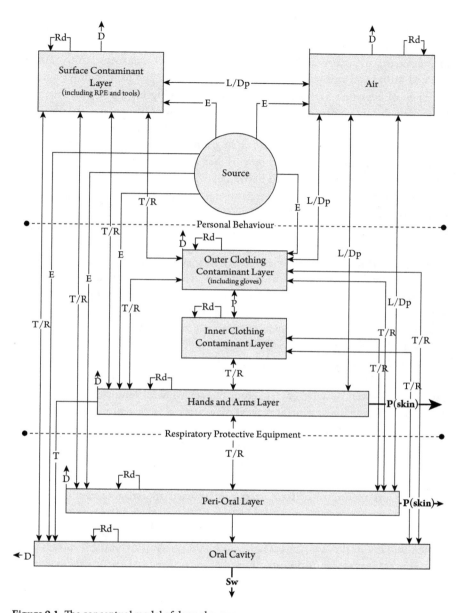

Figure 9.1 The conceptual model of dermal exposure.
For a detailed description refer to Schneider, T., Vermeulen, R., Brouwer, D., Cherrie, J., Kromhout, H., and Fogh, C. (1999). A conceptual model for assessment of dermal exposure. *Occupational and Environmental Medicine*, **56**, 765–773; and Gorman, Ng M, Semple, S., Cherrie, J. W., Christopher, Y., Northage, C., Tielemans, E., et al. (2012). The relationship between inadvertent ingestion and dermal exposure pathways: A new integrated conceptual model and a database of dermal and oral transfer efficiencies. *Annals of Occupational Hygiene*, **56**(9), 1000–1012.

been used to successfully assess exposure among road paving and mastic crews (Agostini et al. 2011). DREAM also provides information on the best methods of measuring exposure and also helps target control measures. CONSEXPO (RIVM 2001) is a software-based model that enables the user to enter data on the type of exposure scenario and the chemical being used and can then provide likely dermal exposure and uptake values. Options for mean and worst-case (95th percentile) predictions are given. CONSEXPO aims to provide full multiroute exposure and uptake data and can be used to aggregate dermal, inhalation, and ingestion exposures. Modeling work has also been carried out to estimate children's residential exposure to pesticides (Zartarian et al. 2000) using observations of typical activity patterns, and data on post-application time period and pesticide application method. The ECETOC Targeted Risk Assessment can be applied to estimate the dermal exposure to consumer products (Delmaar et al. 2013).

RISKOFDERM (Warren et al. 2006) was a large research project to bring together dermal exposure measurements and associated contextual information. This allowed modeling of dermal exposure for dermal exposure operation units, essentially categories of task type that are grouped by exposure determinant and measured levels. Some job-exposure matrices or task-exposure matrices have also been established to provide broad estimates of potential dermal exposure associated with particular tasks. One example of this is TEMPEST—the Task Exposure Matrix for PESTicide exposure in Scotland. This work by Dick and colleagues (2010) used seven decades of data from interviews with long-service employees coupled with estimates made by a group of occupational hygienists to characterise the likely probability and intensity of dermal and inhalation exposure to pesticides during 81 common task types across agricultural and non-agricultural sectors. The authors suggest that the method could be used for epidemiological studies examining the effect of pesticides on health.

There are a number of tools that can be used to estimate dermal absorption for a given exposure event. SkinPerm (Tibaldi et al. 2014) uses quantitative structure–activity relationships to allow the user to assess the potential for dermal uptake in three occupational exposure scenarios including a splash on to bare skin, repeated deposition of a pure liquid to skin, and the uptake produced by exposure to an airborne vapor. This model operates in Microsoft Excel and requires the user to input details of the mass of material deposited on the skin, the duration, and the area of skin exposed. The Excel spreadsheet and associated manual can be freely downloaded from the American Industrial Hygiene Association website (https://www.aiha.org/get-involved/VolunteerGroups/Pages/Exposure-Assessment-Strategies-Committee.aspx).

The skin permeation calculator is available from the US National Institute of Occupational Safety & Health. This online tool (http://www.cdc.gov/niosh/topics/skin/skinPermCalc.html) allows the user to determine the permeation co-efficient for a given chemical within a particular vehicle or mixture. It allows the user to select one of three different datasets and by inputting details of the chemical molecular weight and the octanol–water partition co-efficient, an estimate of the concentration-dependent flux or transfer ability of the chemical through the skin is generated.

9.4 INADVERTENT INGESTION

The mass of material absorbed in to the body through the skin may, under certain conditions, be dwarfed by the mass that is absorbed through inadvertent ingestion due to transfer of contamination from hands and objects to the oral cavity where it is then swallowed. This may be especially true for materials such as heavy metals like lead or cadmium that are poorly absorbed across an intact skin barrier. Cherrie et al. (2006) estimated that inadvertent ingestion may present a nontrivial route of exposure for up to 15% of all workers in the United Kingdom. Consumer exposure to metals in cosmetics is likely to be of even greater importance (Liu et al. 2013).

Dermal and ingestion exposure are often closely related in occupational settings and recent work has brought together new (Gorman Ng et al. 2012) and previously published data on the transfer of materials from surfaces to hands and from hands to the peri-oral area. This database is likely to be of considerable use to those involved in estimating both dermal and ingestion exposures. The Ingestion Exposure Assessment Tool draws upon much of these data together with the conceptual model of dermal exposure to provide-a predictive tool for estimating exposure to liquids, solids and dusts by inadvertent ingestion (http://www.iom-world.org/research/research-expertise/exposure-assessment/ingestion-exposure-assessment-tool/).

9.5 EFFECT OF PERSONAL PROTECTIVE EQUIPMENT

The use of protective clothing and gloves to control dermal exposure is widespread in occupational and non-occupational settings. Most protective clothing, such as overalls, is employed to keep the person relatively clean or prevent normal clothes from becoming contaminated rather than any scientific principle of reducing dermal exposure to or uptake of the chemicals in use. As a result gloves and protective clothing are rarely matched to the exposure scenario and are often poorly managed in workplace settings in terms of cleaning, provision of replacements, or checking when integrity is breached. In addition, although there are a variety of standards for testing protective clothing for professional use (e.g., BSI 2003), none of these tests take into account how the clothing or gloves will perform in workplace conditions. Testing does not usually include repeated exposures, temperature extremes, mechanical effects from stretching, or the effects of chemical mixtures. Work by El-Ayouby et al. (2002) showed that repeated use and decontamination, using alcohol, of nitrile and butyl gloves produced compromised chemical resistance to solvents after only one or two cycles.

Earlier work by Creely and Cherrie (2001) used cotton gloves to assess the effectiveness of a variety of protective glove types when used in a simulated work activity applying a pesticide. By comparing outer glove or "potential exposure" values with inner glove "actual dermal exposure" levels in a method similar to that employed for respiratory protective equipment, this study was able to derive "protection factors" for the gloves used. Geometric mean protection factors between 96 and 470 were reported for three different types of glove. For all glove types protection factors were lowest when workers were classified as "messy" or when the spray equipment was noted to leak. Similar work by Soutar et al. (2000) examined the effectiveness of three different types of protective overalls when spraying pesticides for timber preservation. Penetration of protective clothing was calculated using an inner sampling suit to measure how much material would normally be transferred to the skin. Inner contamination levels ranged from 0% to 36% of the outside exposure quantity. A number of studies have compared dermal exposure measurements made inside and outside protective coveralls (e.g., Tsakirakis et al. 2014), and these generally show a high level of protection. However, studies that have relied on biological monitoring methods to assess the effectiveness of protective clothing have tended to show lower levels of protection. For example, Scheepers and colleagues (2009) studied exposures of dermatology nurses while they were applying ointments containing polycyclic aromatic hydrocarbons, with the aim of evaluating the effectiveness of improved skin protection systems. Nurses performed treatments with loose-fit polyethylene gloves followed by a second treatment without gloves. The use of gloves produced a median reduction of 51% in the excretion of 1-hydroxypyrene in urine compared to not wearing gloves (skin contamination was not measured in this part of the study). They then tested the use of vinyl gloves and Tyvek sleeves, which showed a 97% reduction in skin contamination with pyrene and benzo(a)pyrene but only lowered urinary excretion of 1-hydroxypyrene by 57% compared to no protection.

Although use of protective equipment may help reduce dermal exposure when selected and used properly, there are many situations in which protective overalls or gloves may actually increase the exposure and uptake of chemicals through the skin. First, it may provide the user with a false sense of security and cause him or her to undertake exposure behaviors that they would not previously have carried out. This may be particularly problematic if the gloves or clothing have inadequate resistance to the contaminant substance. Second, there is the problem of wet overalls or gloves acting as a reservoir for contamination and thereby extending the duration of exposure (e.g., Li et al. 2011). Finally, occlusion may also prevent loss of a fluid that might normally evaporate from the skin and so increase the substance available for uptake. It has been argued that personal protective equipment is a poor way of managing dermal exposure (Ogden, 2010).

9.6 USE OF DERMAL MEASUREMENT AND MODELS IN EPIDEMIOLOGY

The explicit consideration of the dermal route of exposure is still rare in epidemiological studies examining the potential health effects of chemicals. A review of the literature indicates that even in studies investigating pesticide exposure, in which in most scenarios the majority of the internalized dose will be from the dermal route, there are few cases in which dermal exposure assessment takes place.

Most studies of pesticide exposure use simple exposure classification methods such as ever/never exposed. These data are either obtained by questionnaire or by simple job-exposure matrices (JEMs) or, in the case of non-occupational exposure, by use of geographical information systems linking residence to records of local pesticide use (Brody et al. 2002). Other methods use semi-quantitative surrogates of "total exposure" such as the number of years working in agricultural industries. More advanced indices may factor in data linked to the frequency and duration of exposure by using the number of hectares on which pesticide was applied, the number of animals treated, or the mass/volume of pesticide mixed.

London and Myers (1998) developed a crop- and job-specific JEM for retrospective assessment of long-term exposure in a study of the neurotoxic effects of organophosphates (OPs). This expert-based system allows estimation of cumulative lifetime exposure measured in kilograms of organophosphate. This study was also able to demonstrate that the generated index was significantly associated with erythrocyte cholinesterase concentrations (a biological effect marker of OP exposure) among a cohort of farmers. Earlier work by Verberk et al. (1990) used a number of work-related parameters such as the pesticide application method, application rate, the use of protective equipment, and the like to generate an exposure index. This general index considered both dermal and inhalation exposure elements and was used to study the health effects of pesticides in the agricultural sector in the Netherlands.

Other studies have examined the dermal exposure of farmers involved in sheep dipping operations. The use of OP-based dips has been implicated in the onset of a range of illnesses such as chronic fatigue syndrome (CFS). It is believed that a significant proportion of the biological dose received during sheep dipping comes via the dermal route. Interestingly, the study by Sewell et al. (1999) suggested that the primary determinant of exposure was handling or mixing sheep dip concentrate. These findings agree with the model of dermal uptake described by Cherrie and Robertson (1995), which describes concentration as the most important factor driving diffusion through the skin.

Tahmaz et al. (2003) also investigated CFS among farmers exposed to OP-based sheep dips. This study developed and applied a new dermal exposure metric to estimate lifetime exposure. This metric was based on the product of concentration, exposure duration, and area of skin exposed. Using questionnaire data on how often farmers carried out sheep dipping, the frequency of contact with concentrate and dilute dip and the use of protective equipment (gloves, overalls, and visors), this work demonstrated that those with higher assessed exposure to OP pesticides reported more symptoms consistent with CFS.

Determination of dermal exposure and uptake in other occupational epidemiological studies is even less common. Dick et al. (2000) and Chen et al. (2002) examined the neurological and neuropsychological effects of solvent use among painters using quantitative measures of lifetime and average annual solvent exposure that were generated using both inhalation and dermal exposure models. The dermal element utilized a predictive model developed by Brouwer et al. (2001) to estimate the amount of paint that would be deposited on a spray painter depending on process and environmental conditions. The degree of dermal uptake was then derived using further modeling methods (Semple et al. 2001) and the fraction of internalized dose received by the dermal route converted to an airborne equivalent value. This work showed that in some working conditions described by painters, in which respiratory protective equipment was used and heat and humidity caused men to wear t-shirts, that the dermal route could provide the majority of absorbed solvent. More typically, however, the dermal route was found to contribute less than 10% of total-body solvent in most painting conditions.

9.7 THE FUTURE

Dermal exposure assessment is clearly of importance in understanding the risk posed by many chemicals. Until recently, assessment of dermal exposure for the purposes of epidemiological investigation has been rare, with few studies employing even simple categorical exposure metrics. There is now a better understanding of the parameters controlling exposure and uptake, and there is a realization of the importance of measuring exposure intensity and the area of skin exposed, together with exposure duration and frequency. For prospective studies there are a range of methods capable of delivering data on these factors, and attempts are being made to build up databases of dermal exposure measurements classified by industry, job, and task. We have also recognized the need to record contextual data about the measurement conditions, skin condition, and the vehicle the substance is contained within, and obtain measures of the exposure variability when gathering dermal exposure data. Advances in modeling, particularly the conceptual model proposed by Schneider et al. (1999) and developed by Gorman Ng et al. (2012), have increased our understanding of how to estimate dermal and inadvertent ingestion exposure patterns, and will prove useful for retrospective assessment purposes. Biological monitoring using blood or urine samples may offer increasing opportunities for assessment of exposure by all routes, including via skin uptake.

Several important challenges remain if we are to further improve the process of dermal exposure assessment. Better methods are still needed for measuring the concentration of material deposited on the skin rather than just mass. Pilot work presented by Lindsay et al. (2006) on a new dermal sampler to measure solvent concentration on the skin holds promise but has yet to be developed. Appropriate exposure metrics are also be required. A metric that considers area exposed, concentration, and duration of exposure will more easily allow exposure to be linked directly to the potential uptake. Additionally, there may be a need for a different type of metric when examining local effects. For example, in the case of irritant dermatitis, the concentration of the material may not be so important and the cyclical nature of "wettedness" and the irritancy potential of the material may be the driving factors in development of dermatitis. Devices such as the prototype wet-work sampler (Cherrie et al. 2007) hold promise in quantifying risk of dermatitis. There is also evidence that the ingestion route may play a significant role in exposure to materials such as pesticides, pharmaceuticals, and heavy metals using a complex path from air to skin to mouth. Work to find methods of controlling the behavioral determinants of hand or object to mouth activity will be important in controlling this pathway, and it is likely that better systems for controlling dermal exposure will assist in limiting ingestion uptake.

Despite these gaps in our knowledge, the progress made in dermal exposure assessment over the past 30 years has been remarkable. The main parameters that should be measured to assess dermal uptake have been identified and there are many good-quality generic and process-specific models that can be used to identify the factors likely to influence potential and actual dermal exposure levels that may be used in epidemiological studies. Even if dermal exposure assessment cannot be carried out on the whole population in an epidemiological study, models can be built in a subpopulation and applied to the whole population (see chapter 5). Epidemiological investigations of a wide variety of skin penetrating substances, from solvents to pesticides, should now be able to incorporate detailed quantitative evaluations of dermal exposure and uptake.

REFERENCES

ACGIH. (2012). *Threshold limit values for chemical substances and physical agents and biological exposure indices.* American Conference of Governmental Industrial Hygienists. Cincinnati, OH.

Agostini, M., Fransman, W., De Vocht, F., Van Wendel de Joode, B., and Kromhout, H. (2011). Assessment of dermal exposure to bitumen condensate among road paving and mastic crews with an observational method. *Annals of Occupational Hygiene, 55,* 578–590.

Bierman, E., Brouwer, D., and van Hemmen, J. (1998). Implementation and evaluation of the fluorescent tracer technique in greenhouse exposure studies. *Annals of Occupational Hygiene, 42,* 467–475.

Boeniger, M., and Nylander-French, L. (2002). Comparison of three methods for determining removal of stratum corneum using adhesive tape strips. Presented at the International Conference on Occupational and Environmental Exposure of Skin to Chemicals: Science and Policy. September 8–11, 2002, Washington, DC.

Boogaard, P. J., van Puijvelde, M. J. P., and Urbanus, J. H. (2014). Biological monitoring to assess dermal exposure to ethylene oxide vapours during an incidental release. *Toxicology Letters, 231*(3), 387–390. doi: 10.1016/j.toxlet.2014.05.014

Bowman, A., and Maibach, H. (2000). Percutaneous absorption of organic solvents. *International Journal of Occupational and Environmental Health*, **6**, 93–95.

Brody, J., Swartz, C., Kennedy, T., and Rudel, R. (2002). Historical pesticide exposure assessment using a geographical information system and self-report in a breast cancer study. *Epidemiology*, **13**, 726.

Brooke, I., Cocker, J., Delic, J., Payne, M., Jones, K., Gregg, N., and Dyne, D. (1998). Dermal uptake of solvents from the vapour phase: An experimental study in humans. *Annals of Occupational Hygiene*, **42**, 531–540.

Brouwer, D., Boeniger, M., and van Hemmen, J. (2000). Hand wash and manual skin wipes. *Annals of Occupational Hygiene*, **44**, 501–510.

Brouwer, D., Brouwer, E., and van Hemmen, J. (1992). Assessment of dermal and inhalation exposure to zaneb/maneb in the cultivation of flower bulbs. *Annals of Occupational Hygiene*, **36**, 373–384.

Brouwer, D., Semple, S., Marquart, J., and Cherrie, J. (2001). A dermal model for spray painters. Part I: Subjective exposure modelling of spray paint deposition. *Annals of Occupational Hygiene*, **45**, 15–23.

BSI. (2003). Protective gloves against chemicals and microorganisms. Determination of resistance to permeation to chemicals. British Standards Institution, London (BS EN 374-3:2003).

Bunge, A. and Ley, E. (2002). Dermal exposure to powdered solids and aqueous solutions: are the risks different? Presented at the International Conference on Occupational and Environmental Exposure of Skin to Chemicals: Science and Policy. September 8–11, 2002. Washington, DC.

Chen, R., Dick, F., Semple, S., Seaton, A., and Walker, L. (2002). Exposure to organic solvents and personality. *Occupational and Environmental Medicine*, **58**, 14–18.

Cherrie, J. W, Apsley, A., and Semple, S. (2007). A new sampler to assess dermal exposure during wet working. *Annals of Occupational Hygiene*, **51**(1), 13–18

Cherrie, J. W., and Robertson, A. (1995). Biologically relevant assessment of dermal exposure. *Annals of Occupational Hygiene*, **39**, 387–392.

Cherrie, J. W., Semple, S., Christopher, Y., Saleem, A., Hughson, G. W., and Philips, A. (2006). How important is inadvertent ingestion of hazardous substances at work? *Annals of Occupational Hygiene*, **50**(7), 693–704.

Cohen Hubal, E., Sheldon, L., Burke, J., McCurdy, T., Beryy, M., Rigas, M., et al. (2000). Children's exposure assessment: a review of factors influencing children's exposure, and the data available to characterize and assess that exposure. *Environmental Health Perspectives*, **108**, 475–486.

Creely, K., and Cherrie, J. (2001). A novel method of assessing the effectiveness of protective gloves-results from a pilot study. *Annals of Occupational Hygiene*, **45**, 137–143.

Davis, J., Stevens, E., and Staff, D. (1983). Potential exposure of apple thinners to azinphos-methyl and comparison of two methods for assessment of hand exposure. *Bulletin of Environmental Contamination and Toxicology*, **31**, 631–638.

Delmaar, J., Bokkers, B. G., ter Burg, W., and van Engelen, J. G. (2013). First tier modeling of consumer dermal exposure to substances in consumer articles under REACH: A quantitative evaluation of the ECETOC TRA for consumers tool. *Regulatory Toxicology and Pharmacology*, **65**(1), 79–86.

Dick, F. D., Semple, S. E., van Tongeren, M., Miller, B. G., Ritchie, P., Sherriff, D, and Cherrie, J. W. (2010) Development of a task-exposure matrix (TEM) for pesticide use (TEMPEST). *Annals of Occupational Hygiene*, **54**(4), 443–452.

Dick, F., Semple, S., Chen, R., and Seaton, A. (2000). Neurological deficits in solvent-exposed painters: a syndrome including impaired colour vision, cognitive defects, tremor and loss of vibration sensation. *Quarterly Journal of Medicine*, **93**, 655–661.

Durham, W., and Wolfe, H. (1962). Measurement of the exposure of workers to pesticides. *Bulletin of the WHO*, **26**, 75–91.

El-Ayouby, N., Gao, P., Wassell, J., and Hall, R. (2002). Effect of cycles of contamination and decontamination on chemical glove performance. Presented at the International Conference on Occupational and Environmental Exposure of Skin to Chemicals: Science and Policy. September 8–11, 2002, Washington, DC.

Fartasch, M., Taeger, D., Broding, H. C., Schöneweis, S, Gellert, B., Pohrt, U., and Brüning, T. (2012). Evidence of increased skin irritation after wet work: Impact of water exposure and occlusion. *Contact Dermatitis*. **67**, 217–228.

Fenske, R., Wong, S., and Leffingwell, J. (1986). A video imaging technique for assessing dermal exposure. II. Fluorescent tracer testing. *American Industrial Hygiene Association Journal*, **47**, 771–775.

Frasch, H. F., Dotson, G. S., Bunge, A. L., Chen, C.-P., Cherrie, J., Kasting, G. B., et al. (2014). Analysis of finite dose dermal absorption data: Implications for dermal exposure assessment. *Journal of Exposure Science and Environtal Epidemiology* **24**, 65–73.

Gordon, S. M., Wallace, L. A., Callahan, P. J., Kenny, D. V., and Brinkman, M. C. (1998). Effect of water temperature on dermal exposure to chloroform. *Environmental Health Perspectives*, **106**, 337–345.

Gorman, Ng M, Semple, S., Cherrie, J. W., Christopher, Y., Northage, C., Tielemans, E., et al. (2012). The relationship between inadvertent ingestion and dermal exposure pathways: A new integrated conceptual model and a database of dermal and oral transfer efficiencies. *Annals of Occupational Hygiene*, **56**(9), 1000–1012.

Grandjean, P. (1990). *Skin penetration: Hazardous chemicals at work*. Taylor & Francis, London.

Hughson, G. and Cherrie, J. (2001). Validation of the EASE expert system for dermal exposure to zinc. *Arbete Och Halsa*, **10**, 17–19.

Kammer, R., Tinnerberg, H., and Eriksson, K. (2011). Evaluation of a tape-stripping technique for measuring dermal exposure to pyrene and benzo(a)pyrene. *Journal of Environmental Monitoring*, **13**, 2165–2171.

Kezic, S., Mohammadi, N., Jakasa, I., Kruse, J., Monster, A., and Verberk, M. (2002). Percutaneous absorption of neat and water solutions of 2-butoxyethanol in man. Presented at the International Conference on Occupational and Environmental Exposure of Skin to Chemicals: Science and Policy. September 8–11, 2002, Washington, DC.

Kezic, S., Monster, A., van de Gevel, I., Kruse, J., Opdam, J., and Verberk, M. (2001). Dermal absorption of neat liquid solvents on brief exposures in volunteers. *American Industrial Hygiene Association Journal*, **62**, 12–18.

Kim, H.-H., Lim, Y.-W., Yang, J.-Y., Shin, D.-C., Ham, H.-S., Choi, B.-S., and Lee, J.-Y. (2013). Health risk assessment of exposure to chlorpyrifos and dichlorvos in children at childcare facilities. *The Science of the Total Environment*, **444**(C), 441–450. doi: 10.1016/j.scitotenv.2012.11.102

Koniecki, D., Wang, R., Moody, R. P., and Zhu, J. (2011). Phthalates in cosmetic and personal care products: Concentrations and possible dermal exposure. *Environmental Research,* **111**(3), 329–336. doi: 10.1016/j.envres.2011.01.013

Lansink, C., van Hensgstum, C., and Brouwer, D. (1997). Dermal exposure due to airless spraying. TNO Report V97.1057.

Li, Y., Chen, L., Chen, Z., Coehlo, J., Cui, L., Liu, Y., et al. (2011). Glove accumulation of pesticide residues for strawberry harvester exposure assessment. *Bulletin of Environmental Contamination and Toxicology,* **86**(6), 615–620. doi: 10.1007/s00128-011-0272-5

Lindsay, F. E., Semple, S., Robertson, A., Cherrie, J. W. (2006). Development of a biologically relevant dermal sampler. *Annals of Occupational Hygiene,* **50**(1), 85–94.

Liu S, et al. (2013). Concentrations and potential health risks of metals in lip products. *Environmental Health Perspectives,* **121**(6), 705–710.

London, L., and Myers, J. (1998). Use of a crop and job specific exposure matrix for retrospective assessment of long term exposure in studies of chronic neurotoxic effects of agrichemicals. *Occupational and Environmental Medicine,* **55**, 194–201.

Mulhausen, J., and Damiano, J. (1998). *A strategy for assessing and managing occupational exposures.* Appendix II. Dermal exposure assessments. American Industrial Hygiene Association, Fairfax, VA.

Nylander-French, L. A. (2000). A tape stripping method for measuring dermal exposure to multifunctional acrylates. *Annals of Occupational Hygiene,* **44**, 645–651.

OECD. (1997). Environmental health and safety publications series on testing and assessment No. 9: Guidance document for the conduct of studies of occupational exposure to pesticides during agricultural application. OECD/GD(97)148y. OECD, Paris.

Ogden, T. (2010). Managing dermal risk: Moving on from gloves. *Annals of Occupational Hygiene,* **54**(2), 131–133. doi: 10.1093/annhyg/mep093

Oliveira, G., Leverett, J. C., Emamzadeh, M., and Lane, M. E. (2014). The effects of heat on skin barrier function and in vivo dermal absorption. *International Journal of Pharmacology,* **464**, 145–151.

Patel, H., and Cronin, M. (2001). Determination of the optimal physico-chemical parameters to use in a QSAR-approach to predict skin permeation rate. Final report: CEFIC-LRI project No. NMALRI-A2.2UNJM-0007. Liverpool John Moores University, Liverpool.

Phillips, A., and Garrod, A. (2000). Assessment of dermal exposure-empirical models and indicative distributions. *Annals of Occupational Hygiene,* **16**, 323–328.

Poland, C., Read, S., Varet, J., Carse, G., Christensen, F., and Hankin, S. (2013). Dermal absorption of nanomaterials. Environmental Project No: 1504. Danish Ministry of the Environment, Environmental Protection Agency. Denmark, ISBN: 978-87-93026-50-6.

Riviere J, and Brooks J. (2011). Predicting skin permeability from complex chemical mixtures: dependency of quantitative structure permeation relationships on biology of skin model used. *Toxicological Science,* **119**(1), 224–232.

RIVM. (2001). CONSEXPO 3.0, consumer exposure and uptake models. RIVM Report 612810011. National Institute of Public Health and the Environment, The Netherlands.

Roff, M. (1994). A novel lighting system for the measurement of dermal exposure using a fluorescent dye and an image processor. *Annals of Occupational Hygiene,* **38**, 903–919.

Sartorelli, P., Aprea, C., Cenni, A., Novelli, M., Orsi, D., Palmi, S., and Matteucci, G. (1998). Prediction of percutaneous absorption from physiochemical data: a model based on data of in-vitro experiments. *Annals of Occupational Hygiene*, **42**, 267–276.

Scheepers PT, van Houtum J, Anzion RB, et al. (2009) The occupational exposure of dermatology nurses to polycyclic aromatic hydrocarbons—evaluating the effectiveness of better skin protection. *Scandinavian Journal of Work, Environment and Health*, **35**, 212–221.

Schneider, T., Vermeulen, R., Brouwer, D., Cherrie, J., Kromhout, H., and Fogh, C. (1999). A conceptual model for assessment of dermal exposure. *Occupational and Environmental Medicine*, **56**, 765–773.

Semple S. (2004). Dermal exposure to chemicals in the workplace: just how important is skin absorption? *Occupational and Environmental Medicine*, **61**, 376–382.

Semple, S., Brouwer, D., Dick, F., and Cherrie, J. (2001). A dermal model for spray painters. Part II: Estimating the deposition and uptake of solvents. *Annals of Occupational Hygiene*, **45**, 25–33.

Sewell, C., Pilkington, A., Buchanan, D., Tannahill, S., Kidd, M., Cherrie, B., and Robertson, A. (1999). Epidemiological study of the relationships between exposure to organophosphate pesticides and indices of chronic peripheral neuropathy, and neuropsychological abnormalities in sheep farmers and dippers. Phase 1. Development and validation of an organophosphate uptake model for sheep dippers. IOM Report TM/99/02a. Institute of Occupational Medicine, Edinburgh.

Soutar, A., Cherrie, B., and Cherrie, J. (2000). Field evaluation of protective clothing against non-agricultural pesticides. IOM Report TM/00/04. Institute of Occupational Medicine, Edinburgh.

Stefaniak, A. B., Duling, M. G., Geer, L., & Virji, M. A. (2014). Dissolution of the metal sensitizers Ni, Be, Cr in artificial sweat to improve estimates of dermal bioaccessibility. *Environmental Science: Processes & Impacts*, **16**(2), 341–351. doi: 10.1039/c3em00570d

Tahmaz, N., Soutar, A., and Cherrie, J. (2003). Chronic fatigue syndrome and organophosphate pesticides in sheep farming: A retrospective study amongst people reporting to a UK pharma-covigilance scheme. *Annals of Occupational Hygiene* **47**(4), 261–267.

Tannahill, S., Robertson, A., Cherrie, B., Donnan, P., MacConnell, E., and Macleod, G. (1996). A comparison of two different methods for assessment of dermal exposure to non-agricultural pesticides in three sectors. IOM Report TM/96/07. Institute of Occupational Medicine, Edinburgh.

Thompson, B., Griffith, W. C., Barr, D. B., Coronado, G. D., Vigoren, E. M., and Faustman, E. M. (2014). Variability in the take-home pathway: Farmworkers and non-farmworkers and their children. *Journal of Exposure Scence and i Environmental Epidemioly* **24**(5), 522–531. doi: 10.1038/jes.2014.12.

Tibaldi, R., Ten Berge W., and Drolet D. (2014). Dermal absorption of chemicals: Estimation by IH SkinPerm. *Journal of Occupational and Environmental Hygiene*, **11**(1), 19–31.

Tsakirakis, A. N., Kasiotis, K. M., Charistou, A. N., Arapaki, N., Tsatsakis, A., Tsakalof, A., and Machera, K. (2014). Dermal & inhalation exposure of operators during fungicide application in vineyards. Evaluation of coverall performance. *The Science of the Total Environment*, **470-471**(C), 282–289. doi: 10.1016/j.scitotenv.2013.09.021

van de Sandt, J. J., van Burgsteden, J. A., Cage, S., Carmichael, P. L., Dick, I., Kenyon, S., et al. (2004). In vitro predictions of skin absorption of caffeine, testosterone, and benzoic acid: A multi-centre comparison study. *Regulatory Toxicology and Pharmacology*, **39**, 271–281.

Van Hemmen, J. (2002). Riskofderm: Risk assessment for occupational dermal exposure. Presented at the International Conference on Occupational and Environmental Exposure of Skin to Chemicals: Science and Policy. September 8–11, 2002, Washington, DC.

van-Wendel-de-Joode, B., Brouwer, D., Vermeulen, R., van Hemmen, J., Heederik, D., and Kromhout, H. (2003). DREAM: A method for semi-quantitative dermal exposure assessment. *Annals of Occupational Hygiene*, **47**, 71–87.

Verberk, M., Brouwer, D., Brouwer, E., Bruyzeel, D., Emmen, H., Van Hemmen, J., et al. (1990). Health effects of pesticides in the flower-bulb culture in Holland. *Medicina del Lavoro*, **81**, 530–534.

Vermeulen, R., Heideman, J., Bos, R., and Kromhout, H. (2000). Identification of dermal exposure pathways in the rubber manufacturing industry. *Annals of Occupational Hygiene*, **44**, 533–541.

Warren, N. D., Marquart, H., Christopher, Y., Laitinen, J., and VAN Hemmen, J. J. (2006). Task-based dermal exposure models for regulatory risk assessment. *Annals of Occupational Hygiene*, **50**(5), 491–503.

Wassenius, O., Jarvholm, B., Engstrom, T., Lillienberg, L., and Medling, B. (1998). Variability in the skin exposure of machine operators exposed to cutting fluids. *Scandinavian Journal of Work, Environment and Health*, **24**, 125–129.

Watkinson, A. C., Bunge, A. L., Hadgraft, J., and Lane, M. E. (2013). Nanoparticles do not penetrate human skin—a theoretical perspective. *Pharmalogical Research.* **30**(8), 1943–1946.

WHO. (1982). *Field survey of exposure to pesticides. Standard protocol: VBC/82.1.* World Health Organisation, Geneva.

Wilkinson, S., and Williams, F. (2001). *In vitro dermal absorption of liquids.* Contract Research Report for HSE (350). HSE Books, Sudbury, UK.

Wolfe, H., Durham, W., and Armstrong, J. (1967). Exposure of workers to pesticides. *Archives of Environmental Health*, **14**, 622–633.

Zartarian, V., Ozkaynak, H., Murke, J., Zufall, M., Rigas, M., and Furtaw, E. (2000). A modelling framework for estimating children's residential exposure and dose to chlorpyrifos via dermal residue contact and nondietary ingestion. *Environmental Health Perspectives*, **108**, 505–514.

10

EXPOSURE MEASUREMENT ERROR
CONSEQUENCES AND DESIGN ISSUES

Ben Armstrong and Xavier Basagaña

10.1 INTRODUCTION

This chapter is concerned with the effects of inaccuracy in exposure assessment (including misclassification of exposure) on results of epidemiological studies. Most readers are aware that such error adversely impacts on studies, but fewer are aware in just what way. Does it add to uncertainty in estimates of measures of effect? If so, is this extra uncertainty reflected in the usual statements of uncertainty, such as confidence intervals? Under what circumstances does it cause bias in a result, and can the direction and extent of bias be known, or even corrected for? Does it compromise the power of the study?

The chapter summarizes, in a manner accessible to the non-statistician, what is known about the effects of measurement error on the results of a study. The chapter is organized in three main and two subsidiary sections in addition to this introduction. The first (10.2) covers the types and contexts of measurement error and how to describe them formally. The second (12.3) describes the effects of error according to its type, first qualitatively and then where possible quantitatively; it also includes an introductory discussion of methods of correcting for these effects. The third main section (10.4) addresses issues in designing epidemiological studies in the presence of measurement error—the resources to be utilized for exposure measurement, and the use of validity or reliability studies. In the last two shorter sections we briefly review the issue in the context of air pollution epidemiology (10.5) and mention those topics related to measurement error that we have not had space to explore in this chapter 10.6.

10.1.1 Terms and Notation

The term *relative risk* (RR) is used here in the statistical tradition, generically to include rate ratios, odds ratios, prevalence ratios, and the like. (This usage is standard in statistics. Some epidemiologists restrict the meaning of RR to be the ratio of cumulative incidence.) The term *effect measure* is used to denote a summary of the association between exposure and outcome, for example, RR or regression coefficient. The true exposure is denoted as T, the approximate measure X, and the error E, with

$$X = T + E \qquad\qquad\qquad\text{(Eq. 10.1)}$$

The standard deviation of T, X, and E are written as σ_T, σ_X, and σ_E, respectively.

10.2 DESCRIBING MEASUREMENT ERROR

The effects of measurement error critically depend on its context and type.

10.2.1 Error in Measuring What?

There are three categories of explanatory variables that may be measured with error:

1. A variable of interest (environmental or occupational exposure)
2. A potential confounder (active smoking, socio-economic status)
3. A potential effectmodifier (markers of vulnerability to the effects of the variable of interest, such as age)

10.2.2 Differential or Non-differential?

1. *Error is called differential if it varies according to the health outcome.* The classic example of this is recall bias in case–control studies, in which cases may recall exposure with error that is different from controls.
2. *Non-differential error does not depend on health outcome.* This can usually be assumed if exposure is measured before outcome is known or deduced from written records, for example, using work histories and a job-exposure matrix.

10.2.3 Scale of Measurement of the Variable(s) with Error

1. *Categorical* (qualitative), comprising:
   • Dichotomous ("exposed" vs. "not exposed")
   • Polytomous (e.g., "high", "medium", "low")
2. *Numerical* (e.g., concentration of particles in air in microgram per cubic metre, number of cigarettes smoked per day).

When occurring in categorical variables, measurement error is termed *misclassification*—study subjects may be classified incorrectly. Numerical variables can be grouped, thus becoming categorical variables. Conversely, ordered polytomous variables sometimes can be treated as numerical.

Two further distinctions apply to error in numerical variables.

10.2.4 Random or Systematic?

1. Systematic. For example, the exposure is overestimated by two units or by 20% in all subjects.
2. Random. In some subjects exposure is overestimated, in others underestimated (the mean error is zero).

Error often has some systematic and some random component. This chapter concentrates on the random component because effects of systematic error are easier to infer and correct by commonsense reasoning. Systematic additive error has no effect on regression coefficients.

10.2.5 Classical or Berkson?

This distinction is not well known and is a little tricky to understand, but it has major implications for the effects of the error.

1. Classical. The average of many replicate measurements of same true exposure would equal the true exposure.
2. Berkson. The same approximate exposure ("proxy") is used for many subjects; the true exposures vary randomly about this proxy, with mean equal to it.

Example: A study investigates the relationship of average lead exposure up to age 10 with IQ in 10-year-old children living in the vicinity of a lead smelter. IQ is measured by a test administered at age 10. Consider two study designs for assessing exposure.

Design 1: Each child has one measurement made for blood lead, at a random time during his or her life. The blood lead measurement will be an approximate measure of average blood lead over life. However, if the investigators were able to make many replicate measurements (at different random time-points), the average would be a good indicator of lifetime exposure. This measurement error is thus classical.

Design 2: The children's place of residence at age 10 (assumed as known exactly) are classified into three groups by proximity to the smelter—close, medium, and far. Random blood leads, collected as described in Design 1, are averaged for each group, and this group average is used as a proxy for lifetime exposure for each child in the group. Here the same approximate exposure ("proxy") is used for all subjects in the same group, and true exposures, although unknown, may be assumed to vary randomly about the proxy. This measurement error is thus a Berkson error.

Often error has both classical and random components, although one usually predominates. Exposures estimated from observed determinants using an exposure prediction model generally have predominantly Berkson error. Indeed, if the determinants are measured and prediction equation coefficients estimated without error, it is entirely Berkson error.

The two types of error are defined statistically as:

1. Classical: $X = T + E$, with E *independent of T* and mean(E) = 0
2. Berkson: $T = X + E$, with E *independent of X* and mean(E) = 0

10.2.6 Describing the Magnitude of Error

Effects of measurement error usually depend on its magnitude. With random error this will vary from measurement to measurement, so more properly one says that the effects of measurement error depend on its distribution. Error distributions are important conceptually, even if there are no data for inference about them. However, it makes this section less abstract if data from a validity study are assumed to be available. A validity study is a study in which for a sample of subjects exposure is measured accurately as well as by the approximate method to be used in the main study. Alternatively, but less usefully, investigators may have data from a reliability study, in which for a sample of subjects exposure is measured two or more times, each time independently. If the same method is used each time, this is called an intra-method reliability study. Otherwise it is an inter-method reliability study. There is more about estimation of magnitude of error from validity and reliability studies later in the chapter, but basic summaries of error magnitude are introduced here.

10.2.6.1 Categorical Variables

The likely extent of misclassification of categorical variables is usually specified as probabilities of misclassification. For dichotomous variables, it is conventional to express these through the sensitivity (the probability of correctly classifying a truly exposed subject as exposed) and the specificity (the probability of correctly classifying a non-exposed subject as non-exposed) of the classification. In the exposure classification illustrated in Table 10.1, sensitivity is 80% (0.8) and specificity is 60% (0.6); so the probability of misclassifying an exposed subject as non-exposed is $1 - 0.8 = 0.2$, and the probability of misclassifying a non-exposed subject as exposed is $1 - 0.6 = 0.4$.

Table 10.1 Describing misclassification of a dichotomous exposure variable

Total		True	
		Unexposed n (%)	Exposed n (%)
According to	Exposed	40 (80%)	20 (40%)
misclassified	Unexposed	10 (20%)	30 (60%)
variable			
	Total	50	50

Table 10.2 Describing misclassification of a polytomous exposure variable

		According to true variable		
		VERY NEAR n (%)	QUITE NEAR n (%)	FAR n (%)
According to missclassified *variable*	very near	80 (80%)	0 (0%)	0 (0%)
	quite near	20 (20%)	100 (100%)	0 (0%)
	far	0 (0%)	0 (0%)	200 (100%)
	Total	100	100	200

Sensitivity and specificity cannot easily be estimated from a reliability study. There are various ways of summarizing agreement between the measurements, the most popular being the kappa (κ) statistic, which takes the value 1 if there is complete agreement and 0 if there is no more agreement than can be explained by chance (White et al. 2008). However for a validity study, sensitivity and specificity are usually a more useful summaries than kappa. The calculation of kappa from the data in Table 10.1 is illustrated below. If the four cell counts are labelled clockwise from top left as n_{00}, n_{01}, n_{11}, and n_{10}, the row totals $n_{0.}$ and $n_{1.}$ and the column totals $n_{.0}$ and $n_{.1}$, then

$$\hat{\kappa} = \frac{2(n_{00}n_{11} - n_{01}n_{10})}{n_{0.}n_{.1} + n_{1.}n_{.0}} = \frac{2(30 \times 40 - 20 \times 10)}{50 \times 60 + 50 \times 40} = 0.4 \tag{Eq. 10.2}$$

For categorical variables of more than two levels, many different sorts of misclassification can occur, which can be specified in a matrix of misclassification probabilities that take the same form as Table 10.1, but with more than two columns and rows. An example is shown in Table 10.2 in which the only misclassification is from the "very near" to "quite near" group. The example is referred to later. Similar tables of agreement can be assembled from reliability studies, but column percentages can no longer be described as misclassification probabilities because column classification is not by true level. Summaries (such as a κ-statistic) are possible, but often are more complex when there are more than two levels, because some types of disagreement are usually more important than others. For example, misclassification into adjacent categories is usually less important than other misclassification. This can be reflected in summaries if different degrees of misclassification are weighted.

10.2.6.2 Numerical Variables

The important aspect of the distribution of random errors (classical or Berkson) in numerical variables are their standard deviation (σ_E) or variance (σ_E^2). This can be estimated directly from a validity study as the sample standard deviation of the observed values of $X-T$. However, other summaries are used often because they are easier to interpret and use for measurement error correction. Classical error is generally described by its coefficient of reliability, which can be defined as the correlation of independent repeated measurements of exposure (ρ_{XX}), such as might be estimated from a reliability study. In theory (in large samples) this may be shown as being equal to the square of the coefficient of validity, which is the correlation between the true and approximate measurements (ρ_{XT}), such as might be estimated from a validity study. The coefficient of reliability is also theoretically equal to many expressions involving standard deviation of errors (σ_E), true exposures (σ_T), and observed approximate exposures (σ_X), for example:

$$\rho_{XX} = \rho_{XT}^2 = \sigma_T^2 / \sigma_X^2 = (\sigma_X^2 - \sigma_E^2) / \sigma_X^2 = 1 - \sigma_E^2 / \sigma_X^2 = 1 - (\sigma_E / \sigma_X)^2$$

$$= \sigma_T^2 / (\sigma_T^2 + \sigma_E^2) = 1/(1 + \sigma_E^2 / \sigma_T^2) = 1/[1 + (\sigma_E / \sigma_T)^2] \qquad \text{(Eq. 10.3)}$$

These values are only theoretically equal (i.e., in large samples when the classical error model is correct). Exact values differ when they are estimated from validity or reliability data. Choice of which summaries to use is discussed further in the following section, after discussion of which of them are important in describing consequences of error.

10.3 THE CONSEQUENCES OF MEASUREMENT ERROR IN EXPOSURE

This section begins with and focuses mainly on the effects of non-differential error or misclassification in the exposure of interest, first on effect measures, followed by the results of significance tests. A brief discussion on effects of errors on confounder control and the investigation of interaction as well as on effects of non-differential errors concludes this section.

10.3.1 Consequences of Error in the Exposure of Interest for Effect Measures

In general, random measurement error or misclassification leads to bias in effect measures (RRs, regression coefficients, differences in means). This bias is usually downward (toward the null), but there are important exceptions. The extent of bias can be estimated with information on type (Berkson or classical), magnitude of measurement error, and exposure variability (or prevalence).

10.3.1.1 Exposure Measured on a Dichotomous Scale

Non-differential misclassification always biases the effect measure toward the null value (there is a technical but unrealistic exception when the sum of sensitivity and specificity of exposure classification is less than 1, implying measurement that tends to reverse exposed and unexposed categories!)

Example: A study of lung cancer in relation to proximity of residence to a coke oven classifies subjects (cases and populations) by distance of residence from the oven at the time of follow-up: NEAR = <4 km from oven; FAR = 4–10 km. The incidence rate is compared in the two groups. Here there is misclassification due to migration—not all persons living NEAR the oven at time of follow-up will have lived there at the etiologically relevant time. Thus if the true RR for subjects living in these areas throughout their lives were 1.5, the observed RR would tend to be less.

The extent of bias is dependent on and can be calculated from the sensitivity and specificity of the classification and the proportion of truly exposed in the non-diseased. This calculation may be by first principles, calculating number of cases and non-cases expected to move between cells of a two-by-two table, or by a formula:

$$OR_{Obs} = \left[p_D * (1 - p_N) \right] / \left[p_N * (1 - p_D) \right], \qquad \text{(Eq. 10.4)}$$

where

p_D = sensitivity * P_D + (1 – specificity) * $(1 - P_D)$;
p_N = sensitivity * P_N + (1 – specificity) * $(1 - P_N)$;
and "P" and "p" =true and observed proportion exposed, "D" = Diseased, "N" = Non-diseased.

Example: Suppose misclassification (migration) in the foregoing example was such that 10% of the NEAR group was in fact FAR at the time of relevant exposure, and vice-versa (i.e., sensitivity = specificity = 0.9), and that 50% of the population overall lived in the NEAR area. The observed RR would then be 1.38.

Further examples are given in Table 10.3. Notice that where exposure is less common than not (<50%), poor specificity biases the odds ratio much more than poor sensitivity.

There is also an approximate formula using the κ-statistic for agreement between two independent classifications with the same instrument (see section 10.4.3.1 Analysis of Validity and Reliability Studies) to link the observed naive and the true odds ratio (White 2008, p. 133):

$$OR_{Obs} \approx (OR_{True})^{\sqrt{\kappa}} \qquad \text{(Eq. 10.5)}$$

For example, if a repeat classification gave κ = 0.7, and OR_T = 1.5, then $OR_{Obs} \approx 1.5^{\sqrt{0.7}} = 1.40$

Table 10.3 The effect of non-differential misclassification on relative risks in two groups

Exposure sensitivity	Exposure specificity	Proportion of exposed in the population	Observed relative risk
1.00	1.00	any	2.00
0.90	0.90	0.01	1.08
0.90	0.90	0.50	1.72
0.90	0.99	0.01	1.47
0.90	0.99	0.50	1.82
0.99	0.90	0.01	1.09
0.99	0.90	0.50	1.89
0.99	0.99	0.01	1.50
0.99	0.99	0.50	1.97

10.3.1.2 Exposure Measured on a Polytomous Scale

Non-differential misclassification biases downward estimates of trend across ordered groups, but comparisons between specific categories can be biased in either direction.

Example: *Assume that in the foregoing example the NEAR group was split into two: VERY NEAR, and QUITE NEAR, with true RRs, relative to FAR, of 2.0 and 1.3. If there is 20% migration from VERY NEAR to QUITE NEAR, but not otherwise (as in Table 10.2), observed risks for VERY NEAR group relative to the FAR group is unchanged on average, but that for the QUITE NEAR group is increased by contamination by the VERY NEAR migrants. The specific value of the misclassified RR was calculated assuming that the NEAR group was divided into two equal-sized groups (25% of total population each), so the misclassified RR is a weighted mean of 1.3 and 2, with weights $w_1 = 25$ and $w_2 = 0.2 \times 25 = 5$ (the migrants from VERY NEAR). Thus RR = {1.3 × 25 + 2 × 5}/{25 + 5)} = 1.42. The RR is increased by misclassification (Table 10.4).*

Table 10.4 The effect on non-differential misclassification on relative risks in three exposure groups—example

	Relative risk		
	VERY NEAR	QUITE NEAR	FAR
True	2.0	1.3	1.0
Misclassified	2.0	1.42	1.0

10.3.1.3 Exposure Measured on a Numerical Scale

Classical errors bias regression coefficients toward zero (equivalently, RR per unit exposure toward 1). The association is described as attenuated. In fact, for linear regression the bias factor is equal to the coefficient of reliability (ρ_{XX}). Thus if

$Y = \alpha_{True} + \beta_{True} T$; then

$$Y = \alpha_{Obs} + \beta_{Obs} X, \text{ with } \beta_{Obs} = \rho_{XX} \times \beta_{True} \tag{Eq. 10.6}$$

The parameter β_{Obs} is sometimes called the "naïve" regression coefficient.

Lead-IQ example—design 1: Suppose that a regression of IQ on true lifetime average blood lead has a regression with coefficient −2 (IQ reduces by 2 points per μg/dl^{-1} blood lead). With classical measurement error with coefficient of reliability 0.5, this would be attenuated, on average, to 0.5 × −2 = −1.

From the alternative expressions for the coefficient of reliability given in section 10.2 ($\rho_{XX} = 1/[1+(\sigma_E/\sigma_T)^2]$), bias in β depends on the average magnitude of measurement error relative to the average magnitude of the true or observed exposure variability (σ_E/σ_T or σ_E/σ_X). This implies that measurement error will have lesser effects if the exposures are more spread out (σ_T or σ_X is greater). Table 10.5 gives attenuation bias as the function of the ratio of the standard deviation of errors to that of true exposures (σ_E/σ_T). This is quite reassuring—error has to be relatively big to give serious bias.

For logistic and log-linear (Poisson) regression coefficients the same qualitative result is true, and the quantitative one approximately so, with the approximation being good except for large error and large RRs. For logistic and log-linear regression RR is linked to the regression coefficient by the formula $RR = \exp(\beta)$, thus

$$RR_{Obs} = (RR_{True})^{\rho_{xx}} \tag{Eq. 10.7}$$

If, in the children exposed to blood lead, investigators were to use as an outcome a child having an IQ below 80, and if the RR (odds ratio) increment per 10 μg/dl^{-1} true blood lead (from logistic regression) was 1.5, then the expected observed RR is given by:

$$RR_{Obs} = 1.5^{0.5} = 1.22 \tag{Eq. 10.8}$$

Berkson errors, however, lead to no bias in linear regression coefficients, and little or no bias in logistic or log-linear regression coefficients. The distinction between classical and Berkson error is thus important.

Table 10.5 The attenuation bias due to exposure measurement error in linear regression

Error σ_E/σ_T[a]	0.0	0.1	0.2	0.3	0.4	0.5	0.75	1.0	1.5	2.0
Error σ_E/σ_X[b]	0.0	0.10	0.20	0.29	0.37	0.45	0.60	0.71	0.83	0.89
Attenuation[c]	1.0	0.99	0.96	0.92	0.86	0.80	0.64	0.50	0.31	0.20

[a] σ_E/σ_T is the ratio of error SD to true exposure SD.

[b] σ_E/σ_X is the ratio of error SD to observedexposure SD.

[c] Attenuation is the factor by which the naïve regression slope will underestimate the true slope.

Lead-IQ Example: Design 2: In this grouped design the error is of Berkson type, so there is no bias in the regression coefficient. However, precision would be lost (width of confidence interval would be wider), and power would not be as great as without measurement error, or as in the biased Design 1.

10.3.2 Consequences for Significance Tests and Power

All types of non-differential random measurement errors or misclassifications reduce study power—the chance that a study will find a statistically significant association if one is truly present. This is true for Berkson as well as classical error, and for misclassification. The extent of power loss can be quantified if magnitude of measurement error and exposure variability (or for a dichotomous measure, prevalence) are known.

Example: A cohort study is designed to have 80% power to detect a RR of 2.0 between truly exposed and truly unexposed persons (80% of similar-sized studies would find the association), by inclusion of sufficient subjects (10% exposed) to expect 14 cases in the exposed group under the null hypothesis (Breslow and Day 1987). If approximate measurements were used, the power would be less. If the measure of exposure has sensitivity = specificity = 0.9 and 10% of the population are exposed, then a true RR of 2.0 would be attenuated, on average, to 1.48 (formula in 10.3.1.). Power to detect this reduced RR is only 30% (Breslow and Day 1987). To restore 80% power would require a study about four times bigger.

For numerical exposure variables (and approximately for dichotomous exposures if coded as 0 and 1) power loss is based on the result that the effective loss in sample size is equal to the coefficient of reliability of the measure (Lagakos 1988).

Example: A study with exposure measured with a coefficient of reliability 0.5 will have similar power to one with accurate exposure assessment and half the number of subjects.

10.3.3 Confounders

10.3.3.1 Errors in Confounders

The general rule is that errors in confounders compromise our ability to control for their effect, leaving "residual" confounding. The effect measure adjusted using the approximate confounder will on average lie between the crude, unadjusted effect measure and the effect measure adjusted using the true (unknown) confounder. The validity of significance tests on the effect of exposure is compromised.

Example: *A study of the relationship of lung cancer to air pollution adjusts for smoking using a crude estimate of pack-years for each subject. Any confounding of the RR for lung cancer versus air pollution will be only partially controlled. For example, if crude $RR_{(crude)} = 1.50$ (95% CI 1.20–1.88; p < 0.001), and $RR_{(adjusted\ for\ true\ pack-years)} = 1.04$ (95% CI 0.86–1.24; p = 0.67), then the partially adjusted $RR_{(adjusted\ for\ approximate\ pack-years)}$ will in general lie between 1.50 and 1.04 and the partially adjusted p-value will lie between 0.001 and 0.67.*

The degree of residual confounding depends on the coefficient of reliability of the measure of the confounder. A coefficient of reliability of 0.5 will imply that about half the confounding present will be controlled, in the sense that the observed log(RR) (more generally the regression coefficient) will on average lie about half-way between the crude unadjusted log(RR) and the fully adjusted log(RR).

Continuing the same example, if the coefficient of reliability of measured pack-years is 0.5, then $log(RR_{(adjusted\ for\ approximate\ pack-years)})$ will lie about halfway between $log(RR_{(crude)})$ and $log(RR_{(adjusted\ for\ true\ pack-years)})$, which gives $RR_{(adjusted\ for\ approximate\ pack-years)} = 1.25$ (95% CI 1.03–1.52; p = 0.03).

There are a few exceptions. Entirely systematic error (everyone under-reporting their smoking by 20%) will not usually compromise control of confounding. In special situations (when the effects of the confounder and the exposure of interest are strictly additive) Berkson error (e.g., use of group mean rather than individual pack-years of smoking) also leaves no residual confounding. Most important, if the variable suspected of confounding is in fact not associated with the exposure of interest (smoking is not associated with air pollution), then there is no confounding or residual confounding, however strongly the variable is associated with the outcome (however bad the smoking data, the observed association of lung cancer with air pollution is not biased).

Correlation between errors in measuring confounders with errors in measuring the exposure of interest or with exposure itself further complicates the situation, although the same broad conclusion—that error compromises control of confounding—remains.

10.3.3.2 Presence of Confounders Measured Without Error

Having to control for confounders, whether measured with error or not, somewhat increases the effect of error in the variable of interest on the RR of interest. The formulae for the simple situation without confounders can be extended to cover this situation by replacing the validity coefficient or quantities from which it may be derived with their value conditional on the presence of the confounder (Carrol 2006, p. 52). For example, the reliability coefficient of an exposure measure conditional on age is the partial correlation between independent repeat measures after control for age, which is typically lower.

10.3.4 Effect Modifiers

An effect modifier is a variable that modifies the effect of the exposure of interest (e.g., identifying subgroups vulnerable or resistant to the exposure). In statistical terms, this is described as an interaction between the effect modifier and the exposure.

10.3.4.1 Error in the Effect Modifiers

Error in measuring effect modifiers tends to diminish effect modification. Vulnerable subgroups are thus harder to identify.

Lead-IQ Example: *Suppose diet modified the effect of lead on IQ, children with vitamin-deficient diets have a regression slope of −3 and others a slope of −1. If diet is measured with error (misclassified), the apparent modification will tend to be less, for example, the slope in vitamin-deficient children might be −2.5 and that in others −1.5.*

10.3.4.2 Error in the Exposure of Interest

Even if the putative effect-modifier is measured without error, error in the variable of interest can distort effect modification, and even create spurious modification. This may happen because the magnitude of error, and hence bias, depends on the putative modifier. Even if this is not the case, the variation of exposure may depend on the putative modifier, in which case the bias due to measurement error will again depend on the putative modifier.

Lead-IQ Example: *Suppose now that interest is in modification of the effect of lead on IQ by sex, which is measured without error, but lead is again measured with (classical) error. Suppose also that although the average error was the same for boys and girls, boys had more varied lead exposures than girls (σ_T is higher in boys than in girls). In this case, if the true regression slope of IQ on lead is −2 for both boys and girls, the estimated slope will tend to be more attenuated for girls (say to −0.5) than for boys (say to −1.5). (For girls the standard deviation σ_T is lower, and hence the attenuation bias $\sigma_T^2/(\sigma_T^2 + \sigma_E^2)$ is more extreme.) Thus sex appears to modify the effect of lead on IQ, but does not in fact do so.*

10.3.5 Differential Error

Differential error can cause bias in the effect measure either upward or downward, depending on whether adverse outcomes are associated with over- or underestimation of exposure. Significance tests are not valid in the presence of differential error. For dichotomous exposure, the bias can be quantified if the sensitivity and specificity of the approximate classification in cases and in non-cases are known.

Example: *The association of exposure to VDU use with spontaneous abortion is investigated by means of a case-control study in which women are interviewed after a live birth* *or abortion, and asked about the number of hours per week that they spent using a VDU. The RR of spontaneous abortion in women using VDUs for 15 or more hours per week was 1.20 (95% CI 1.06–1.34). Due to media attention to the hypothesized association, women who had experienced spontaneous abortions may have been more likely to recall their VDU use fully. In this case, some or all of the excess of VDU users in the cases relative to the controls would be spurious, so that the true RR would be less than 1.20, possibly 1.00.*

10.3.6 Correcting for Measurement Error

If there is information on the magnitude and type of error it is possible (but not always easy!) to allow for it in estimating the effect measure, at least for reasonably simple forms of measurement error. Sometimes it is sufficient to invert the formulae for deriving the effects of measurement error, for example

$$\beta_{True} = \beta_{Obs} / \rho_{xx}, \ RR_{True} = \left(RR_{Obs}\right)^{(1/\rho_{xx})}. \tag{Eq. 10.9}$$

In the Lead-IQ study, if investigators had observed a regression coefficient (β_{Obs}) of -1, and known that the coefficient of reliability of measurement (ρ_{XX}) was 0.5, then they could estimate

$$\beta_{True} = -1/0.5 = -2 \tag{Eq. 10.10}$$

Similarly, if investigators observed an increment in RR of low IQ per 10 μg dl⁻¹ observed blood lead: $RR_{Obs} = 1.22$, then approximately

$$RR_{True} = 1.22^{(1/0.5)} = 1.5 \tag{Eq. 10.11}$$

Corrections will not in general affect the *p*-value of a test of the null hypothesis of no association, nor will the power of the test be improved. However, confidence intervals normally get wider.

Example:*In the lead-IQ study mentioned earlier, suppose the regression coefficient of −1 had a 95% CI (−1.8, −0.2), with p = 0.01. Assuming coefficient of reliability 0.5, the corrected coefficient is −2, the 95% CI (−3.6, −0.4), and p = 0.01, as before. If there was uncertainty in the coefficient of reliability, then a more sophisticated approach that reflected this would give a wider confidence interval, but its lower limit would remain below zero, consistent with the p-value, for which a correction is not required.*

Other methods are available that refine and generalize this approach. The aim of these more sophisticated methods is usually to use other sorts of information on measurement error, more precisely to eradicate bias, or to reflect in the estimate and confidence intervals uncertainty as to the magnitude of the error. A review is given by Carrol (2000).

Probably the most popular group of methods is called regression calibration. In general, these seek to correct an observed effect measure by applying to it a calibration factor, typically obtained from a validity or reliability study. For example, from validity study data one can estimate the calibration factor λ as the regression coefficient of true accurate exposure (Y variable) on approximate exposure (X variable)—this estimates the average change in the accurate exposure corresponding to unit change in the approximate variable. Observed regression coefficients from the main study are divided by λ to obtain an unbiased estimate of the true coefficient: $\beta_T = \beta_{Obs}/\lambda$. Using the formulae given earlier with ρ_{XX} or ρ_{XY} estimated from reliability of validity studies are also examples of regression calibration.

Example: Zeger et al. (2000) applied the regression calibration method when correcting estimates of increased mortality per μgm^{-3} PM$_{10}$ from a time-series mortality study in Riverside, California, which used a central site monitor to estimate exposure. The study found mortality to increase by 0.84% per 10 μgm^{-3} PM$_{10}$ (95% CI −0.06, 1.76). A validity study had been carried out in which 49 people from Riverside had worn personal monitors for a total of 178 sampling days. Regressing personal measure (Y variable) on ambient exposure (X variable) gave a regression calibration slope of 0.60 (SE 0.08). (Thus each 1 μgm^{-3} change in PM$_{10}$ in ambient exposures was on average reflected in a 0.6 μgm^{-3} change in personal levels.) This allowed the observed regression slope of 0.84 to be corrected by dividing by 0.60: true regression slope = 0.84/0.60 = 1.40. Confidence limits were obtained by applying the same correction to the naïve limits, thus (−0.11, 2.95). These confidence limits are slightly too narrow, because they do not reflect uncertainty in the calibration factor. As Zeger discusses, the measurement error in this situation is a mixture of the Berkson and classical types. Regression calibration making direct use of the calibration slope provided a way of correcting for bias without having to assume either all-Berkson or all-classical error.

The "method of moments" estimator is an alternative correction procedure. For this, one estimates just the variance of the error distribution—(σ_E^2) from a reliability study (half the variance of differences in measurements) or validity study. This estimate can be transported to the main study with fewer assumptions than needed for λ, ρ_{XX}, or ρ_{XY} (see the following). The variance of observed exposures (σ_X^2) is then estimated from the main study and the naïve regression slope is corrected using the expression

$$\beta_{True} = \beta_{Obs} / \left\{ (\sigma_{X^2} - \sigma_{E^2}) / \sigma_{X^2} \right\} \qquad \text{(Eq. 10.12)}$$

For an example showing two methods of correction for measurement error applied to occupational epidemiology, see Spiegelman and Valanis (1998).

Other methods are also gaining popularity. One of them is multiple imputation, a technique to deal with missing data that is now implemented in most statistical software packages. Indeed, in the context of studies that include a validity study, measurement error can be seen as a missing data problem—the true exposure is missing in those participants not included in the validation sample. The idea is to predict the true exposure in the full dataset using a regression model that includes as predictors the approximate exposure variable and possibly additional variables. Once the true exposure is predicted for all participants, this predicted variable can be used in the planned analysis (e.g., linear or logistic regression) to obtain corrected estimates. In order to obtain correct standard errors that account for the uncertainty in exposure prediction, the full process (true exposure prediction and data analysis using the predicted exposure) needs to be repeated several times. The results of all iterations are then combined using some specific rules, in a process that is usually done automatically by the software. Multiple imputation is a very flexible technique, as it can easily be used to correct for differential measurement error, it works for both continuous and categorical variables, it can be used for more than one variable measured with error, and it works in studies with a validation sample obtained by stratified random sampling.

More details on multiple imputation for measurement error correction can be found in Cole et al. (2006). Other methods, such as moment reconstruction or simulation extrapolation, are also used in practice. Freedman et al. (2008) provides more details on using these methods in the context in which a validity study is available, whereas Keogh and White (2014) describes their use in reliability studies, that is, when there are repeated measures of the exposure.

10.3.6.1 Limitations of Corrections for Measurement Error

Information on the magnitude of measurement error is needed. This requires reliability studies (a sample of repeated independent measurements) or validity studies (a sample of gold standard measurements in parallel with the approximate measurements). These are not often available, and even if they are, much uncertainty remains unless they are large. If corrections are carried out on the basis of incorrect information on error magnitude, bias may be increased, rather than decreased. "Corrections" for attenuation can also magnify confounding or other information bias, rather than a true association. Researchers should give the naïve effect measure (using the approximate exposure in a regular analysis), even if including effect measures corrected for measurement error. Also worth considering is the calculation of corrections under a variety of assumptions, in the spirit of a sensitivity analysis.

10.4 DESIGN ISSUES

10.4.1 What Resources Should Be Utilized for Estimating Exposure?

Random exposure measurement error reduces the power of a study and (except Berkson error) biases effect measures. To avoid these problems, it is desirable to design studies with minimum measurement error. However, making exposure measurement more accurate may be costly and must be considered against alternative uses for the resources. Thus the practical question is usually, "What proportion of resources should be put into exposure measurement in order to improve accuracy?"

When a study aims to add to evidence as to whether an exposure causes an outcome, study power is the main consideration. For these studies, Lagakos's result cited previously can be used to address this question, by justifying the following principle.

To maximize study power, resources should be spent on improving accuracy until the proportional increase in the square of the validity coefficient ρ_{XT}^2 is less than the proportional increase in total study costs per subject that is required to achieve it.

For example, if it is possible to increase ρ_{XT}^2 from 0.6 to 0.9 (i.e., by a factor of 1.5) by spending 30% more per subject, it is worth it. If it costs 100% more, it is not—the money would be better spent recruiting more subjects. As usual in such design decisions, input information (ρ_{XT}^2 or equivalent) may have to be obtained from pilot studies if it is not available. More details and examples are given by Armstrong (1996).

10.4.1.1 Deciding on the Number of Repeat Exposure Measurements

A special case in this problem occurs whenincrease in precision is possible by making independent repeat measurements of exposure for each study subject, and the question is "How many replicates?" With costs of each exposure measurement C_Z, other marginal study costs per subject (e.g., outcome measurement) C_I, and the reliability of the measurement ρ_{XX}, the aforementioned principle yields the optimal number n of replicates:

$$n = \frac{C_I(1-\rho_{XX})}{C_Z \rho_{XX}}$$

(Eq. 10.13)

For example, if ρ_{XX} is 0.6, C_Z is \$20, and C_I is \$100, then $n = 100(1 - 0.6)/(20 \times 0.6) = 40/12 = 3.3$; that is, about three repeat exposure measurements per subject. The square of the validity coefficient, or another of the equivalent expressions can be substituted for reliability coefficient in this expression.

10.4.1.2 Limitations to Designing for Maximum Power

When a study aims not only to add evidence to whether an exposure causes an outcome, but also to quantify how much risk is consequent to a measured level of exposure (the absolute dose–response relationship), then the bias in effect measure assumes an added importance, and power is an inadequate criterion for choice of resources to go into exposure measurement. Increasing the sample size does not reduce measurement error bias, although it does increase power. Formal approaches to this problem require more assumptions. Less formal trade-offs between bias and power, perhaps informed by the power criterion, are likely to be necessary. The sections that follow address this situation.

10.4.2 Designing for Berkson Rather Than Classical Error

If bias in effect measure is the major consideration (rather than study power), there is sometimes scope to design exposure measurement to utilize the fact that Berkson error causes little bias. This can be achieved two ways:

1. By using mean exposure over groups of subjects. The lead-IQ study can provide an example. Using each child's blood lead measurement gave rise to classical error, biasing the regression coefficient, but if investigators grouped children according to proximity to smelter, this error would be changed to mainly Berkson type, not biasing the coefficient. (Mainly rather than entirely Berkson, because any error in the mean as an estimate of true group mean remains classical, but this will be small unless the number of measurements per group is small.) Using the group mean thus eliminates or greatly reduces bias. Remaining bias can be reduced by making groups larger. However, this procedure does not improve power. In fact, using group means in this way usually reduces power. Thus, there is a choice between retaining power and reducing bias.

2. By using a prediction model. This is a generalization of the grouping method. Individual measures are used to estimate coefficients of a model for predicting exposure given some easily measured predictor variables. Then, predicted values from the prediction model are used in place of the individual measures when investigating the association of exposure with outcome. The resulting error is again mainly Berksonian. Some classical error will remain if the sample in the prediction model is small, as when using group means, and also if the predictor variables are measured with error. Again, bias will be reduced, but usually at the cost of power.

In fact, both grouping and prediction models are usually used when not all subjects in the study have individual exposure measures, so their use is forced and there is no choice. Nevertheless, it may be useful when deciding between strategies to be aware that the resulting primarily Berkson-type error will bias effect measures little if at all, but will reduce power. The use of grouping and of prediction models is discussed further in chapters 7 and 13,

10.4.3 Validity, Reliability, and Two-Stage Studies

As an alternative to or in addition to improving exposure assessment for every study subject, investigators can use a cheap approximate method for the main study and supplement this by a smaller validity study (a sample of gold standard measurements in parallel with the approximate measurements) or reliability substudy (a sample of repeated independent approximate measurements). In this section we discuss analysis of such substudies, and how parameters estimated from the substudy can be used to inform interpretation of the main study and sometimes to correct the effect measure in the main study for measurement error. It is usually best if the validity or reliability study samples can be drawn from among the main study subjects. This is partly to improve portability of error parameters (see section 10.4.3.2), and partly so that the additional information on exposure in the subsample can be used to improve the power of the main study (see section 10.4.3.4).

10.4.3.1 Analysis of Validity and Reliability Studies

Data from a validity or reliability substudy should be analyzed first to describe agreement, rather than immediately focusing on estimation of parameters required for correction of attenuation of exposure–response relationships under specific assumptions. A few key features of standard analysis of agreement between two numerical measurements are given here. Fuller treatment is available in Shoukri (2000) and Bland and Altman (1986).

1. The mean (and CI) of differences between numerical measurements displays the extent to which one instrument measures consistently higher than another.
2. The standard deviation of the differences in measurements displays the extent of variation in agreement (random error). The mean and standard deviation can be brought together to define "limits to agreement," for example, mean ±1.96SD estimates the limits within which the difference will lie 95% of the time. In a validity study, the standard deviation of differences estimates the standard deviation of measurement error σ_E. In an intra-method reliability study, the standard deviation estimates $(\sqrt{2})\sigma_E$. (The variance of differences estimates twice the variance of errors.)
3. Various plots can be used to explore whether agreement depends on other factors. For example, plotting differences against the mean or sum of the two measurements identifies whether agreement varies according to the magnitude of exposure, and will suggest departure from additivity if present.
4. With data from a validity study, classical and Berkson error can be distinguished by examining whether differences are correlated with true or approximate measurements, for example, by plotting.

These analyses allow evaluation of some assumptions of measurement error models and correction techniques (additivity, Berkson/classical distinction). Also, most investigators will wish to be aware of features of error, for example, additive bias, even if it does not affect study power or bias effect measures. Once a general description of agreement is obtained, it is reasonable to focus on the parameters that determine the extent of attenuation due to measurement error, and hence are needed to correct it. The standard deviation (σ_E) or variance of errors (σ_E^2) may be the most useful parameter for this purpose (see discussion in section 10.4.3.2). However, the parameters most directly related to attenuation are the validity and reliability coefficients.

If there are two repeats of each measurement the validity or reliability coefficient can be estimated directly as the Pearson correlation coefficient from the paired measurements. However, it is more efficient to estimate them as "intra-class" correlation coefficients (ICC) or equivalently from variance components. When there are several repeat measurements, the ICC/variance component method is the only one.

The ICC can be expressed as a function of the ratio of variances within (σ_W^2) to between (σ_B^2) pairs (or triplets, etc.): ICC=$1/[1+(\sigma_W^2/\sigma_B^2)]$ (Shoukri 2000; White et al. 2008), if these variances are estimated from the measurements in the substudy as "variance components." Variance components and ICC are obtainable from most statistical software. Interpretation of the ICC depends on context. With data from a reliability study, the ICC estimates the reliability coefficient ρ_{XX}, which in simple models is the attenuation factor and loss in effective sample size and hence power (see section 10.3.1). With data from a validity study, the ICC estimates the validity coefficient, which estimates the square root of the reliability coefficient. If the mean for a subject is the true exposure, and repeated measurements are taken on a sample of subjects, the variance components become those between- and within-subjects. If the main study relating exposure to outcome uses just one exposure measure per subject, the formula for ICC again estimates reliability coefficient and attenuation. If means of exposures from m repeats are used in the main study, the attenuation reduces to $1/[1+(\sigma_W^2/\sigma_B^2)/m]$ (Liu et al. 1978). Variance components are discussed further in chapter 5.

In general, it is not possible to use measures of agreement from inter-method reliability studies to estimate the bias that use of either method might produce in an epidemiological study. The problem is in apportioning the lack of agreement between the two methods. However, the regression calibration method can be used if the errors of the two measures are independent (Wacholder et al. 1993).

10.4.3.2 Portability of Coefficients from Substudies to Main Studies

Using results from a validity or reliability substudy to inform a main study requires "transporting" estimates of agreement, for example, a validity coefficient from one to the other. This should be done cautiously, with a view to possible factors that might make the underlying values of the coefficients different in the two contexts. For example, a reliability coefficient depends not only on the variance of the error distribution, but also on the variance of true exposures. Thus even if the measurement instrument used in the main and reliability studies are identical, if the distribution of true exposures differ, the reliability coefficient is not portable. The same applies to calibration regression coefficients and to κ-statistics.

This problem can be minimized by randomly choosing the reliability or validity sample from the main study subjects. Alternatively, more portable coefficients can be used. For example, the method of moments correction requires only the variance of the error from a validity or reliability study, which is usually more portable than the reliability coefficient.

10.4.3.3 Sample Size of Validity and Reliability Studies

Given that the motivation for conducting validity and reliability studies usually goes beyond their use for correcting exposure–response relationships, it is useful to consider simple general-purpose aids to decide their sample size. Perhaps most important is the following frequently misunderstood point.

Sample size determinations for identifying the presence of an association between true and imperfectly measured exposures or two imperfectly measured exposures (e.g., by a χ^2-test, or test of a correlation being zero) are of no interest when determining sizes of validity or reliability studies. Such tests merely assess evidence for the two measurements being associated. This would not advance us much—even very poor measurements are associated somewhat with the true exposure.

The requirement is to quantify the strength and features of the association. Depending on the context, the parameter or parameters of interest may be any of many, for example, sensitivity and specificity (proportions), validity of reliability coefficients (correlation coefficients), a regression coefficient, a mean difference, or a κ coefficient. Usually, the most straightforward and adequate approach is to show how the precision of an estimate to be made from the proposed study depends on the sample size. Choosing a sample size reflects the trade-off between the advantages of a precise estimate and the cost of obtaining it.

For example, a validity coefficient of 0.5 estimated from a validity study would have confidence intervals depending on sample size as displayed in Table 10.6. The method of estimating confidence intervals is given in most intermediate-level statistical methods textbooks, and they may be obtained from many statistical software (e.g., stata's "ci2" command). The results are quite sobering, suggesting that with less than say 100 pairs of measurements the validity coefficient would be rather imprecisely estimated. Of course, investigators do not know that the correlation coefficient will be 0.5, but the pattern of widths of confidence intervals does not usually depend very strongly on such guessed values. To check, the calculations can always be repeated using a range of values.

Table 10.6 Effect of reliability study sample size on estimate of reliability coefficient.

Sample size (pairs)	10	25	50	100	250	500
Confidence interval	−0.19,0.86	0.13,0.75	0.26,0.69	0.34,0.63	0.40,0.59	0.43,0.56

10.4.3.4 Two-Stage Studies

Epidemiological studies with more accurate exposure assessment on a subsample are sometimes called "two-stage" studies. Careful choice of which subjects to include in the subsample can improve precision and power, although analysis to achieve this becomes more complicated (Zhao and Lipsitz 1992). The optimal design of two-stage and other studies with validation substudies has been discussed by Greenland (1988), who concludes that unless the cost of the better measurement is many times that of the approximate one, a "fully validated" study (using the better measure or replicate measures on all subjects) is frequently the optimal one. Where differential error is a concern, validation studies must be particularly large.

10.5 MEASUREMENT ERROR IN AIR POLLUTION EPIDEMIOLOGY

Air pollution is the most commonly studied environmental risk factor, and raises some specific measurement error issues. The studies can be broadly classified into two groups: those that investigate the health effects of short-term exposure (same day or a few previous days) and those that investigate the effects of long-term exposure (years). Short-term effects studies often use Poisson regression models to link the daily counts of mortality or hospital admissions in a city or region with the daily outdoor air pollution levels (obtained from a single monitor or using the average of several monitors in the study area). Often, these studies are only interested in the health effects of outdoor levels, as they are the ones being regulated. In that case, two main error components affect these models, a Berkson error component, resulting from assigning an average concentration to all participants in the region, and a classical error component, resulting from the fact that only a sample of locations are used to calculate the average. Berkson error is believed to be the dominant part, and therefore relatively little bias due to exposure measurement error is expected in time series studies. When one uses outdoor levels but aims to estimate the effects of personal exposure to air pollution, including indoor exposure, the difference between ambient and personal levels comes into play as an extra error component (Sheppard et al. 2012). Dominici et al. (2000) shows how validation studies with personal measurements can be used to correct the estimators obtained using outdoor levels via regression calibration or Bayesian models.

Studies on long-term effects capitalize mostly on spatial rather than temporal variations in exposure. More and more, these studies attempt to estimate the spatial surface of outdoor pollution levels at a very fine scale, capturing also within-city variations. This is achieved by using emission-dispersion models (Chapter 4), spatial interpolation models (Chapter 4), or the so-called "land use regression models"(Chapter 13) that use predictors that can be derived in any point of a city via geographical information systems (GIS) (Chapter 3). The predicted exposure resulting from these models suffers from Berkson-like error, due to smoothing the exposure surface using a model that does not include all sources of variation, and from classical-like error, that arises from having to estimate the model parameters (Szpiro et al. 2011). Although most of the error is again believed to be of Berkson type, which introduces little bias in health effect estimates, in situations in which-models are derived using a small number of measurements and a large number of potential predictors, the classical-like error is substantial and the estimated health effects can be significantly biased (Basagaña et al. 2013). As in studies on short-term effects, one can use validation studies with personal measures and regression calibration to account for differences between outdoor and personal levels (Van Roosbroeck et al. 2008).

10.6 ISSUES NOT COVERED IN THIS CHAPTER

For simplicity of presentation some assumptions and points of interpretation have been passed over. The most important of these are described here.

10.6.1 Outcomes

This chapter has not dealt with errors in measuring outcomes. Where outcomes are numerical (e.g., lung function), these do not cause bias in effect measures, but do cause loss of power and precision. Where outcomes are categorical, misclassifying them non-differentially (with respect to exposure) biases effect measures toward the null. All our results have assumed that errors in measuring exposure are unrelated to errors in measuring outcome. Such associations can cause bias in any direction.

10.6.2 Bias

Many of the results concern bias in an effect estimate. Bias is an average effect if the study were to be repeated many times. In a large study the effect of measurement error will be close to this average "bias." However, in a single small sample, the effect may differ appreciably from this average (Sorahan and Gilthorpe 1994). In these cases random error can sometimes even lead to an effect measure estimated from approximate exposures that is more extreme than that with the true exposure. It remains more likely, however, that if true exposure has an effect it is stronger than the estimate using the approximate measurement (Wacholder et al. 1995).

10.6.3 Prediction

It has been assumed in this chapter that it is the relationship between the true exposure and health outcome that is of interest. Sometimes this is not the case. If you wish to use the study to predict risks in subjects using the same approximate measure of exposure and drawn from the same population, then the naïve effect estimate (e.g., β_{Obs}) is appropriate.

10.6.4 Shape

Exposure measurement error can distort the shape of exposure–outcome associations as well as bias estimates of slope of linear associations. Apart from the specific effect of multiplicative error noted below, in general random error tends to make non-linear associations appear more linear (Carroll et al. 2006; Keogh et al. 2012; sections 1.1 and 8.7.2).

10.6.5 Multiplicative Error

Multiplicative error (proportional to the true exposure), with lognormal distribution of true exposures, is common in environmental and occupational epidemiology. Here measurement error changes the shape of the regression, for example, from a quadratic curve to a straight line (Doll and Peto 1978; Pierce et al. 1991).

10.6.6 Ecologic Studies

Ecological studies, which have groups as the unit of analysis, have some unexpected error effects. If the exposure is proportion of individuals in the area with an attribute(e.g., proportion of smokers) and the individual measure is subject to misclassification, then the slope of the regression of outcome against proportion with the attribute will be greater than the true individual effect of the attribute on the outcome, that is, bias is away from the null (Greenland 1992). Where the group exposure measure is a good approximation to the mean true exposure across individuals in the group, then error is Berksonian, as discussed earlier, and little or no bias results.

10.6.7 Directed Acyclic Graphs

Directed acyclic graphs (DAGs), a set of tools based on causal diagrams that is increasingly used in epidemiological research, has been used to represent measurement error settings. Directed acyclic graphs can be used to conclude about the presence and direction of causal effects, even in some situations involving differential errors (VanderWeele and Hernán 2012).

10.6.8 Causality

The impact of random non-differential exposure measurement error on inference about the size of an effect is fairly clear once a causal relationship is assumed—the true effect of exposure is most likely to be greater than that estimated. The impact of measurement error on the evidence that such a study brings on whether a causal relationship exists is more problematic. The following points should be considered:

1. One should usually be more cautious, if there is measurement error, in concluding from a "negative" study that no causal association exists. The reduced power implies that it is more likely that a true underlying association has been missed.

2. One should not use the (uncorrected) confidence interval for RR (or other measure of effect) to indicate the highest risk that is compatible with the data. For example, an uncorrected confidence interval for RR of (0.80, 1.25) suggests that relative risks in excess of 1.25 can be excluded. With exposure measurement error, however, the true uncertainty is greater, so that a higher RR is possible.

3. Random non-differential measurement error should not lead us to discount an observed association of exposure with disease—observing a positive association is no more likely with measurement error. On the other hand, one cannot assume that a small non-significant or even significant estimated effect of exposure would be larger and more significant in the absence of exposure measurement error. Such small associations could be due to chance or to uncontrolled bias or confounding, in which case they would not be larger, on average, in the absence of measurement error.

10.7 FURTHER READING

Most textbooks in epidemiology discuss the effect of misclassification of exposure on estimates of RR, and some give methods for calculating and correcting for bias due to measurement error. The book by White et al. (2008) on exposure measurement in epidemiology is the most accessible source for most of the results discussed in this chapter. The statistical literature continues to include quite large numbers of papers on this topic, mainly focused on methods for correction of bias from measurement error. Carroll et al. (2006) is an excellent review monograph with a particular focus on logistic regression, and with most examples from epidemiology. Also, by Carroll (2000) is a briefer review, somewhat more accessible to non-statisticians. More limited recent reviews given by Keogh (2014) and Spiegelman (2010), and Hutcheon et al. (2010) offer a basic introduction. Earlier reviews include Armstrong (1990) (especially useful for further discussion of and references on Berkson errors and errors in confounders), De Klerk et al. (1989) (especially useful for results on the impact of error on comparisons of risk in quantiles of the exposure distribution), and Armstrong (1998) (a precursor to this chapter!).

REFERENCES

Armstrong, B. G. (1990). The effects of measurement errors on relative risk regressions. *American Journal of Epidemiology*, **132**(6), 1176–1184.

Armstrong, B. G. (1996). Optimizing power in allocating resources to exposure assessment in an epidemiologic study. *American Journal of Epidemiology*, **144**(2), 192–197.

Armstrong, B. G. (1998). Effect of measurement error on epidemiological studies of environmental and occupational exposures. *Occupational and Environmental Medicine*, **55**(10), 651–656.

Basagaña, X., Aguilera, I., Rivera, M., Agis, D., Foraster, M., Marrugat, J., Elosua, R., and Künzli, N. (2013). Measurement error in epidemiologic studies of air pollution based on land-use regression models. *American Journal of Epidemiology*, **178**(8), 1342–1346.

Bland, M., and Altman, D. (1986). Statistical methods for assessing agreement between two methods of clinical measurement. *The Lancet*, **327**(8476), 307–310.

Breslow, N., and Day, N. (1987). *Statistical methods in cancer research. Vol II. The design and analysis of cohort studies. IARC Science Publication*. International Agency for Research on Cancer, Lyon, France.

Carroll, R. (2000). Measurement error in epidemiologic studies. In *Encyplopedia of epidemiologic method* (eds. M. H. Gail, and J. Benichou), 530–557. Wiley, New York.

Carroll, R. J., Ruppert, D., Stefanski, L. A., and Crainiceanu, C. M. (2006). *Measurement error in nonlinear models: A modern perspective*. CRC Press, Boca Raton.

Cole, S. R., Chu, H., and Greenland, S. (2006). Multiple-imputation for measurement-error correction. *International Journal of* Epidemiology, **35**(4), 1074–1081.

de Klerk, N. H., English, D. R., and Armstrong, B. K. (1989). A review of the effects of random measurement error on relative risk estimates in epidemiological studies. *International Journal of Epidemiology*, **18**(3), 705–712.

Doll, R., and Peto, R. (1978). Cigarette smoking and bronchial carcinoma: Dose and time relationships among regular smokers and lifelong non-smokers. *Journal of Epidemiology and Community Health*, **32**(4), 303–313.

Dominici, F., Zeger, S. L., and Samet, J. M. (2000). A measurement error model for time-series studies of air pollution and mortality. *Biostatistics*, **1**(2), 157–175.

Freedman, L. S., Midthune, D., Carroll, R. J., and Kipnis, V. (2008). A comparison of regression calibration, moment reconstruction and imputation for adjusting for covariate measurement error in regression. *Statistics in Medicine*, **27**(25), 5195–5216.

Greenland, S. (1988). Statistical uncertainty due to misclassification: Implications for validation substudies. *Journal of Clinical Epidemiology*, **41**(12), 1167–1174.

Greenland, S. (1992). Divergent biases in ecologic and individual-level studies. *Statistics in Medicine*, **11**(9), 1209–1223.

Hutcheon, J. A., Chiolero, A., and Hanley, J. A. (2010). Random measurement error and regression dilution bias. *British Medical Journal*, **340**, 1406–1402.

Keogh, R. H., Strawbridge, A. D., and White, I. R. (2012). Effects of classical exposure measurement error on the shape of exposure-disease associations. *Epidemiologic Methods*, **1**(1), 13–32.

Keogh, R. H., and White, I. R. (2014). A toolkit for measurement error correction, with a focus on nutritional epidemiology. *Statistics in Medicine*, **33**, 2137–2155.

Lagakos, S. (1988). Effects of mismodelling and mismeasuring explanatory variables on tests of their association with a response variable. *Statistics in Medicine*, **7**(1-2), 257–274.

Liu, K., Stamler, J., Dyer, A., McKeever, J., and McKeever, P. (1978). Statistical methods to assess and minimize the role of intra-individual variability in obscuring the relationship between dietary lipids and serum cholesterol. *Journal of Chronic Diseases*, **31**(6), 399–418.

Pierce, D. A., Preston, D. L., Stram, D. O., and Vaeth, M. (1991). Allowing for dose-estimation errors for the A-bomb survivor data. *Journal of Radiation Research (Tokyo)*, **32**, 108–121.

Sheppard, L., Burnett, R. T., Szpiro, A. A., Kim, S.-Y., Jerrett, M., Pope III, C. A., and Brunekreef, B. (2012). Confounding and exposure measurement error in air pollution epidemiology. *Air Quality, Atmosphere & Health*, **5**(2), 203–216.

Shoukri, M. M. (2000). Agreement, measurement of. In *Encyplopedia of epidemiologic method*. (eds. M. H. Gail and J. Benichou), 35–48. Wiley, New York.

Sorahan, T., and Gilthorpe, M. S. (1994). Non-differential misclassification of exposure always leads to an underestimate of risk: An incorrect conclusion. *Occupational and Environmental Medicine*, **51**(12), 839.

Spiegelman, D. (2010). Approaches to uncertainty in exposure assessment in environmental epidemiology. *Annual Review of Public Health*, **31**, 149–163.

Spiegelman, D., and Valanis, B. (1998). Correcting for bias in relative risk estimates due to exposure measurement error: A case study of occupational exposure to antineoplastics in pharmacists. *American Journal of Public Health*, **88**(3), 406–412.

Szpiro, A. A., Sheppard, L., and Lumley, T. (2011). Efficient measurement error correction with spatially misaligned data. *Biostatistics*, **12**, 610–623.

Van Roosbroeck, S., Li, R., Hoek, G., Lebret, E., Brunekreef, B., and Spiegelman, D. (2008). Traffic-related outdoor air pollution and respiratory symptoms in children: The impact of adjustment for exposure measurement error. *Epidemiology*, **19**(3), 409–416.

VanderWeele, T. J., and Hernán, M. A. (2012). Results on differential and dependent measurement error of the exposure and the outcome using signed directed acyclic graphs. *American Journal of Epidemiology*, **175**(12), 1303–1310.

Wacholder, S., Armstrong, B., and Hartge, P. (1993). Validation studies using an alloyed gold standard. *American Journal of Epidemiology*, **137**(11), 1251–1258.

Wacholder, S., Hartge, P., Lubin, J. H., and Dosemeci, M. (1995). Non-differential misclassification and bias towards the null: A clarification. *Occupational and Environmental Medicine*, **52**(8), 557–558.

White, E., Armstrong, B. K., and Saracci, R. (2008). *Principles of exposure measurement in epidemiology: Collecting, evaluating and improving measures of disease risk factors*: Oxford University Press, New York.

Zeger, S. L., Thomas, D., Dominici, F., Samet, J. M., Schwartz, J., Dockery, D., and Cohen, A. (2000). Exposure measurement error in time-series studies of air pollution: Concepts and consequences. *Environmental Health Perspectives*, **108**(5), 419–426.

Zhao, L., and Lipsitz, S. (1992). Designs and analysis of two-stage studies. *Statistics in Medicine*, **11**(6), 769–782.

SECTION II

Current Topics

11

EXPOSURE ASSESSMENT FOR BIOLOGICAL AGENTS IN ENVIRONMENTAL EPIDEMIOLOGY

Dick Heederik and Heike Schmitt

11.1 INTRODUCTION

Biological agents include microorganisms such as fungi, bacteria, viruses, and their associated constituents such as allergens and toxins. Some definitions are wider and also include plant and animal matter. Exposure to biological agents often occurs in the form of bio-aerosols. Bio-aerosols are usually defined as aerosols or particulate matter of microbial, plant, or animal origin. Bio-aerosols contain constituents of micro-organisms, such as high molecular weight (HMW) allergens, bacterial endotoxins, mycotoxins, peptidoglycans, $\beta_{(1\rightarrow3)}$ or $\beta_{(1\rightarrow6)}$ glucans, and so on.

The interest in bio-aerosol exposure has increased over the last decades. This is largely because it is recognized that exposures to biological agents in the outdoor, occupational, and residential indoor environment are associated with a wide range of health effects with potentially major public health impact. These effects include infectious diseases, acute toxic effects, allergies, and cancer. Potential protective effects of microbial exposure have also been described and are often referred to as the hygiene hypothesis (Strachan 2000; Braun-Fahrlander et al. 2002).

Despite the recognition of the importance of bio-aerosol exposure for human health, the precise role of biological agents in the development and aggravation of symptoms and diseases is often only poorly understood. With the exception of specific pathogens in relation to infectious diseases, and a few individual components such as bacterial endotoxin and specific allergens, little insight exists into which specific micro-organisms or their component(s) primarily account for health effects. As an example, indoor humidity is consistently associated with increased occurrence of respiratory symptoms (Fisk et al. 2007). Biological agent exposure has been associated with indoor humidity and water damage. However, a direct association between biological agent exposure and respiratory health effects has only been established in a few studies and results are conflicting (Zock et al. 2002; Belanger et al. 2003). Few dose–response relationships have been described and knowledge on threshold exposure levels is limited (Eduard 2008). The lack of accurate quantitative exposure assessment methods likely contributed to the lack of knowledge. New assays and molecular technologies are rapidly changing this perspective. In this chapter an overview is given of exposure assessment methods for biological agents and applications in environmental epidemiological studies are presented.

11.2 HISTORIC PERSPECTIVE

Louis Pasteur was the first who assessed environmental microbial exposure using flasks containing growth media and can be considered one of the first aero-biologists (Ariatti and Comptois 1993). Around 1860 he aerosolized dust samples from different origins and established the principle of volumetric sampling. He observed a clear heterogeneity of the bacterial species distribution in the air and described dispersal and deposition through the air. He analyzed samples using the microscope. Major improvements were reached after the introduction of active microbial samplers that contained petri dishes facilitating easy processing of samples after sampling in the 20th century (Eduard and Heederik, 1998). Nowadays, different types of so-called "viable samplers" exist and these can be differentiated into impactors, filter methods, and impingers. A general problem is the sampling stress exerted on micro-organisms, leading to reduced viability. This complicates sampling and potentially results in a biased exposure estimate. There is a tendency to avoid long sampling times because of viability issues. Another constraint is that impactors, which contain nutrient agar plates, have an upper limit of detection because of potential overgrowth and this limits sampling duration. Short sampling times are associated with a high variability in measured concentrations and high exposure variability limits the application of viable sampling techniques in environmental studies. An illustration is given by a study in humid homes (Verhoeff et al. 1992). The presence of viable molds in indoor air was investigated using the widely used N6-Andersen sampler in combination with DG18-agar agar plates. Repeated measurements were performed and this allowed evaluation of the variability over time and the correlation between repeats. The variability in time was high and the correlation between repeated total colony-forming unit (CFU) measurements on the two occasions varied between 0.05 and 0.8. Especially low correlations between consecutive measurement requires intensive repeated sampling in order to obtain stable estimates for long-term average exposure in a home (Table 11.1).

For viable sampling, over short sampling times, theoretical calculations lead to 8 to 200 repeated measurements, depending on the measure of exposure, required to avoid underestimation of an exposure response relation by maximally 10%. Thus variability over time limits the use of CFU measurements in studies that explore associations between exposure to molds and health effects. Only when considerable contrast in exposure exists, for instance in occupational environments, or severely water damaged buildings, a limited number of measurements can be sufficient to document differences in microbial exposure among different environments and pick up existing contrasts in exposure (Rao et al. 2007).

Around the same time Pasteur worked on sampling bacteria, Charles Blackley sampled and counted spores from the air with a simple passive sampling device and

Table 11.1 Correlations between repeated CFU measurements using the Andersen sampler in a study in Dutch homes and the number of repeated measurements k required to obtain an accurate estimate of long-term average CFU exposure to avoid bias in an exposure response relation to 10% maximally

	ρ	k to limit bias to 10% in observed relation relative to true relation
Total CFU/m³	0.28	35
Aspergillus sp.	0	$+\infty$
Claudosporium sp.	0.23	43
Penicillium sp.	0.8	8
Wallemia sp.	0.05	200

Verhoeff, A. P., van Wijnen, J. H., Brunekreef, B., Fischer, P., van Reenen-Hoekstra, E. S., and Samson, R. A. (1992). Presence of viable mould propagules in indoor air in relation to house damp and outdoor air. *Allergy*, **47**, 83–91.

a microscope as part of his work on hay fever, published in 1873 (Blackley 1873). He considered that "... the number as well as the kind of germs and other organic bodies found in the dust ..." was of crucial importance. He also made interesting observations on the effect of measurement position on the amount of deposited dust, the effect of hedges and forests, meteorological conditions such as wind speed and rain, and differences between rural and urban areas.

Modern non-viable measurement techniques often make use of direct counting and identification of microorganisms by (electron) microscope, and were considered an alternative for viable sampling (Eduard 1996). An additional advantage of non-viable sampling is that modern dust sampling techniques can be used, which sample according to health-based size selective distributions. Early non–culture-based methods made use of staining techniques with fluorescent agents that facilitated counting by light microscopy (Palmgren, Strom, Blomquist, and Malmberg 1986). More advanced methods made use of electron microscopy for determination. Although useful for characterization of a small number of samples, these techniques are too laborious and costly for quantitative exposure assessment in population-based studies (Karlsson and Malmberg 1989). Early molecular techniques, such as fluorescent in situ hybridization (FISH), enabled taxonomic determinations at the genus or species level (Lange et al. 1997). However, these techniques could only identify a limited number of species at a time, required highly skilled personnel, and hardly found an application. Since the 1980s other non-viable techniques have been developed based on bioassays, immunoassays, and chemical methods. These methods have been used to measure markers of microbial exposure, such as endotoxins and a range of other molecules. These methods, together with methods to measure micro-organisms by DNA-based methods, are discussed in greater detail in the following paragraphs.

11.3 SAMPLING METHODS FOR NON-VIABLE BIOLOGICAL AGENTS

When the respiratory organ is the port of entry, ideally, exposure to bio-aerosols should be assessed by taking air samples. Many reviews describe the available sampling devices and their pros and cons (Eduard and Heederik 1998; Eduard et al. 2012; Raulf et al. 2014). Static and personal sampling techniques have been used to take such samples, but for bio-aerosols, few personal samplers exist. The specification of an air sampler, with regard to particle sizes sampled, is an important element that should be evaluated carefully. As mentioned, viable sampling of micro-organisms has major limitations. In indoor air research, many studies have relied on reservoir samples from floors, mattresses, or upholstered furniture. Reservoir samples are believed to be more stable over time and the concentration estimated per gram of dust may vary considerably less than the concentration of a short-term air sample measured at a single occasion. This has in particular been studied for endotoxin and some allergens in the home environment (Hirsch et al. 1998; Topp et al. 2003; Abraham et al. 2005; Crisafulli et al. 2007). However, reservoir samples are considered poor proxies for inhalatory exposure because reservoir samples also contain particles that are too large to become airborne for a prolonged period of time. The reservoirs sampled may not be the only relevant sources for personal exposure of inhabitants of these houses (Tovey et al. 2013). Nowadays, some good experiences have been reported with passive samplers in exposure and epidemiological studies (Wurtz et al. 2005; Noss et al. 2008, 2010). These techniques can be used to sample deposition of particulates over longer periods of time. These low-tech devices can be placed in houses, classrooms, or even stables to accumulate dust and can be sent by surface mail to the laboratory after dust collection. The dust load is relatively low, but by optimizing extraction, samples can be used to even measure viable micro-organisms under some conditions, endotoxins, allergens, glucans, and a range of genetic targets (Noss et al. 2008; Normand et al. 2011; Krop et al. 2014). Reproducibility of measurements taken with these dust collectors is relatively good because of the longer sampling times, so that a few measurements over time give a reasonable estimate of longer-term average exposure (Topp et al. 2003; Noss et al. 2008; J. H. Jacobs et al. 2014).

11.4 ASSESSMENT METHODS FOR MICROBIAL CONSTITUENTS AND MARKERS

Instead of counting culturable or non-culturable micro-organisms, constituents or metabolites of microorganisms can be measured (Eduard 1996; Raulf et al. 2014). Toxic (e.g., mycotoxins) or pro-inflammatory (e.g., endotoxin) components can be measured, but non-toxic molecules may also serve as markers of either large groups of microorganisms or specific microbial genera or species. Molecules such as endotoxins, extracellular polysaccharides (EPS), glucans, and muramic acid, which originate from cell walls of micro-organisms, are recognized by the innate and humoral immune system and referred to as "pathogen or micro-organism associated molecular patterns" (PAMPs or MAMPS). Many PAMPs are recognized by cellular receptors of the innate immune system, such as so called Toll-like receptors (TLRs), and are known potent pro-inflammatory agents (Palma et al. 2006; Taylor et al. 2007; Mogensen 2009). Toll-like receptors have been identified in humans and recognize ligands from different micro-organisms ranging from endotoxin from Gram-negative bacteria, heat shock proteins, lipoproteins, lipopeptides, or flagellin from bacteria, bacterial DNA, or viral RNA. Toll-like receptors signaling pathways have been unravelled to a large extent and play a role in explaining health effects resulting from PAMP or MAMP exposure. Mycotoxins in particular have been associated with a variety of toxic effects and mechanisms, although few attempts have been described to measure these agents in indoor environments (Jarvis 1990).

Important advantages of measuring these agents are the stability of most of the measured components, allowing longer sampling times, and frozen storage of samples before analysis. Only few of the mentioned agents or markers are discussed in somewhat more detail.

Endotoxin is most often measured by using a *Limulus* amoebocyte lysate (LAL) test prepared from cells of the horseshoe crab, *Limulus Polyphemus* (LPS; Bang 1956). Analytical chemistry methods for quantification of LPS have also been developed employing gas chromatography-mass spectrometry (GC-MS) (Sonesson et al. 1988, 1990). However, these methods require special LPS extraction procedures and are less widely used. They have found application in studies in which LPS molecules with different chain lengths were measured (Hines et al. 2000; Park et al. 2004). Some markers for the assessment of fungal biomass include ergosterol measured by GC-MS or fungal extracellular polysaccharides measured with specific enzyme immunoassays, allowing partial identification of the mold genera present (Miller and Young, 1997; Douwes et al. 1999). Agents such as $\beta(1\rightarrow3)$-glucans and bacterial endotoxin are being measured because of their toxic potency (Aketagawa et al. 1993; Nagi et al. 1993; Douwes et al. 1996, 1997). $\beta(1\rightarrow3)$-glucans can be measured using a method based on the LAL assay and by immunoassays (Aketagawa et al. 1993; Douwes et al. 1996). N-acetyl-muramic acid, a major component of bacterial peptidoglycan, part of the cell wall of extracellular polysaccharides of mainly Gram-positives, is often measured as a marker. Ergosterol and $\beta(1-3)$- and $\beta(1-6)$-glucans are markers of fungal mass (Zhiping et al. 1996; Saraf et al. 1997; Douwes et al. 1999; Heederik et al. 1999; Laitinen et al. 2001; Tischer et al. 2011). Most of the methods to measure microbial constituents (with the exception of the method to measure bacterial endotoxins) have not been standardized and are not commercially available. Even for some well-established methods (e.g., the LAL assay to measure bacterial endotoxin) significant variations exist in exposure assessment among laboratories, but differences are mainly related to sample treatment and analysis (Thorne et al. 1997; Spaan et al. 2007, 2008) (Table 11.2).

Although earlier studies mainly addressed the work environment, later studies studied the indoor environment related to humidity and moldy houses and protective effects of microbial exposure in particular in farming communities

Table 11.2 Some well-known and commonly applied markers for microbial exposure

Microbial marker name	Microbial marker for
Endotoxin or LPS	Gram-negative bacteria
Peptidoglycan (muramic acid)	Gram-positive bacteria
Ergosterol	Molds
$\beta_{(1\rightarrow3)}$ and $\beta_{(1\rightarrow6)}$ Glucans	Molds
Extracellular polysaccharides (EPS)	Different groups of fungi (*Aspergillus* and *Penicillium* sp.)
Volatile organic compounds	Any micro-organism

(Braun-Fahrlander et al. 2002; van Strien et al. 2004; Schram-Bijkerk et al. 2005; Douwes et al. 2006; Gehring et al. 2008; Sordillo et al. 2011; J. Jacobs et al. 2014). There are numerous studies that have now associated exposure to microbial markers in the home environment to health effects. Endotoxin is associated with protective effects for eczema (Perzanowski et al. 2006) and asthma, the latter in cross-sectional (Gereda, Leung, and Liu 2000; Gereda, Leung, Thatayatikom, et al. 2000; Gehring et al. 2007, 2008) and longitudinal (Douwes et al. 2006; Tischer et al. 2011) studies. In some studies these signals are present after mutual adjustment, indicating that several independent microbial signals, from bacteria and molds, can exert protective effects (Douwes et al. 2006; Sordillo et al. 2010). However, it has been suggested that continued exposure may be required to maintain optimal protection (Douwes et al. 2008). Studies among occupationally exposed adults without early childhood exposures have shown clear protective effects associated with endotoxin exposure, albeit at exposures that were orders of magnitude higher than usually encountered in the home environment (Smit, Heederik, Doekes, Lammers, and Wouters 2010).

11.5 DNA/RNA-BASED MOLECULAR METHODS FOR MEASURING SPECIES

Several useful references exist on the recent technological revolution with regard to measurement techniques for DNA/RNA and also their application in ecological studies, exposure studies, and (environmental) epidemiology (Thomas, Gilbert, and Meyer 2012; Kelley and Gilbert 2013). The spectrum of techniques available is extremely wide and still growing.

The most commonly used molecular technique to measure micro-organisms in the environment is based on PCR amplification by use of primers that are complementary to the target gene or target sequence. For this approach all DNA is directly extracted from all cells, including from dead material, in the sample. With quantitative polymerase chain reaction (qPCR) the concentration of DNA template molecules in a sample can be assessed. The concentration is calculated from the C_T value of a sample in the amplification process, which describes the cycle during which fluorescence in the PCR reaction exceeds a detection threshold. Quantification is reached by use of a standard curve of C_T values against the concentration of the target micro-organism in a dilution series. Quantitative PCR is a rapid analytical procedure compared with culturing and can handle large numbers of samples in a short period of time. Quantitative PCR has been used for analysis of broad microbial markers, pathogens, or specific genes such as antibiotic resistance genes in indoor and outdoor dust samples (Nehme et al. 2009; Letourneau et al. 2010; Gilbert et al. 2012; J. Jacobs et al. 2014). In the infectious disease field these PCR techniques can open up the black box of transmission and exposure (Foxman 2011).

During the last few years, molecular methods based on amplification and detection of DNA or RNA sequences in micro-organisms led to a revolution in epidemiological studies on infectious and chronic diseases in which microbial exposures play a role. For studies on infectious diseases they contribute to exact measurement of the outcomes by reducing misclassification of disease and thus improving outbreak studies or longer-term epidemiologccal studies (Foxman 2011). In exposure assessment, they facilitate measurement of the specific causal agent in the environment. For instance, the species *Coxiella burnetii*, the causative agent of Q-fever that is responsible for major outbreaks, can be measured in inhalable or PM10 dust samples using two unique target sequences (*com1 and IS1111*) (Hogerwerf et al. 2012). Similarly, these techniques can also be used to attempt to measure specific strains. An example is methicillin-resistant *Staphylococcus aureus* of the sequence type ST398 (MRSA-ST398), a microorganism resistant to antimicrobials. This strain emerged a decade ago and circulates in livestock animals because of the high usage of antimicrobials in for instance pig and poultry production. It has been measured in the environment and in nasal swab samples of people handling dead or alive animals at the farm and in slaughterhouses (Gilbert et al. 2012). Two DNA targets were used to measure *Staphylococcus aureus* ST398 directly in environmental samples; the *C01* fragment specific for *Staphylococcus aureus* ST398 and the *mecA* gene that codes for methicillin resistance of MRSA (Francois et al. 2003; van Wamel et al. 2010). Multiple primers have to be used for the *mecA* gene, because of its heterogeneity. These two targets would identify a cultured strain of *Staphylococcus aureus* ST398 when both would be found simultaneously in the DNA a colony. However, when these targets are directly measured in a dust sample, both signals might come from different micro-organisms present in the sample. Thus the presence of *Staphylococcus aureus* ST398 cannot be established with absolute certainty. First, the *mecA* gene can be found in other species than *Staphylococcus aureus* ST398. Thus parallel presence of these two signals in a dust sample does not necessarily mean MRSA ST398 is present in a sample. Second, some *Staphylococcus aureus* ST398 are sensitive for methicillin because they do not have the *mecA* gene, whereas other do possess the *MecA* gene and as a result are methicillin resistant. However, studies in which these two signals have been measured directly in large numbers of environmental samples do show a relatively high correlation between the two targets, which seems indicative of the presence of MRSA ST398. Air levels of these markers were associated with nasal carriage of MRSA ST398, the latter assessed after plating and colonization and identification of the isolated strain and not directly assessed in the nasal sample as done for the dust sample (Gilbert et al. 2012; Bos et al. 2014). This example clearly illustrates that when one is interested in a very specific strain, it might not always be possible to identify this strain with certainty, using multiple DNA targets and direct PCR analysis of environmental samples.

A public health issue is whether ST398 MRSA can be transmitted through the environment to humans living near farms. To explore this issue, the same molecular markers were measured in PM10 samples taken in a region with intensive livestock farming in the Netherlands to obtain insight in the MRSA ST398 air levels (Table 11.3). Repeated PM10 samples were taken over 2-week periods. The number of livestock farms were assessed in a 1000-meter radius around the sampling points.

MecA could be measured in all PM10 samples, whereas CO1 often could not be detected, but the number of positive samples per location out of all samples was associated with the number of livestock farms present. The mecA level in air was positively correlated with the number of livestock farms around the sampling location in a regression analysis (β 1.07; $p = 0.017$). MecA and CO1 levels correlated significantly (0.40; $p < 0.05$). These results indicated that people living around livestock farms are likely exposed to elevated Staphylococcus aureus ST398 levels. Other studies, at shorter distances, have assessed that Staphylococcus aureus colonies can still be viable (Gibbs et al. 2006). Population surveys have not been able to find an elevated risk for nasal carriage of Staphylococcus aureus ST398 in people living near livestock farms (van Cleef et al. 2010; Bisdorff et al. 2012).

DNA-based techniques have the advantage that organisms can be measured that are extremely difficult to grow, such as Coxiella burnetii or Legionella pneumophila (Sirigul et al. 2006). Molecular fingerprinting techniques can also be used to explore whether Legionella sp. found in infected patients are similar to the species found in environmental samples and thus enable assessing highly specific epidemiological associations (Ishimatsu et al. 2001) Another intriguing example

Table 11.3 Levels of mecA and CO1 targets for measuring Staphylococcus aureus ST398 in PM10 samples in an areas with intensive livestock production in the Netherlands

Location	# livestock farms in 1000 m radius from air sampling location	Molecular markers for MRSA ST398			
		mecA		CO1	
Background	0	13/13	100%	1/13	8%
A	3	13/13	100%	2/13	15%
B	7	12/12	100%	10/12	83%
C	18	12/12	100%	6/12	50%
D	18	13/13	100%	6/13	46%
E	23	11/11	100%	10/11	91%

Wouters, I. M., Schmitt, H., Smit, L. A., van Rotterdam, B., De Bruin, A., and Heederik, D. (2015). Microbial agents and bacterial resistance in PM10 in air in areas with intensive livestock production: A potential source of human exposure. Submitted for publication.

are organisms from the domain Archaea, formerly classified as Archaea-bacteria. Archaea can be extreme anaerobes, can be extremely difficult to culture, and some live in the gut of ruminants. Levels in stable air have been measured and are as high as $10^8/m^3$ on the basis of qPCR measurements. Some Archaea species have been suggested to have protective properties with regard to allergy and asthma development (Nehme et al. 2009).

Detection of DNA does not imply that the investigated organisms were viable. Thus, overestimations of pathogen presence can occur if environmental stress largely reduces the number of viable and thus infective pathogens in a sample, as PCR also detects DNA from dead microbial cells.

Quantitative polymerase chain reaction can be used to assess moldiness. Based on qPCR analysis of 35 indicator mold species, attempts have been undertaken to classify indoor environments using the indoor environmental moldiness index with some success (Vesper et al. 2007). A study from a large European study in schools performed in different European countries, shows that mold levels vary within and between countries, possibly complicating the use of a simple generic mold indicator (Jacobs et al. 2014). Dust from settled dust boxes was pooled for predefined clusters of classrooms in the same area of a school. In these pooled dust samples DNA was measured by qPCR from *Cladosporium herbarum, Eurotium amstelodami, Stachybotrys chartarum, Wallemia sebi, Penicillium chrysogenum,* group *Trichoderma viride/atroviride/koningii,* group *Penicillium* spp./*Aspergillus* spp./ *Paecilomyces variotii, Mycobacterium* spp., *Streptomyces* spp., Gram-positive bacteria, and Gram-negative bacteria. The lowest levels were generally seen in Finland, often below the detection limit, in particular during the winter. Levels of microbial markers in classrooms differed strongly among countries and were higher in Spain and the Netherlands compared with Finland. *Cladosporium herbarum* levels showed some seasonal trend in all three countries, with highest levels during spring/early summer and low levels during the winter. Other microbial markers showed no seasonal trends in Spain and the Netherlands, with clearly lower levels in Finland during winter compared with spring. *Penicillium chrysogenum* levels were higher in classrooms of schools with dampness problems, compared with reference schools in all three countries, although differences were not always statistically significant. The majority of PCR markers were higher in schools with dampness problems, but differences were generally not statistically significant. Associations with respiratory endpoints were most pronounced in Finland, despite lower microbial levels compared with Spanish and Dutch schools. Results suggested that associations among moisture, microbial exposure, and health may vary among countries. Possibly, the particular exposure pattern in Finland (low and intermittent) contributes to symptom occurrence.

An important issue with these genetic markers is that some species occur at relatively low levels in the environment. This results in many samples with non-detectable levels and requires modeling of the exposure after imputation, or use of statistical techniques, which can deal with left censored data or zero-inflated regression models (Lubin et al. 2004; Zeileis et al. 2014).

11.6 MICROBIAL DIVERSITY AND HEALTH

Over the last decades, a rapid increase in diseases associated with inflammation has been observed (Bach 2002; von Hertzen et al. 2011). This increase has been assumed to be associated with a decrease in infectious diseases and reduced presence of micro-organisms in the living environment, leading to a less diverse microbial exposure of humans with westernized lifestyles. This concept is referred to as the *hygiene* or *microbial deprivation* hypothesis and triggers interest in the diversity of microbial exposure in relation to the human microbiome, the microbial interface between human cells and the environment. The composition of the human microbiome is believed to play an important role in the development of different chronic immunological diseases (Foxman and Goldberg 2010).

As an example, breastfeeding is associated with a different microbial community of the upper airways in infants than formula feeding and this may contribute to the protective effect of breastfeeding to the development of allergy and asthma (Biesbroek et al. 2014). The respiratory microbiome is different in asthmatics, individuals with chronic obstructive pulmonary disease and smokers, suggesting a role of microbial diversity in the development of disease (Charlson et al. 2010; Hilty et al. 2010; Dickson, Martinez, and Huffnagle 2014).

The role of the environmental microbial exposure in these diseases has also seen growing interest. Studies of soil and water samples reveal the presence of thousands of different species, many of which are novel (Tringe and Rubin 2005; Tringe and Hugenholtz 2008; Tringe et al. 2008). Bacterial diversity in outdoor air is variable over time and dependent on meteorological conditions and higher in areas with agriculture than suburban areas and forests (Brodie et al. 2007; Bowers, McLetchie et al. 2011). Indoor diversity is smaller than found outdoors and often human related (Tringe et al. 2008; Taubel et al. 2009). Similarly, fungal diversity seems also strongly driven by environmental selection and is more diverse in temperate zones (Amend et al. 2010). The relevance for human health needs to be established.

Diversity information can be obtained directly from environmental samples after DNA extraction. Most previously mentioned studies made use of PCR amplification of parts of the 16S ribosomal rRNA gene for bacteria and ITS or 18S genes for fungi. "Universal" PCR primers are being used to amplify these genes from the genomic material extracted. By comparing the sequences obtained from these highly conserved regions with databases, they can be used for genus/species identification and for characterization of microbial communities and community–host interactions. Early methods like denaturing gradient gel electrophoresis (DGGE), single strand confirmation polymorphisms (SSCP), and terminal restriction fragment length polymorphism (tRFLP), separated the pool of amplified pieces of DNA ("amplicons") on gels. The band pattern that emerges on the gels gives information about the community of micro-organisms. By excision of bands, re-amplification, and sequencing and comparing with databases, identification of micro-organisms is possible. Limitations of these methods are that at best they are semi-quantitative and not very sensitive because they are only able to detect the most dominant taxa, and may have a more limited resolution. An example of an application in an epidemiological context is a study among German farmers' children. Exposure to higher numbers of species was inversely related to asthma risk, and this result triggers new studies with technologically more advanced molecular methods that can characterize microbial diversity (see Ege et al. 2011) (Figure 11.1).

Direct sequencing of DNA from environmental samples has created a revolution in 16S RNA analysis (Tringe and Rubin 2005; Tringe and Hugenholtz 2008). Phylogenetic analysis by comparing sequences obtained with external databases, gives an impression of the microbial diversity of the sample. This method is extremely powerful, but concerns exist that different DNA extraction protocols lead to different outcomes. In addition, primers are not "completely universal," which potentially introduces biases in the observed community composition. Further, the copy number of target genes such as 16S varies among bacterial species, complicating the analysis of the absolute composition of a sample.

Analysis of taxonomic marker genes were initially performed in clone libraries. Next generation sequencing analyses made analyses of much higher amounts of sequences economically feasible. In meta-genomic analyses, the total genetic

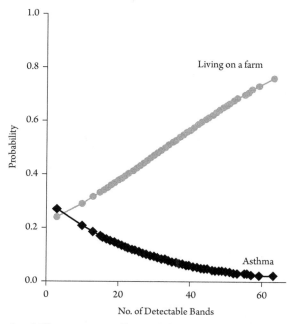

Figure 11.1 Farming children were generally exposed to more microorganisms in their mattress dust than non-farming children as assessed by SSCP. The likelihood of asthma decreased clearly with increasing numbers of species in mattress dust.

From Ege, M. J., Mayer, M., Normand, A. C., Genuneit, J., Cookson, W. O., Braun-Fahrlander, C., et al. (2011). Exposure to environmental microorganisms and childhood asthma. *The New England Journal of Medicine*, **364**, 701–709.

content of samples is investigated without pre-amplification. This approach allows for an identification of functional genes, including virulence genes, and reduces the bias introduced through PCR pre-amplification if used for taxonomic profiling.

Microbial diversity data can be analyzed in different ways. Descriptive results are often presented in the form of phylogenetic trees, which can be produced with specialized software. Sequences are usually grouped into one species if their 16S rRNA genes are 95% to 99% identical, although species can still vary considerably at a similarity threshold as high as 99% (Konstantinidis and Tiedje 2005). One straightforward approach is to express diversity in a single parameter, reflecting how many different species are present in a sample and how individuals are distributed over these species. Some examples are richness and evenness, α-diversity, and the Shannon Diversity Index (Boon et al. 2002; Ege et al. 2011). These variables can then be used as dependent variables in a conventional multiple regression analysis, adjusting for confounders. This approach ignores that associations with environmental determinants may differ for (sub-)populations of micro-organisms or individual micro-organisms. To take the full richness of the collected diversity data into account, and to enable analysis of associations with environmental variables, multivariate statistical techniques are required. Techniques that can deal with multiple dependent (microbiome) and independent (metadata comprising potential confounding variables and environmental determinants) have been applied such as Canonical Correlation analysis, Principal Coordinate or Principal Component analysis, and other multidimensional scaling techniques, with different levels of refinement (Lozupone and Knight 2005; Ramette 2007; Wang et al. 2012; Morris et al. 2013; Biesbroek et al. 2014; Buttigieg and Ramette 2014).

11.7 METHODOLOGICAL ISSUES

Optimal exposure assessment by measuring an individual's environmental exposure with similar accuracy and precision as an individual's genome has been mentioned as a requirement for future studies (Wild 2005). This is not likely to be achieved easily because up to now, relatively simple proxies of inhalatory exposure are being used (Horick et al. 2006; Noss et al. 2008), and environmental exposure is highly variable (Horick et al. 2006) for many microbial agents (Verhoeff et al. 1992; Topp et al. 2003; Giovannangelo et al. 2007). Variability in the composition of the environmental microbiome can lead to different types of errors (Foxman and Goldberg 2010). These errors in the exposure assessment may lead to bias of exposure–response relations, but can also create other difficulties in the interpretation of studies and may require novel data-analytical approaches and statistical techniques and replication (Vineis et al. 2009). Type 1 errors refer to false positive results from the large number of comparisons. Potential analytical errors will be superimposed on top of the large environmental variability over time and space. To be able to distinguish between microorganisms that are transiently and permanently present, repeated measurement studies are required in powerful longitudinal studies. It is important to realize that non-commensal pathogens are in most cases transiently present by definition. Type II errors refer to lack of sensitivity of measurement techniques, resulting in false negative results. Levels for some of the individual species in environmental samples are expected to be low and the available material for analysis is often limited. Some of the early analytical molecular techniques, like SSCP and DGGE, have relatively high detection limits (Korthals et al. 2008). Thus, the likelihood that these errors may arise is high. Polymerase chain reaction, which is one of the most sensitive molecular methods, still has limits of detection that are often higher than culture techniques. Moreover, the longer sampling times that are applicable for DNA analysis partly overcome this limitation. Meta-genomic analysis of dust samples can also be sensitive but still has its limitations. Type III errors refer to the lack of biological relevance of some microorganisms detected in statistical analyses. This is a crucial issue because the underlying mechanisms are not unraveled and the role of individual micro-organisms or microbial communities in the etiology of disease is only poorly understood. Presence of different microbial signals is likely to be correlated when they come from the same samples. Analysis of (highly) correlated data becomes a major issue in the interpretation of findings. Replication of associations with environmental exposures seems essential, but may be more difficult because of inherent high variability in exposure (Fierer et al. 2008; Vineis et al. 2009; Foxman and Goldberg 2010).

Molecular methods create exposure assessment opportunities where classical techniques failed. Both universal and specific primers and probes for bacteria and molds have found application in studies in the agricultural, work, and indoor environment. The recent development of molecular techniques to study the microbiome has opened new avenues that will help researchers to understand the contribution of environmental exposure to microorganisms and their diversity to human health. The microbiome does not only relate to human body habitats, but also to a human's exposure to diverse microbial communities in the exterior environment and its potential impact on human health. These developments may require application of new concepts, such as the investigation of microbial ecological systems rather than the identification of individual pathogens. Many questions relating to the best methodologies to assess exposures and their impact on human health are still open and need to be explored in a new generation of large interdisciplinary studies.

REFERENCES

Abraham, J. H., Gold, D. R., Dockery, D. W., Ryan, L., Park, J. H., and Milton, D. K. (2005). Within-home versus between-home variability of house dust endotoxin in a birth cohort. *Environmental Health Perspectives*, **113**, 1516–1521.

Aketagawa, J., Tanaka, S., Tamura, H., Shibata, Y., and Saito, H. (1993). Activation of limulus coagulation factor G by several (1-->3)-beta-D-glucans: Comparison of the potency of glucans with identical degree of polymerization but different conformations. *Journal of Biochemistry*, **113**, 683–686.

Amend, A. S., Seifert, K. A., Samson, R., and Bruns, T. D. (2010). Indoor fungal composition is geographically patterned and more diverse in temperate zones than in the tropics. *Proceedings of the National Academy of Science of the U S A*, **107**, 13748–13753.

Ariatti, A., and Comptois, P. (1993). Louis pasteur: The first experimental aerobiologist. *Aerobiologica*, **9**, 5–14.

Bach, J. F. (2002). The effect of infections on susceptibility to autoimmune and allergic diseases. *The New England Journal of Medicine*, **347**, 911–920.

Bang, F. B. (1956). A bacterial disease of Limulus polyphemus. *Bulletin of the Johns Hopkins Hospital*, **98**, 325–351.

Belanger, K., Beckett, W., Triche, E., Bracken, M. B., Holford, T., Ren, P., et al. (2003). Symptoms of wheeze and persistent cough in the first year of life: Associations with indoor allergens, air contaminants, and maternal history of asthma. *American Journal of Epidemiology*, **158**, 195–202.

Biesbroek, G., Bosch, A. A., Wang, X., Keijser, B. J., Veenhoven, R. H., Sanders, E. A., and Bogaert, D. (2014). The impact of breastfeeding on nasopharyngeal microbial communities in infants. *American Journal of Respiratory and Critical Care Medicine*, **190**, 298–308.

Bisdorff, B., Scholholter, J. L., Claussen, K., Pulz, M., Nowak, D., and Radon, K. (2012). MRSA-ST398 in livestock farmers and neighbouring residents in a rural area in Germany. *Epidemiology & Infection*, **140**, 1800–1808.

Blackley, C. (1873). *Experimental researches on the causes of catarrhus astivus (hay-fever or hay-asthma)*. Balliere, Tyndall and Cox, London. https://archive.org/details/experimentalres00blacgoog

Boon, N., Windt, W., Verstraete, W., and Top, E. M. (2002). Evaluation of nested PCR-DGGE (denaturing gradient gel electrophoresis) with group-specific 16S rRNA primers for the analysis of bacterial communities from different wastewater treatment plants. *FEMS Microbiology Ecology*, **39**, 101–112.

Bos, M., Verstappen, K. M., van Cleef, B., Dohmen, W., Dorado-Garcia, A., Graveland, H., et al. (2014). Transmission through air as a possible route of exposure for MRSA. *Journal of Exposure Science and Environmental Epidemiology*, accepted for publication. See http://www.ncbi.nlm.nih.gov/pubmed/25515375

Bowers, R. M., McLetchie, S., Knight, R., and Fierer, N. (2011). Spatial variability in airborne bacterial communities across land-use types and their relationship to the bacterial communities of potential source environments. *ISME Journal*, **5**, 601–612.

Braun-Fahrlander, C., Riedler, J., Herz, U., Eder, W., Waser, M., Grize, L., et al. (2002). Environmental exposure to endotoxin and its relation to asthma in school-age children. *The New England Journal of Medicine*, **347**, 869–877.

Brodie, E. L., DeSantis, T. Z., Parker, J. P., Zubietta, I. X., Piceno, Y. M., and Andersen, G. L. (2007). Urban aerosols harbor diverse and dynamic bacterial populations. *Proceedings of the National Academy of Science of the U S A*, **104**, 299–304.

Buttigieg, P. L., and Ramette, A. (2014). A guide to statistical analysis in microbial ecology: A community-focused, living review of multivariate data analyses. *FEMS Microbiology and Ecology*, **90**. See http://www.ncbi.nlm.nih.gov/pubmed/25314312. doi: 10.1111/1574-6941.12437

Charlson, E. S., Chen, J., Custers-Allen, R., Bittinger, K., Li, H., Sinha, R., et al. (2010). Disordered microbial communities in the upper respiratory tract of cigarette smokers. *PLoS One*, **5**, e15216.

Crisafulli, D., Almqvist, C., Marks, G., and Tovey, E. (2007). Seasonal trends in house dust mite allergen in children's beds over a 7-year period. *Allergy*, **62**, 1394–1400.

Dickson, R. P., Martinez, F. J., and Huffnagle, G. B. (2014). The role of the microbiome in exacerbations of chronic lung diseases. *Lancet*, **384**, 691–702.

Douwes, J., Cheng, S., Travier, N., Cohet, C., Niesink, A., McKenzie, J., et al. (2008). Farm exposure in utero may protect against asthma, hay fever and eczema. *European Respiratory Journal*, **32**, 603–611.

Douwes, J., Doekes, G., Montijn, R., Heederik, D., and Brunekreef, B. (1996). Measurement of beta(1-->3)-glucans in occupational and home environments with an inhibition enzyme immunoassay. *Applied Environmental Microbiology*, **62**, 3176–3182.

Douwes, J., Doekes, G., Montijn, R., Heederik, D., and Brunekreef, B. (1997). An immunoassay for the measurement of (1-->3)-beta-D-glucans in the indoor environment. *Mediators of Inflammation*, **6**, 257–262.

Douwes, J., van der Sluis, B., Doekes, G., van Leusden, F., Wijnands, L., van Strien, R., et al. (1999). Fungal extracellular polysaccharides in house dust as a marker for exposure to fungi: Relations with culturable fungi, reported home dampness, and respiratory symptoms. *The Journal of Allergy and Clinical Immunology*, **103**, 494–500.

Douwes, J., van Strien, R., Doekes, G., Smit, J., Kerkhof, M., Gerritsen, J., et al. (2006). Does early indoor microbial exposure reduce the risk of asthma? The Prevention and Incidence of Asthma and Mite Allergy birth cohort study. *The Journal of Allergy and Clinical Immunology*, **117**, 1067–1073.

Eduard, W. (1996). Measurement methods and strategies for non-infectious microbial components in bioaerosols at the workplace. *Analyst*, **121**, 1197–1201.

Eduard, W. (2008). A health-based criteria document on fungal spore exposure in the working population. Is it relevant for the general population? *Indoor Air*, **18**, 257–258.

Eduard, W., and Heederik, D. (1998). Methods for quantitative assessment of airborne levels of noninfectious microorganisms in highly contaminated work environments. *American Industrial Hygiene Association Journal*, **59**, 113–127.

Eduard, W., Heederik, D., Duchaine, C., and Green, B. J. (2012). Bioaerosol exposure assessment in the workplace: The past, present and recent advances. *Journal of Environmental Monitoring*, **14**, 334–339.

Ege, M. J., Mayer, M., Normand, A. C., Genuneit, J., Cookson, W. O., Braun-Fahrlander, C., et al. (2011). Exposure to environmental microorganisms and childhood asthma. *The New England Journal of Medicine*, **364**, 701–709.

Fierer, N., Liu, Z., Rodriguez-Hernandez, M., Knight, R., Henn, M., and Hernandez, M. T. (2008). Short-term temporal variability in airborne bacterial and fungal populations. *Applied Environmental Microbiology*, **74**, 200–207.

Fisk, W. J., Lei-Gomez, Q., and Mendell, M. J. (2007). Meta-analyses of the associations of respiratory health effects with dampness and mold in homes. *Indoor Air*, **17**, 284–296.

Foxman, B. (2011). *Molecular tools and infectious disease epidemiology*. Academic Press, New York.

Foxman, B., and Goldberg, D. (2010). Why the human microbiome project should motivate epidemiologists to learn ecology. *Epidemiology*, **21**, 757–759.

Francois, P., Pittet, D., Bento, M., Pepey, B., Vaudaux, P., Lew, D., and Schrenzel, J. (2003). Rapid detection of methicillin-resistant *Staphylococcus aureus* directly from sterile or nonsterile clinical samples by a new molecular assay. *Journal of Clinical Microbiology*, **41**, 254–260.

Gehring, U., Heinrich, J., Hoek, G., Giovannangelo, M., Nordling, E., Bellander, T., et al. (2007). Bacteria and mould components in house dust and children's allergic sensitisation. *European Respiratory Journal*, **29**, 1144–1153.

Gehring, U., Strikwold, M., Schram-Bijkerk, D., Weinmayr, G., Genuneit, J., Nagel, G., et al. (2008). Asthma and allergic symptoms in relation to house dust endotoxin: Phase Two of the International Study on Asthma and Allergies in Childhood (ISAAC II). *Clinical & Experimental Allergy*, **38**, 1911–1920.

Gereda, J. E., Leung, D. Y., and Liu, A. H. (2000). Levels of environmental endotoxin and prevalence of atopic disease. [Letter]. *Journal of the American Medical Association*, **284**, 1652–1653.

Gereda, J. E., Leung, D. Y., Thatayatikom, A., Streib, J. E., Price, M. R., Klinnert, M. D., and Liu, A. H. (2000). Relation between house-dust endotoxin exposure, type 1 T-cell development, and allergen sensitisation in infants at high risk of asthma. *Lancet*, **355**, 1680–1683.

Gibbs, S. G., Green, C. F., Tarwater, P. M., Mota, L. C., Mena, K. D., and Scarpino, P. V. (2006). Isolation of antibiotic-resistant bacteria from the air plume downwind of a swine confined or concentrated animal feeding operation. *Environmental Health Perspectives*, **114**, 1032–1037.

Gilbert, M. J., Bos, M. E., Duim, B., Urlings, B. A., Heres, L., Wagenaar, J. A., and Heederik, D. J. (2012). Livestock-associated MRSA ST398 carriage in pig slaughterhouse workers related to quantitative environmental exposure. *Occupational and Environmental Medicine*, **69**, 472–478.

Giovannangelo, M., Nordling, E., Gehring, U., Oldenwening, M., Bellander, T., Heinrich, J., et al. (2007). Variation of biocontaminant levels within and between homes—the AIRALLERG study. *Journal of Exposure Science and Environmental Epidemiology*, **17**, 134–140.

Heederik, D., Doekes, G., and Nieuwenhuijsen, M. J. (1999). Exposure assessment of high molecular weight sensitisers: Contribution to occupational epidemiology and disease prevention. *Occupational and Environmental Medicine*, **56**, 735–741.

Hilty, M., Burke, C., Pedro, H., Cardenas, P., Bush, A., Bossley, C., et al. (2010). Disordered microbial communities in asthmatic airways. *PLoS One*, **5**, e8578.

Hines, C. J., Milton, D. K., Larsson, L., Petersen, M. R., Fisk, W. J., and Mendell, M. J. (2000). Characterization and variability of endotoxin and 3-hydroxy fatty acids in an office building during a particle intervention study. *Indoor Air*, **10**, 2–12.

Hirsch, T., Kuhlisch, E., Soldan, W., and Leupold, W. (1998). Variability of house dust mite allergen exposure in dwellings. *Environmental Health Perspectives*, **106**, 659–664.

Hogerwerf, L., Borlee, F., Still, K., Heederik, D., van Rotterdam, B., de Bruin, A., et al. (2012). Detection of *Coxiella burnetii* DNA in inhalable airborne dust samples from goat farms after mandatory culling. *Applied Environmental Microbiology*, **78**, 5410–5412.

Horick, N., Weller, E., Milton, D. K., Gold, D. R., Li, R., and Spiegelman, D. (2006). Home endotoxin exposure and wheeze in infants: Correction for bias due to exposure measurement error. *Environmental Health Perspectives*, **114**, 135–140.

Ishimatsu, S., Miyamoto, H., Hori, H., Tanaka, I., and Yoshida, S. (2001). Sampling and detection of *Legionella pneumophila* aerosols generated from an industrial cooling tower. *Annals of Occupational Hygiene*, **45**, 421–427.

Jacobs, J., Borras-Santos, A., Krop, E., Taubel, M., Leppanen, H., Haverinen-Shaughnessy, U., et al. (2014). Dampness, bacterial and fungal components in dust in primary schools and respiratory health in schoolchildren across Europe. *Occupational and Environmental Medicine*, **71**(10), 704–712. See http://www.ncbi.nlm.nih.gov/pubmed/25035116. doi: 10.1136/oemed-2014-102246.

Jacobs, J. H., Krop, E. J., Borras-Santos, A., Zock, J. P., Taubel, M., Hyvarinnen, A., et al. (2014). Endotoxin levels in settled airborne dust in European schools: The HITEA school study. *Indoor Air*, **24**, 148–157.

Jarvis, B. B. (1990). Mycotoxins and indoor air quality. In *Biological contaminants in indoor environments*. (eds. P. R. Morey, J. C. Feeley, and J. A. Otten) 201–214. ASTM, Philidelphia.

Karlsson, K., and Malmberg, P. (1989). Characterization of exposure to molds and actinomycetes in agricultural dusts by scanning electron microscopy, fluorescence microscopy and the culture method. *Scandinavian Journal of Work, Environment & Health*, **15**, 353–359.

Kelley, S. T., and Gilbert, J. A. (2013). Studying the microbiology of the indoor environment. *Genome Biology*, **14**, **202**.

Konstantinidis, K. T., and Tiedje, J. M. (2005). Towards a genome-based taxonomy for prokaryotes. *Journal of Bacteriology*, **187**, 6258–6264.

Korthals, M., Ege, M. J., Tebbe, C. C., von Mutius, E., and Bauer, J. (2008). Application of PCR-SSCP for molecular epidemiological studies on the exposure of farm children to bacteria in environmental dust. *Journal of Microbiological Methods*, **73**, 49–56.

Krop, E. J., Jacobs, J. H., Sander, I., Raulf-Heimsoth, M., and Heederik, D. J. (2014). Allergens and beta-Glucans in dutch homes and schools: Characterizing airborne levels. *PLoS One*, **9**(2), e88871.

Laitinen, S., Kangas, J., Husman, K., and Susitaival, P. (2001). Evaluation of exposure to airborne bacterial endotoxins and peptidoglycans in selected work environments. *Annals of Agricultural and Environmental Medicine*, **8**, 213–219.

Lange, J. L., Thorne, P. S., and Lynch, N. (1997). Application of flow cytometry and fluorescent in situ hybridization for assessment of exposures to airborne bacteria. *Applied Environmental Microbiology*, **63**, 1557–1563.

Letourneau, V., Nehme, B., Meriaux, A., Masse, D., Cormier, Y., and Duchaine, C. (2010). Human pathogens and tetracycline-resistant bacteria in bioaerosols of swine confinement buildings and in nasal flora of hog producers. *International Journal of Hygiene and Environmental Health*, **213**, 444–449.

Lozupone, C., and Knight, R. (2005). UniFrac: a new phylogenetic method for comparing microbial communities. *Applied Environmental Microbiology*, **71**, 8228–8235.

Lubin, J. H., Colt, J. S., Camann, D., Davis, S., Cerhan, J. R., Severson, R. K., et al. (2004). Epidemiologic evaluation of measurement data in the presence of detection limits. *Environmental Health Perspectives*, **112**, 1691–1696.

Miller, J. D., and Young, J. C. (1997). The use of ergosterol to measure exposure to fungal propagules in indoor air. *American Industrial Hygiene Association Journal*, **58**, 39–43.

Mogensen, T. H. (2009). Pathogen recognition and inflammatory signaling in innate immune defenses. *Clinical Microbiology Reviews*, **22**, 240–273.

Morris, A., Beck, J. M., Schloss, P. D., Campbell, T. B., Crothers, K., Curtis, J. L., et al. (2013). Comparison of the respiratory microbiome in healthy nonsmokers and smokers. *American Journal of Respiratory and Critical Care Medicine*, **187**, 1067–1075.

Nagi, N., Ohno, N., Adachi, Y., Aketagawa, J., Tamura, H., Shibata, Y., et al. (1993). Application of limulus test (G pathway) for the detection of different conformers of (1-->3)-beta-D-glucans. *Biological and Pharmaceutical Bulletin*, **16**, 822–828.

Nehme, B., Gilbert, Y., Letourneau, V., Forster, R. J., Veillette, M., Villemur, R., and Duchaine, C. (2009). Culture-independent characterization of archaeal biodiversity in swine confinement building bioaerosols. *Applied Environmental Microbiology*, **75**, 5445–5450.

Normand, A. C., Sudre, B., Vacheyrou, M., Depner, M., Wouters, I. M., Noss, I., et al. (2011). Airborne cultivable microflora and microbial transfer in farm buildings and rural dwellings. *Occupational and Environmental Medicine*, **68**, 849–855.

Noss, I., Doekes, G., Sander, I., Heederik, D. J., Thorne, P. S., and Wouters, I. M. (2010). Passive airborne dust sampling with the electrostatic dustfall collector: Optimization of storage and extraction procedures for endotoxin and glucan measurement. *Annals of Occupational Hygiene*, **54**, 651–658.

Noss, I., Wouters, I. M., Visser, M., Heederik, D. J., Thorne, P. S., Brunekreef, B., and Doekes, G. (2008). Evaluation of a low-cost electrostatic dust fall collector for indoor air endotoxin exposure assessment. *Applied Environmental Microbiology*, **74**, 5621–5627.

Palma, A. S., Feizi, T., Zhang, Y., Stoll, M. S., Lawson, A. M., Diaz-Rodriguez, E., et al. (2006). Ligands for the beta-glucan receptor, Dectin-1, assigned using "designer" microarrays of oligosaccharide probes (neoglycolipids) generated from glucan polysaccharides. *Journal of Biological Chemistry*, **281**, 5771–5779.

Palmgren, U., Strom, G., Blomquist, G., and Malmberg, P. (1986). Collection of airborne micro-organisms on Nuclepore filters, estimation and analysis—CAMNEA method. *Journal of Applied Bacteriology*, **61**, 401–406.

Park, J. H., Szponar, B., Larsson, L., Gold, D. R., and Milton, D. K. (2004). Characterization of lipopolysaccharides present in settled house dust. *Applied Environmental Microbiology*, **70**, 262–267.

Perzanowski, M. S., Miller, R. L., Thorne, P. S., Barr, R. G., Divjan, A., Sheares, B. J., et al. (2006). Endotoxin in inner-city homes: Associations with wheeze and eczema in early childhood. *The Journal of Allergy and Clinical Immunology*, **117**, 1082–1089.

Ramette, A. (2007). Multivariate analyses in microbial ecology. *FEMS Microbiology Ecology*, **62**, 142–160.

Rao, C. Y., Riggs, M. A., Chew, G. L., Muilenberg, M. L., Thorne, P. S., Van Sickle, D., et al. (2007). Characterization of airborne molds, endotoxins, and glucans in homes in New Orleans after Hurricanes Katrina and Rita. *Applied Environmental Microbiology*, **73**, 1630–1634.

Raulf, M., Buters, J., Chapman, M., Cecchi, L., de Blay, F., Doekes, G., et al. (2014). Monitoring of occupational and environmental aeroallergens—EAACI Position Paper: Concerted action of the EAACI IG Occupational Allergy and Aerobiology & Air Pollution. *Allergy*, **69**(10), 1280–1299.

Saraf, A., Larsson, L., Burge, H., and Milton, D. (1997). Quantification of ergosterol and 3-hydroxy fatty acids in settled house dust by gas chromatography-mass spectrometry: Comparison with fungal culture and determination of endotoxin by a Limulus amebocyte lysate assay. *Applied Environmental Microbiology*, **63**, 2554–2559.

Schram-Bijkerk, D., Doekes, G., Douwes, J., Boeve, M., Riedler, J., Ublagger, E., et al. (2005). Bacterial and fungal agents in house dust and wheeze in children: The PARSIFAL study. *Clinical & Experimental Allergy*, **35**, 1272–1278.

Sirigul, C., Wongwit, W., Phanprasit, W., Paveenkittiporn, W., Blacksell, S. D., and Ramasoota, P. (2006). Development of a combined air sampling and quantitative real-time PCR method for detection of *Legionella* spp. *Southeast Asian Journal of Tropical Medicine and Public Health*, **37**, 503–507.

Smit, L. A., Heederik, D., Doekes, G., Lammers, J. W., and Wouters, I. M. (2010). Occupational endotoxin exposure reduces the risk of atopic sensitization but increases the risk of bronchial hyperresponsiveness. *International Archives of Allergy and Immunology*, **152**, 151–158.

Sonesson, A., Larsson, L., Fox, A., Westerdahl, G., and Odham, G. (1988). Determination of environmental levels of peptidoglycan and lipopolysaccharide using gas chromatography with negative-ion chemical-ionization mass spectrometry utilizing bacterial amino acids and hydroxy fatty acids as biomarkers. *Journal of Chromatography*, **431**, 1–15.

Sonesson, A., Larsson, L., Schutz, A., Hagmar, L., and Hallberg, T. (1990). Comparison of the limulus amebocyte lysate test and gas chromatography-mass spectrometry for measuring lipopolysaccharides (endotoxins) in airborne dust from poultry-processing industries. *Applied Environmental Microbiology*, **56**, 1271–1278.

Sordillo, J. E., Alwis, U. K., Hoffman, E., Gold, D. R., and Milton, D. K. (2011). Home characteristics as predictors of bacterial and fungal microbial biomarkers in house dust. *Environmental Health Perspectives*, **119**, 189–195.

Sordillo, J. E., Hoffman, E. B., Celedon, J. C., Litonjua, A. A., Milton, D. K., and Gold, D. R. (2010). Multiple microbial exposures in the home may protect against asthma or allergy in childhood. [Research Support, N.I.H., Extramural]. *Clinical & Experimental Allergy*, **40**, 902–910.

Spaan, S., Doekes, G., Heederik, D., Thorne, P. S., and Wouters, I. M. (2008). Effect of extraction and assay media on analysis of airborne endotoxin. *Applied Environmental Microbiology*, **74**, 3804–3811.

Spaan, S., Heederik, D. J., Thorne, P. S., and Wouters, I. M. (2007). Optimization of airborne endotoxin exposure assessment: Effects of filter type, transport conditions, extraction solutions, and storage of samples and extracts. *Applied Environmental Microbiology*, **73**, 6134–6143.

Strachan, D. P. (2000). Family size, infection and atopy: The first decade of the "hygiene hypothesis." *Thorax*, **55 Suppl 1**, S2–10.

Taubel, M., Rintala, H., Pitkaranta, M., Paulin, L., Laitinen, S., Pekkanen, J., et al. (2009). The occupant as a source of house dust bacteria. *The Journal of Allergy and Clinical Immunology*, **124**, 834–840 e847.

Taylor, P. R., Tsoni, S. V., Willment, J. A., Dennehy, K. M., Rosas, M., Findon, H., et al. (2007). Dectin-1 is required for beta-glucan recognition and control of fungal infection. *Nature Immunology*, **8**, 31–38.

Thomas, T., Gilbert, J., and Meyer, F. (2012). Metagenomics—a guide from sampling to data analysis. *Microbial Informatics and Experimentation*, **2**, 3.

Thorne, P. S., Reynolds, S. J., Milton, D. K., Bloebaum, P. D., Zhang, X., Whitten, P., and Burmeister, L. F. (1997). Field evaluation of endotoxin air sampling assay methods. *American Industrial Hygiene Association Journal*, **58**, 792–799.

Tischer, C., Gehring, U., Chen, C. M., Kerkhof, M., Koppelman, G., Sausenthaler, S., et al. (2011). Respiratory health in children, and indoor exposure to (1,3)-beta-D-glucan, EPS mould components and endotoxin. *European Respiratory Journal*, **37**, 1050–1059.

Topp, R., Wimmer, K., Fahlbusch, B., Bischof, W., Richter, K., Wichmann, H. E., and Heinrich, J. (2003). Repeated measurements of allergens and endotoxin in settled house dust over a time period of 6 years. *Clinical & Experimental Allergy*, **33**, 1659–1666.

Tovey, E. R., Willenborg, C. M., Crisafulli, D. A., Rimmer, J., and Marks, G. B. (2013). Most personal exposure to house dust mite aeroallergen occurs during the day. *PLoS One*, **8**, e69900.

Tringe, S. G., and Hugenholtz, P. (2008). A renaissance for the pioneering 16S rRNA gene. *Current Opinions in Microbiology*, **11**, 442–446.

Tringe, S. G., and Rubin, E. M. (2005). Metagenomics: DNA sequencing of environmental samples. *Nature Reviews Genetics*, **6**, 805–814.

Tringe, S. G., Zhang, T., Liu, X., Yu, Y., Lee, W. H., Yap, J., et al. (2008). The airborne metagenome in an indoor urban environment. *PLoS One*, **3**, e1862.

van Cleef, B. A., Verkade, E. J., Wulf, M. W., Buiting, A. G., Voss, A., Huijsdens, X. W., et al. (2010). Prevalence of livestock-associated MRSA in communities with high pig-densities in The Netherlands. *PLoS One*, **5**, e9385.

van Strien, R. T., Engel, R., Holst, O., Bufe, A., Eder, W., Waser, M., et al. (2004). Microbial exposure of rural school children, as assessed by levels of N-acetyl-muramic acid in mattress dust, and its association with respiratory health. *The Journal of Allergy and Clinical Immunology*, **113**, 860–867.

van Wamel, W. J., Hansenova Manaskova, S., Fluit, A. C., Verbrugh, H., de Neeling, A. J., van Duijkeren, E., and van Belkum, A. (2010). Short term micro-evolution and PCR-detection of methicillin-resistant and -susceptible *Staphylococcus aureus* sequence type 398. *European Journal of Clinical Microbiology and Infectious Diseases*, **29**, 119–122.

Verhoeff, A. P., van Wijnen, J. H., Brunekreef, B., Fischer, P., van Reenen-Hoekstra, E. S., and Samson, R. A. (1992). Presence of viable mould propagules in indoor air in relation to house damp and outdoor air. *Allergy*, **47**, 83–91.

Vesper, S., McKinstry, C., Haugland, R., Wymer, L., Bradham, K., Ashley, P., et al. (2007). Development of an Environmental Relative Moldiness index for US homes. *J Occupational and Environmental Medicine*, **49**, 829–833.

Vineis, P., Khan, A. E., Vlaanderen, J., and Vermeulen, R. (2009). The impact of new research technologies on our understanding of environmental causes of disease: The concept of clinical vulnerability. *Environmental Health*, **8**, 54.

von Hertzen, L., Hanski, I., and Haahtela, T. (2011). Natural immunity. Biodiversity loss and inflammatory diseases are two global megatrends that might be related. *EMBO Reports*, **12**, 1089–1093.

Wang, X., Eijkemans, M. J., Wallinga, J., Biesbroek, G., Trzcinski, K., Sanders, E. A., and Bogaert, D. (2012). Multivariate approach for studying interactions between environmental variables and microbial communities. *PLoS One*, **7**, e50267.

Wild, C. P. (2005). Complementing the genome with an "exposome": The outstanding challenge of environmental exposure measurement in molecular epidemiology. *Cancer Epidemiology, Biomarkers & Prevention*, **14**, 1847–1850.

Wouters, I. M., Schmitt, H., Smit, L. A., van Rotterdam, B., De Bruin, A., and Heederik, D. (2015). Microbial agents and bacterial resistance in PM10 in air in areas with intensive livestock production: A potential source of human exposure. Submitted for publication.

Wurtz, H., Sigsgaard, T., Valbjorn, O., Doekes, G., and Meyer, H. W. (2005). The dustfall collector—a simple passive tool for long-term collection of airborne dust: A project under the Danish Mould in Buildings program (DAMIB). *Indoor Air*, **15 Suppl 9**, 33–40.

Zeileis, A., Kleiber, C., and KJackman, S. (2014). *Regression models for count data in R. CRAN.* Retrieved September 19, 2014. http://www.jstatsoft.org/v27/i08/paper.

Zhiping, W., Malmberg, P., Larsson, B. M., Larsson, K., Larsson, L., and Saraf, A. (1996). Exposure to bacteria in swine-house dust and acute inflammatory reactions in humans. *American Journal of Respiratory and Critical Care Medicine*, **154**, 1261–1266.

Zock, J. P., Jarvis, D., Luczynska, C., Sunyer, J., Burney, P., and European Community Respiratory Health, S. (2002). Housing characteristics, reported mold exposure, and asthma in the European Community Respiratory Health Survey. *The Journal of Allergy and Clinical Immunology*, **110**, 285–292.

12

PARTICULATE MATTER
EXPOSURE ASSESSMENT AND HEALTH

Helen H. Suh

12.1 INTRODUCTION

Exposure assessment is a critical and central component of environmental epidemiological studies, characterizing chemical, biological, or other environmental exposures to examine their relationship with health. For any environmental epidemiology study, the best exposure assessment approaches balance the needs for accurate and precise exposure measures with the needs for an efficient and cost-effective study design. This balance recognizes that imperfect exposure measures may be sufficient to detect exposure-effect associations for many study designs and that individual-specific measures of personal exposures may be cost inefficient, limiting the size and thus statistical power of the study.

For epidemiological studies of fine particulate matter ($PM_{2.5}$), this balance has historically resulted in the use of $PM_{2.5}$ concentrations measured at stationary ambient monitoring (SAM) sites as the exposure measure, with individual measures of exposure used seldomly. Recent development of new exposure assessment methods and approaches for $PM_{2.5}$, however, has substantially enhanced the ability of epidemiological studies to examine $PM_{2.5}$-associated health impacts using individual measures of exposure or to apply individual-specific information to inform health risks. These advances have resulted in epidemiological studies that are able to measure exposures with less error, estimate health risks more accurately, and examine susceptibility for individuals with potentially high $PM_{2.5}$ exposures (Pope 2000; US EPA 2010—http://www.epa.gov/ttn/naaqs/standards/pm/data/PM_RA_FINAL_June_2010.pdf). This chapter provides examples of these gains using selected findings from research studies.

12.2 EXPOSURE CHARACTERIZATION AND ERROR

Personal exposures to $PM_{2.5}$ can vary widely for the same ambient concentration, with this variation dependent on numerous factors, including the age and activity patterns of the exposed person, the composition of $PM_{2.5}$, the strength and proximity of the individual to $PM_{2.5}$ sources, the season and time of day, the region of the country, and the ventilation characteristics of the home and other indoor environments.

Using exposure data for older adults from nine US cities, Kioumourtzoglou et al. (2014) showed monthly personal $PM_{2.5}$ were on average higher than concentrations at both the nearest ambient monitor and outdoor home predictions, with mean monthly personal $PM_{2.5}$ exposures equaling 24.54 (±18.97) ug/m³ as compared with 15.86 (±5.58) and 15.47 (±4.77) ug/m³, respectively. Although not directly comparable, mean personal $PM_{2.5}$ concentrations in the nine cities were shown to vary substantially by city, ranging for example between 12.5 (±7.1) ug/m³ in Seattle, WA and 45.6 (±30.3) ug/m³ in Elizabeth, NJ. Between-city differences in mean nearest monitor ambient $PM_{2.5}$ concentrations were smaller than those for personal exposures, for example with ambient concentrations lowest in Seattle at 11.2 (±3.9) ug/m³ as compared to Los Angeles, CA which had the highest concentrations at 21.1 (±7.7) ug/m³.

Ambient $PM_{2.5}$ concentrations measured at SAM sites are often used as proxies of personal $PM_{2.5}$ exposures. These estimates are imperfect measures of personal exposures, as they are unable to account for spatial variation in outdoor concentrations, differential infiltration of $PM_{2.5}$ from outdoor to indoor environments, and movement of individuals or populations as they go about their day (Armstrong 1990, 2004; Bateson et al. 2007). The impact of this exposure error on observed health risks is important to consider, as it can distort associations and interactions between covariates and outcomes, reduce the power to detect effects, and lead to invalid inference (Thomas, Stram, and Dwyer 1993; Zeger et al. 2000; Bateson et al. 2007). To minimize exposure error, exposures to $PM_{2.5}$ and its constituents would ideally be measured in epidemiological studies using personal monitors. Such methods, however, are both expensive and intrusive and thus not feasible for studies conducted over long time periods and/or with many subjects.

Zeger et al. (2000) identified three major components of exposure error for time series studies, using particulate matter as a case study. These error components include 1) the difference between the average population exposure and the true ambient concentration; 2) the difference between the exposures of the population and people within the population, which can be considered to be a measure of the inter-individual variation in exposure; and (3) spatial variability in ambient concentrations. Analyses of the PTEAM study suggested that the difference between population exposures and true ambient concentrations is the largest contributor to overall exposure error, with the magnitude of its error varying by the $PM_{2.5}$ component (Zeger et al. 2000). More recent evidence, however, indicates that error from all three components can be substantial depending on the study design and study population.

12.2.1 Relationship Between Mean Population Exposures and Ambient Concentrations

Numerous exposure studies have examined the relationship between personal $PM_{2.5}$ exposures and corresponding ambient concentrations (Janssen et al. 1997; Ebelt et al. 2000; Evans et al. 2000; Janssen et al. 2000; Rojas-Bracho et al. 2000,

2002; Sarnat et al. 2000, 2006; Williams et al. 2000; Brown et al. 2008; Suh and Zanobetti 2010). In these studies, some combination of 12-hour or 24-hour personal, indoor, and outdoor concentrations of PM_{10} and $PM_{2.5}$ were measured repeatedly for a cohort of sensitive individuals. Data from these studies were used to examine the individual-specific associations between ambient particulate concentrations and personal exposures, with study findings generally discussed relative to the median, individual-specific personal-ambient correlation coefficient for the study cohort.

Results from these studies have consistently shown 24-hour personal $PM_{2.5}$ concentrations to be strongly associated with corresponding ambient concentrations over time. Results from the Janssen et al. study of senior citizens (Janssen et al. 2000), for example, showed mean personal, indoor, and outdoor concentrations in the Netherlands to equal 24.3, 28.6, and 20.6 ug/m³, respectively. Higher personal and indoor concentrations were attributed to environmental tobacco smoke. Because ETS exposure was limited to few homes, however, its ability to affect the association between personal and outdoor concentrations was limited, as the personal-ambient correlation remained high (median $r = 0.79$). Strong personal-ambient associations for $PM_{2.5}$ have been attributed to a) its spatially uniform concentrations across large geographic areas (Burton et al. 1996; Suh et al. 1997) and b) its relatively high effective penetration efficiencies from outdoor to indoor environments (Abt et al. 2000; Long et al. 2001; Sarnat et al. 2002). Further, for elderly individuals in St. Louis, it has been shown that associations between indoor and outdoor air pollution are strong over time periods of a day or longer (Dubowsky et al. 2006), with the findings consistent with other exposure studies of elderly individuals in Baltimore, MD (Sarnat et al. 2000), Steubenville, OH (Sarnat et al. 2006), and Fresno, CA [105].

As shown in Table 12.1, the ability of ambient concentrations to act as a proxy of personal exposures over time is independent of location and particle composition, as similarly strong personal-ambient associations have been shown for studies conducted in the eastern United States (Rojas-Bracho et al. 2000; Sarnat et al. 2000; Williams et al. 2000), midwestern United States (Sarnat et al. 2006), western United States (Evans et al. 2000), Canada (Ebelt et al. 2000), and Western Europe (Janssen et al. 1997; Janssen et al. 2000). Even in more polluted environments correlations between personal and ambient concentrations are also strong, as shown in Santiago Chile, where a crude r value of 0.80 was found (Rojas-Bracho et al. 2002).

For PM_{10}, a pollutant with more indoor sources and greater spatial variability, the results are less consistent. In Mexico City, where PM_{10} levels are much higher, the correlation between personal and ambient PM_{10} levels was low, with a value of only 0.26 (pooled r value) (Santos-Burgoa et al. 1998), whereas in Japan in a study with minimal indoor sources, an r value close to 1 was found (Tamura et al. 1996). These findings suggest that the presence of local particulate sources, either indoors or outdoors, may reduce the ability of ambient concentrations to act as exposure surrogates.

For potentially sensitive subgroups, such as children, the elderly, or those with pre-existing disease, it is possible that the relationship between personal and ambient exposures over time may differ from those of the general population. These differences may reflect the influence of activity patterns, in which children, for example, may spend more time outdoors than adults. Conversely, senior citizens, especially those with pre-existing disease, may be less active as compared with the general population and as a result, may participate in fewer activities that generate particles, such as cooking, cleaning, or tobacco smoking, and may spend less time outdoors. Despite these differences in activity patterns, the association between personal exposures and ambient concentrations, as reflected by the median personal-ambient correlation coefficient, tends to be comparable across sensitive subgroups (Table 12.1), with perhaps the exception of individuals with chronic obstructive pulmonary disease, for whom the median correlation coefficients are somewhat lower.

For these and other populations, scientific studies provide convincing evidence that ambient $PM_{2.5}$ concentrations are reasonable proxies of population personal exposures over time. Given this, it has been possible for numerous epidemiological time-series and chronic exposure studies to find associations between ambient $PM_{2.5}$ concentrations and health effects using SAM ambient concentrations alone. For studies of individuals or smaller groups, however, it is possible that exposure error may be substantial, contributing to bias and reduced power.

Table 12.1 Median subject-specific correlation coefficients for the comparison of personal versus ambient $PM_{2.5}$ levels: by study cohort and location

Cohort	No. Subjects	Days/Subject	Correlation Coefficient	
			Median	Range
Children:				
Netherlands[1]	13	6	0.86	−0.11−0.99
Santiago, Chile[2]	20	5	0.80	
Elderly:				
Fresno, CA[3]	16	24	0.84	
Baltimore, MD[4]	15	12	0.76	−0.21−0.95
Baltimore, MD[5]	21	5−22	0.80	−0.38−0.98
COPD:				
Vancouver, BC[6]	16	7	0.48	−0.68−0.83
Boston, MA[7]	18	12−18	0.61	0.10−0.93
Elderly w/CVD:				
Netherlands[8]	36	22	0.79	−0.41−0.98
Finland[8]	46	27	0.76	−0.12−0.97

[1]Janssen et al. 1997; [2]Rojas-Bracho et al. 2002; [3]Evans et al. 2000; [4]Sarnat et al. 2000; [5]Williams et al. 2000; [6]Ebelt et al. 2000; [7]Rojas-Bracho et al. 2000; [8]Janssen et al. 2000.

12.2.2 Inter-Individual Variation in Exposure

Personal exposures to $PM_{2.5}$ can vary substantially by person, even for people living in the same community. This inter-personal variation is reflected in the fact that associations between personal exposures and ambient concentrations vary substantially by person, as evidenced by the range in observed correlation coefficients (Table 12.1). Results indicate that personal exposures are strongly associated with corresponding outdoor concentrations for some but not all individuals. This inter-individual variability in the personal-ambient association suggests that although ambient $PM_{2.5}$ may be an appropriate surrogate for population exposures, it may be less able to reflect the exposures of individuals adequately.

Results from recent exposure studies have shown that this variation may be systematic, which suggests that the effect of this error component on risk estimates may be important to consider. Systematic variation in personal exposures has been attributed to a variety of factors, with increased exposure to motor vehicle pollution and home ventilation being the best studied of these factors. Both have been shown to modify personal $PM_{2.5}$ exposures, their relationship with ambient concentrations, and through these impacts, $PM_{2.5}$ health risks.

12.2.2.1 Motor Vehicle Pollution

In urban areas, road traffic is a major source of $PM_{2.5}$ (Health Effects Institute 2010). Exposures to motor vehicle-related $PM_{2.5}$ for a given person or population cannot be measured directly, given the number of motor vehicles that may contribute to an individual's or population's motor vehicle exposures, each of which may emit or generate pollution at a different rate that may vary throughout the day. As a result, exposure assessment and epidemiology studies have generally examined the impact of motor vehicle-related $PM_{2.5}$ pollution using indirect methods, such as source apportionment, distance from road measures, or tracers of motor vehicle-related pollution, including $PM_{2.5}$ components such as ultrafine particles (UFPs) and elemental (EC) and black carbon (BC). Estimates from $PM_{2.5}$ source apportionment studies suggest that mobile sources comprise on average approximately 10% of 24-hour total $PM_{2.5}$ concentrations (Hopke et al. 2006a) and 7% of total $PM_{2.5}$ exposures (Larson et al. 2004).

Results from exposure assessment studies show that outdoor motor vehicle concentrations exhibit substantial spatial variability outdoors. The mobile source pollutants UFP, EC, and BC show steep concentrations gradients near roadways, with levels increasing with proximity to roadways (Zhu et al. 2002; Ntziachristos et al. 2007; Baldauf et al. 2008). Correspondingly, annual average particulate mass concentrations have been shown to be higher at urban as compared to rural sites in the Northeastern United States (Salmon et al. 1997). Observed differences between urban and rural particulate levels were attributed to corresponding differences in their concentrations of EC, as urban EC levels were considerably higher than corresponding rural levels whereas urban and rural sulfate concentrations were comparable (Salmon et al. 1997). Within a city outdoor EC concentrations and filter blackness—an indicator of EC—have also been shown to vary substantially in relation to local traffic (Nitta et al. 1993; Brunekreef et al. 1997). In a Harlem, New York City study, for example, Kinney et al. (2000) measured 8-hour ambient PM$_{2.5}$ and EC concentrations on four geographically distinct sidewalks and collected corresponding diesel truck, bus, car, and pedestrian count data for each of these sites. Although mean PM$_{2.5}$ concentrations at the four sites varied only slightly, EC concentrations varied widely, with a fourfold difference observed between the sites (Figure 12.1). This difference was associated with bus and truck counts on adjacent streets. Similarly, Roorda-Knape and colleagues (1998) reported strong within-city variations in outdoor traffic particle concentrations in Europe. Similarly, Belander et al. (2001) reported an 11-fold range of variation in estimated exposure to NO$_2$, a pollutant that originates outdoors predominantly from traffic, across 11,000 residential addresses in Stockholm.

Motor vehicle-related PM$_{2.5}$ exposures reflect this observed variability in motor vehicle–related outdoor concentrations. In inner city Boston, Levy and colleagues (2001) examined personal exposure to PM$_{2.5}$ in subjects living near a major bus depot. There was considerable variation in exposure to traffic particles, which was related to proximity to the bus depot and diesel traffic. Consistent with these findings, Adar et al. (2007) reported substantially higher motor vehicle related PM$_{2.5}$, BC, and UFP exposures for elderly individuals aboard a diesel bus. Exposures to BC, for example, were on average nine-times higher than PM$_{2.5}$ exposures when the individuals were at their living facilities. These findings

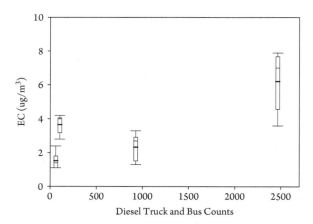

Figure 12.1 Impact of diesel traffic on elemental carbon concentrations: Harlem, NY. Kinney, P. L., Aggarwal, M., Northridge, M. E., Janssen, N. A. H., and Shepard, P. (2000). Airborne concentrations of (PM$_{2.5}$) and diesel exhaust particles on Harlem sidewalks: A community-based pilogt study. *Environmental Health Perspectives*, **108**, 213–218.

suggest that individuals living closer to major roads or spending time in motor vehicles will have higher motor-vehicle related exposures as compared with other individuals.

These higher motor vehicle-related $PM_{2.5}$ exposures have important implications for health, as combustion-generated $PM_{2.5}$ is thought to be more harmful to health than other types of $PM_{2.5}$ (WHO 2007). In a Health Effects Institute literature review (2010), for example, traffic-related air pollution was found to be causally related to asthma exacerbation. Suggestive evidence of a causal relationship was also found for a variety of other health outcomes, including childhood asthma onset, nonasthma respiratory symptoms, impaired lung function, total and cardiovascular mortality, and cardiovascular morbidity (HEI, 2010). These associations have generally been found using BC or NO_2 or using source apportionment techniques, with both methods usually based on measurements made at central monitoring sites.

As has been shown for $PM_{2.5}$, these central monitoring site–based exposures are estimated with error. However, the magnitude and impact of this error on health risk estimates is not well understood, given that few epidemiological studies have assessed traffic-related exposures using personal exposure measures. In one such study, Kramer and colleagues (2000) examined 317 children at risk of asthma in three German communities. Measurements of NO_2 were made outside the homes of each of the children, and personal NO_2 exposures were measured for each child. Outdoor NO_2 concentrations at the homes were shown to vary with traffic density, with the highest levels found at homes with the highest traffic density. The outdoor NO_2 measurements, but not the personal exposures (which reflect indoor generated NO_2 as well), were significant predictors of hay fever, symptoms of allergic rhinitis, wheezing, and sensitization against pollen, house dust mites, or cats. Because traffic is a major source of outdoor NO_2 it is possible that NO_2 is acting as a proxy measure for toxic components of traffic pollution, which may in turn be associated with atopy and wheezing.

Correspondingly, in a panel study of the elderly living in Altanta, GA, exposures to $PM_{2.5}$ and the traffic pollutants BC and NO_2 were related to changes in heart rate variability (HRV) (Suh and Zanobetti 2010). Exposures were assessed for each participant using personal, indoor, outdoor, and ambient measurements. Results from this study showed that changes in HRV, particularly those associated with parasympathetic control, were significantly and negatively associated with the traffic pollutants EC and, to a lesser extent, NO_2, when personal measurements were used to assess exposures. Although associations were also negative, associations with HRV were no longer significant when ambient concentrations were used as the exposure measure. These insignificant findings for ambient concentrations were attributed to the fact that ambient EC and NO_2 concentrations were poorly associated with their corresponding personal exposures, and were thus poor proxies of personal exposures.

12.2.2.2 Ventilation

Ventilation modifies the ability of ambient particles to penetrate indoors. For $PM_{2.5}$, the fraction of particles that penetrate indoors has been shown to range between 0.3 and 1.0 depending on home ventilation rates. As a result of this variable penetration, corresponding personal $PM_{2.5}$ exposures for individuals living even within the same city may differ substantially for a given ambient concentration.

In a study by Sarnat et al. (2000), for example, personal particulate and gaseous exposures were measured repeatedly for a cohort of senior citizens living in Baltimore, MD. In addition to these exposure measurements, participants kept detailed diaries in which they documented information about their activities, including the nature and location of each activity. For activities located indoors, participants were asked to record whether the windows were open. Measured personal particulate and gaseous exposures were subsequently compared with ambient concentrations measured at federal and state SAM sites to examine the influence of various factors on the personal-ambient relationship. Results from this study showed that ventilation, expressed as the fraction of time spent in indoor environments with open windows (f_v), was a significant predictor of inter-individual variability in personal exposures, wherein the association between ambient and personal $PM_{2.5}$ was strongest for individuals spending most of their time in well-ventilated environments (Figure 12.2a) and weakest for individuals spending their time in poorly ventilated environments (Figure 12.2b). Weaker associations for individuals in the poor ventilation category were attributed to lower effective penetration efficiency of $PM_{2.5}$ and to increased influence of indoor particle sources.

The relative importance of these factors was investigated further using the corresponding ambient-personal relationship for sulfate (SO_4^{2-}), a pollutant that has few indoor sources (Koutrakis et al. 1992; Tolocka et al. 2001) and can therefore be considered a tracer of fine particles of outdoor origin. Unlike $PM_{2.5}$, the strength of the personal-ambient associations for SO_4^{2-} were comparable across ventilation categories (Figures 12.3a,b), suggesting that ambient concentrations are strong exposure surrogates of $PM_{2.5}$ of ambient origin. However, the effective penetration efficiency of SO_4^{2-}, as shown by the slope of the personal on ambient regression lines, did vary with ventilation, with the lowest effective penetration efficiencies observed for individuals spending time in poorly ventilated environments. These results suggest that the $PM_{2.5}$ exposures of ambient origin will increase by a smaller amount for people spending time in poorly as compared to well-ventilated homes for the same increase in outdoor $PM_{2.5}$ concentrations.

These differences have important implications for epidemiological studies of ambient $PM_{2.5}$, suggesting that exposure error can be reduced by accounting for ventilation when ambient concentrations are used to assess exposures. In an analysis of data from the National Morbidity, Mortality, and Air Pollution Study (NMAPS), Janssen and colleagues (2002) found differences in ventilation to explain some of the observed variation in the city-specific risk coefficients for hospital admissions and ambient PM_{10} from

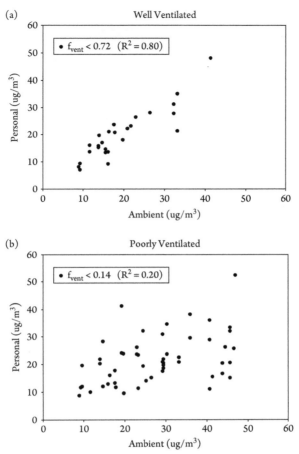

Figure 12.2 Personal versus Ambient PM$_{2.5}$: Baltimore, MD. **A:** Well ventilated. **B:** Poorly ventilated.

Adapted from Sarnat, J., Koutrakis, P., and Suh, H. H. (2000). Assessing the relationship between personal particulate and gaseous exposures of senior citizens living in Baltimore, MD. *Journal of Air Waste Management Association*, **50**, 1184–1198.

14 US cities. In their analyses, risk coefficients from each of the 14 cities were regressed against a population indicator of ventilation—the percentage of air conditioners used in each of these cities—to examine whether ventilation conditions modify the risk posed by outdoor particles. Cities were stratified by whether their PM$_{10}$ levels peaked in the winter or nonwinter months.

For both winter- and nonwinter peaking cities, the risk coefficients were found to decrease with increasing prevalence of air conditioners (Figure 12.4). This finding is consistent with exposure studies that have shown air conditioner use to be associated with lower air exchange rates, which are in turn associated with lower effective penetration efficiencies for fine particles. As a result, for the same outdoor concentration, exposures will be lower in cities in which air conditioner use is more

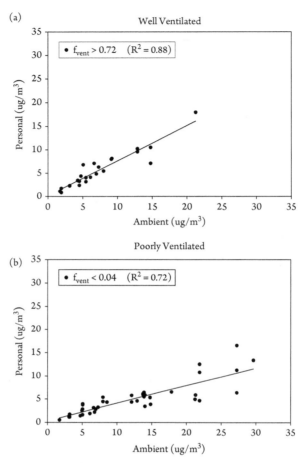

Figures 12.3 Personal versus Ambient SO_4^{2-}: Baltimore, MD. **A:** Well ventilated. **B:** Poorly ventilated. Adapted from Sarnat, J., Koutrakis, P., and Suh, H. H. (2000). Assessing the relationship between personal particulate and gaseous exposures of senior citizens living in Baltimore, MD. *Journal of Air Waste Management Association*, **50**, 1184–1198.

prevalent as compared to other cities, thus resulting in lower observed risk coefficients for ambient particles. Correspondingly, cities with winter-peaking PM_{10} concentrations were found to have lower risks as compared to other cities.

Again, these lower risks may be attributed to home ventilation, where for a given increase in outdoor levels, exposures are lower during the winter months when homes are more tightly sealed. Importantly, these findings have been confirmed in numerous subsequent studies (Levy et al. 2005; O'Neill et al. 2005; Franklin et al. 2007; Bell et al. 2009).

12.2.3 Spatial Variation in $PM_{2.5}$ Exposures

Spatial variability in ambient $PM_{2.5}$ concentrations—described by Zeger et al. (2000) as the difference between the true and measured ambient concentrations—is

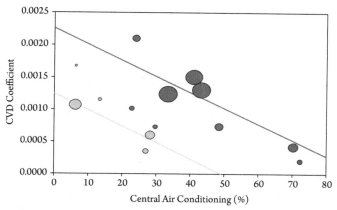

Figure 12.4 Percentage of homes with AC versus regression coefficients for CVD-related hospital admissions. Red circles represent cities with non–winter-peaking PM_{10} concentrations; yellow circles cities with winter-peaking PM_{10} concentrations. Circle area is proportional to the inverse of the variance of the effect estimate. Lines represent inverse variance weighted regression equations (fixed effect model).
Adapted from Janssen, N. A. H., Schwartz, J., Zanobetti, A., and Suh, H. H. (2002). Air conditioning and source-specific particles as modifiers of the effect of PM_{10} on hospital admissions for heart and lung disease. *Environmental Health Perspectives*, **110**, 43–49.

a potential source of error when $PM_{2.5}$ exposures are assessed using SAM site measurements. For $PM_{2.5}$, this component has historically been thought to contribute little to overall exposure error, because ambient $PM_{2.5}$ concentrations are relatively uniform across large areas (Burton et al. 1996).

A growing body of evidence from exposure and health studies, however, indicates that the contribution of spatial variability to exposure error for $PM_{2.5}$ may be more substantial than previously thought. Using data for 27 US urban areas for 1999 and 2000, Pinto et al. (2004), for example, found that spatial variability in daily $PM_{2.5}$ concentrations could be substantial within an urban area depending on season and location, with correlation coefficients for sites within an urban area ranging between 0.28 and 0.98 for the examined 27 MSAs. Of note, 24-hour $PM_{2.5}$ concentrations were found to differ within an urban area, even when the intra-urban correlations were high, due to the influence of local $PM_{2.5}$ sources, topography, and other location specific issues.

To account for this intra-urban spatial variation as well as variation between cities, researchers have used a variety of models to predict exposures outside participant residences, including land-use regression, kriging and other statistical smoothing models, and satellite-based or geographical information system (GIS)-based spatio-temporal models (Jerrett et al. 2005; Hoek et al. 2008; Liu et al. 2009; Yanosky et al. 2008, 2009). An example of one such model is provided by a GIS-based spatio-temporal exposure models that was developed and validated to predict monthly PM_{10}, $PM_{2.5}$, and coarse particle ($PM_{10-2.5}$) exposures for any location within the conterminous United States (all states save Alaska and

Hawaii) (Yanosky et al. 2008, 2009; Paciorek et al. 2009). Briefly, these models use monthly-average measured concentrations of either PM_{10} or $PM_{2.5}$, GIS-derived covariates, and monthly time-varying meteorological data to estimate separate monthly PM prediction surfaces by geographic region, which allows the effects of GIS-derived and meteorological covariates to differ by region and to capture important patterns of variation in space and time. Model covariates include distance to nearest roads by class, urban land use, tract- and county-level population density, point-source $PM_{2.5}$ or PM_{10} emissions density within 7.5 km, elevation, wind speed, temperature, precipitation, and number of air stagnation days per month. The GIS-based spatio-temporal models for PM_{10} and $PM_{2.5}$ have been shown to perform extremely well.

The models yielded individual-specific, highly resolved spatial and temporal exposure information. As shown by cross-validation techniques, nationwide models indicated high predictive accuracy, with cross-validation R^2 values of 0.59, 0.76, and 0.77 for PM_{10}, pre-1999 $PM_{2.5}$, and post-1999 $PM_{2.5}$, respectively. High model performance is due in large part to the inclusion of GIS- and meteorological covariates, which allows the model to reflect local spatial patterns (such as the effects of individual roads and emissions sources) that are not captured using purely spatial modeling as with standard kriging techniques.

The utility of these GIS-based spatio-temporal models for particulate matter was demonstrated in the Nurses' Health Study, a prospective cohort of 121,700 female nurses (Puett et al. 2008, 2009). Using the GIS-based spatio-temporal models, we showed that yearly $PM_{2.5}$ exposures were significantly associated with all-cause mortality (HR: 1.45, 95% CI: 1.19, 1.78) in models adjusted for age, calendar time, and state of residence (Puett et al. 2009). $PM_{10-2.5}$ was also associated with increased risk (HR: 1.13, 95% CI: 0.98, 1.30). Importantly, the spatio-temporal models were better predictors of exposure as compared with simpler estimation approaches (Paciorek et al. 2009). These results provide convincing support for the use of GIS–based spatio-temporal models in chronic health studies.

12.2.4 Particle Composition and Sources

Particle composition may vary substantially by location. In the eastern United States, for example, sulfate is the major component of $PM_{2.5}$, accounting for approximately 38% of fine particulate mass (USEPA 2002). By contrast, sulfate constitutes on average only 11% of $PM_{2.5}$ in the western United States (USEPA 2002). Similar differences in composition can be found for other $PM_{2.5}$ components, such as crustal materials and elemental carbon. Both components contribute approximately 4% and 15% to $PM_{2.5}$ in the eastern and western United States, respectively (USEPA 2002). Results from exposure studies have shown that these differences in particle composition may also modify the impact of particle exposures on health, and have provided information that better define the roles of particles as potential causative factors of respiratory and cardiovascular disease (CVD).

Table 12.2 Percent increase in daily deaths by specific $PM_{2.5}$ sources: six cities study (1979–1988)

Source Factor	% Increase	95% CI
Crustal (Si)	−2.3	−5.8–1.2
Motor Vehicles (Pb)	3.4	1.7–5.2
Coal (Se)	1.1	0.3–2.0

% Increase in daily deaths associated with 10 ug/m³ increase in mass concentration from source. Cities: Boston, MA; St. Louis, MO; Knoxville, TN; Madison, WI; Steubenville, OH; Topeka, KS. Adapted from Laden, F., Neas, L. M., Dockery, D. W., and Schwartz, J. (2000). Association of fine particulate matter from different sources with daily mortality in six US cities. *Environmental Health Perspectives*, **108**, 941–947.

The impact of particle composition on health has been examined using a variety of techniques, including the use of specific particle components as source tracers, particle emission inventories to examine the impact of particle sources on health, and source apportionment and other statistical methods to quantify source contributions. Using source apportionment methods, for example, Laden et al. (2000) showed that traffic particles were associated with daily deaths, independent of particles from coal or residual oil burning, and that their effect was triple that of the coal-derived particles (Table 12.2). Janssen and colleagues (2002) used particle emission inventories from the US Environmental Protection Agency to examine the contribution of particle sources to variability in the cardiovascular health risks in their 14-city re-analysis of NMAPS data (Table 12.3). Results from this re-analysis showed that the city-specific effect size for heart disease admissions (adjusted for the proportion of homes with central air conditioning) increased with the fraction of PM_{10} emissions from traffic and oil combustion. PM_{10} hospital admission coefficients increased by 55% (std. error 10%) and 38% (std. error 9%) for traffic and oil combustion emissions, respectively, for an interquartile range increase in the proportion of PM_{10} emissions from traffic.

12.2.5 Confounding

Exposure assessment research has been able to address directly whether confounding by gaseous pollutants is possible in epidemiological studies of particulate matter. Traditionally, the issue of confounding has been examined in epidemiological studies indirectly using multi-pollutant statistical models and by examining correlations among ambient $PM_{2.5}$ and ambient co-pollutant concentrations. The recent development of the multi-pollutant monitor, however, has allowed the relationship between personal $PM_{2.5}$ exposures and personal gaseous pollutant exposures to be assessed for the first time.

Table 12.3 Percent change in ambient PM_{10} on CVD-hospital admissions coefficients by source type

| Source parameter | β CVD, Lag 0/1 | |
	% Change	Standard error (%)
% PM_{10} from:		
Highway vehicles	55.3*	9.9
Highway diesels	52.8*	9.4
Coal combustion	0.6	2.6
Oil combustion	37.5*	9.3
Wood burning	2.7	3.2
Metal processing	29.0*	13.0
Fugitive dust	−49.4*	16.5

% change for interquartile increase in source parameter, adjusted for central AC. * $p < 0.05$.

Adapted from Janssen, N. A. H., Schwartz, J., Zanobetti, A., and Suh, H. H. (2002). Air conditioning and source-specific particles as modifiers of the effect of PM_{10} on hospital admissions for heart and lung disease. *Environmental Health Perspectives*, **110**, 43–49.

Over the past 5 year, several studies have been conducted that measure personal particulate and gaseous exposures simultaneously; however, results from most of these studies have not yet been finalized. In one of the earliest of these studies (Sarnat et al. 2000), associations among personal exposures to $PM_{2.5}$, coarse

Table 12.4 Relationship between ambient concentrations and personal exposures to $PM_{2.5}$ and ozone

| Comparison | Total $PM_{2.5}$ | | | $PM_{2.5}$ of Ambient Origin | | |
	n	Slope	t-value	n	Slope	t-value
Ambient $PM_{2.5}$ vs:						
Ambient O_3:						
Summer	48	0.84	5.98			
Winter	37	−0.67	−5.56			
Personal O_3:						
Summer	24/193	0.21	1.31	15/130	0.22	1.56
Winter	45/434	−0.05	−0.20	30/282	−0.18	−1.66
Ambient O_3:						
Summer	24/225	**0.28**	**4.00**	15/150	**0.37**	**6.23**
Winter	45/487	**−0.29**	**−4.86**	30/301	**−0.36**	**−14.04**

Boldface represents statistically significant values at the 0.05 level.

Adapted from Sarnat, J. A., Schwartz, J., Catalano, P. J., Suh, H. H. (2001). Gaseous pollutants in particulate matter epidemiology: Confounders or surrogates? *Environmental Health Perspectives*, **109**, 1053–1061.

particles, ozone, sulfur dioxide, and nitrogen dioxide were examined for a cohort of senior citizens living in Baltimore, MD. Their exposures were compared with those among the ambient concentrations and with those between the ambient concentrations and personal exposures for the individual pollutants (Sarnat et al. 2001).

As shown in part on Table 12.4, results from this study showed that ambient $PM_{2.5}$ concentrations were strongly associated with corresponding ambient concentrations of several gaseous co-pollutants, including ozone, although the strength and direction of these associations differed by season. For example, ambient ozone was positively associated with ambient $PM_{2.5}$ in the summer and negatively associated with ambient $PM_{2.5}$ in the winter. Based on ambient results alone, then, it is reasonable to assume that confounding by gaseous co-pollutants may impact observed associations between ambient $PM_{2.5}$ and health. With the exception of $PM_{2.5}$, however, ambient pollutant concentrations were weak indicators of their respective personal exposures. Similarly, the associations among the personal $PM_{2.5}$ and gaseous pollutant exposures were also weak. These weak associations among personal $PM_{2.5}$, ozone, nitrogen dioxide, and sulfur dioxide, together with the strong personal–ambient associations for $PM_{2.5}$, provide evidence that the observed $PM_{2.5}$-associated health effects are not due to confounding by the gaseous pollutants, at least for individuals with similar exposure profiles and living in similar urban locations. Although exposures to the gaseous co-pollutants are unlikely to be potential confounders of $PM_{2.5}$, ambient co-pollutants concentrations were surrogates of personal $PM_{2.5}$. Ambient ozone was significantly correlated with personal $PM_{2.5}$, with the same seasonal pattern observed as in the associations between their ambient levels.

The generalizability of the Baltimore study findings to other cities and to other cohorts is not yet known, but should become clearer as results from more multi-pollutant exposures studies become available. Despite this, results from the Baltimore study have already helped explain results from epidemiological air pollution studies, as illustrated by Sarnat and colleagues (2001) using ozone mortality results from NMAPS (Samet et al. 2000). In NMAPS, data from 90 cities were compiled to assess the percentage change in mortality associated with changes in ambient air pollutant concentrations. Among other findings, ozone was found to be positively associated with mortality in the summer but to have a seemingly protective effect in the winter months. This wintertime protective relationship was "puzzling and (may) reflect some unmeasured confounding factor." The Baltimore study findings suggest that the wintertime ozone finding may be due to ambient ozone acting as a surrogate for $PM_{2.5}$ exposures, in which the observed negative wintertime associations between ambient ozone and mortality reflect a corresponding negative association between ambient ozone and personal $PM_{2.5}$ exposures."

12.3 CONCLUSION

Particulate matter provides just one example of how exposure assessment research is a critical and necessary component of health effect studies. Similar examples of the importance of exposure assessment research can also be found using other pollutants as case studies, including gaseous air pollutants such as ozone and nitrogen dioxide, as well as other single- or multi-media pollutants such as lead and polychlorinated biphenyls.

Exposure assessment has multiple roles. It is a tool to measure and characterize exposures for study populations. It also plays an important role in the quantification of exposure error, in the identification of factors that may modify exposure–disease relationships, and in the examination of the potential for confounding by other ambient pollutants. Moreover, together with epidemiological and toxicological studies, results from future exposure studies will help to answer current questions about particle health effects regarding sensitive populations, biological mechanisms, and chemical composition. The benefits provided by these advances will likely be far reaching, as they will ultimately be used to develop sound and cost-effective regulatory policies to protect public health.

REFERENCES

Abt, E. Suh, H., Catalano, P., and Koutrakis, P. (2000). Relative contribution of outdoor and indoor particle sources to indoor concentrations. *Environmental Science Technology*, **34**, 3579–3587.

Adar, S. D., Gold, D. R., Coull, B. A., Schwartz, J., Stone, P. H., and Suh, H. (2007). Focused exposures to airborne traffic particles and heart rate variability in the elderly. *Epidemiology*, **18**, 95.

Armstrong, B. A. (1990). The effects of measurement errors on relative risk regressions. *American Journal of Epidemiology*, **132**(6), 1176–1184.

Armstrong, B. A. (2004). Exposure measurement error: consequences and design issues. In *Exposure assessment in occupational and environmental epidemiology*. New York, NY: Oxford University Press.

Baldauf, R. W., Thomas, E., Hays, M., Shores, R., Kinsey, J., Gullett, B., et al. (2008). Traffic and meteorological impacts on near road air quality: Summary of methods and trends from the Raleigh near road study. *Journal of Air Waste Management Association*, **58**, 865–878.

Bateson, T. F., Coull, B. A., Hubbell, B., Ito, K., Jerrett, M., Lumley, T., et al. (2007). Panel discussion review: session three—issues involved in interpretation of epidemiologic analyses—statistical modeling. *Journal of Exposure Science and Environmental Epidemiology*, **17**, S90–S96.

Belander, T., Berglind, N., Gustavsson, P., Jonson, T., Nyberg, F., Pershagen, G., and Jarup, L. (2001). Using geographic information systems to assess individual historical exposure to air pollution from traffic and house heating in Stockholm. *Environmental Health Perspectives*, **109**, 633–639.

Bell, M. L., Ebisu, K., Peng, R. D., and Dominici, F. (2009). Adverse health effects of particulate air pollution: modification by air conditioning. *Epidemiology*, **20**, 682–686. doi: 10.1097/EDE.0b013e3181aba749.

Brown, K. W., Sarnat, J. A., Suh, H. H., Coull, B. A., Spengler, J. D., and Koutrakis, P. (2008). Ambient site, home outdoor and home indoor particulate concentrations as proxies of personal exposures. *Journal of Environmental Monitoring*, **10**, 1041–1051.

Brunekreef, B., Janssen, N. A. H., deHartog, J., Hassema, H., Knape, M., and vanVliet, P. (1997). Air pollution from truck traffic and lung function in children living near motorways. *Epidemiology*, **8**, 298–303.

Burton, R. M., Suh, H. H., and Koutrakis, P. (1996). Characterization of outdoor particle concentrations within metropolitan Philadelphia. *Environmntal Science and Technology*, **30**, 400–407.

Chang, L. T., Sarnat, J., Wolfson, J. M., Rojas-Bracho, L., Suh, H. H., and Koutrakis, P. (1999). Development of a personal multi-pollutant exposure sampler for particulate matter and criteria gases. *Pollution Atmosphérique*, **10**, 31–39.

Chang, L. T., Suh, H. H., Wolfson, J. M., Misra, K., Allen, G. A., Catalano, P., and Koutrakis, P. (2001). Laboratory and field evaluation of measurement methods for one-hour exposures to O_3, $PM_{2.5}$ and CO. *Journal of Air Waste Management Association*, **51**, 1414–1422.

Chang L. T., and Suh, H. H. (2002). Characterization of the composition of personal, indoor, and outdoor particulate exposures. Report to the California Air Resources Board. Contract No. 98-330.

Dubowsky, S. D., Suh, H. H., Coull, B. A., Schwartz, J., and Gold, D. R. (2006). Diabetes, obesity, and hypertension may enhance the acute inflammatory response to air pollution. *Environmental Health Perspectives*, **114**, 992–998.

Ebelt, S. T., Petkau, A. J., Vedal, S., Fisher, T. V., and Brauer, M. (2000). Exposure of chronic obstructive pulmonary disease patients to particulate matter: Relationships between personal and ambient air concentrations. *Journal of Air Waste Management Association*, **50**, 1081–1094.

Evans, G. F., Highsmith, R. V., Sheldon, L. S., Suggs, J. C., Williams, W. R., Zweidinger, R. B., et al. (2000). The 1999 Fresno particulate matter exposure studies: comparison of community, outdoor, and residential PM mass measurements. *Journal of Air Waste Management Association*, **50**, 1700–1703.

Franklin, M., Zeka, A., and Schwartz, J. (2007). Association between PM and all-cause and specific-cause mortality in 27 US communities. *Journal of Exposure Science and Environmental Epidemiology*, **17**, 279–387.

Health Effects Institute. (2010). Traffic-related air pollution: A critical review of the literature on emissions, exposure, and health effects. Special Report 17.

Hoek, G., Beelen, R., de Hoogh, K., Vienneau, D., Gulliver, J., Fischer, P., and Briggs, D. (2008). A review of land-use regression models to assess spatial variation of outdoor air pollution. *Atmospheric Environment*, **42**, 7561–7578.

Hopke, P. K., Ito, K., Mar, T., Christensen, W. F., Eatough, E. J., Henry, R. C., et al. (2006a). PM source apportionment and health effects: 1. Intercomparison of source apportionment results. *Journal of Exposure Science and Environmental Epidemiology*, **16**, 275–286. doi: 10.1038/sj.jea.7500458.

Howard-Reed, C., Rea, A. W., Zufall, M. J., Burke, J. M., Williams, R. W., Suggs, J. C., et al. (2002). Use of a continuous nephelometer to measure personal exposure to particles during the U.S. Environmental Protection Agency Baltimore and Fresno panel studies. *Journal of Air Waste Management Association*, **50**, 1125–1132.

Janssen, N. A. H., De Hartog, J. J., Hoek, G., Brunekreef, B., Lanki, T., Timonen, K. L., and Pekkanen, J. (2000). Personal exposure to fine particulate matter in elderly subjects: relation between personal, indoor, and outdoor concentrations. *Journal of Air Waste Management Association*, **50**, 1133–1143.

Janssen, N.A.H., Hoek, G., Harssema, J., and Brunekreef, B. (1997). Childhood exposure to PM_{10}: Relation between personal, classroom, and outdoor concentrations. *Occupational Environmental Medicine*, **54**, 888–894.

Janssen, N. A. H., Schwartz, J., Zanobetti, A., and Suh, H. H. (2002). Air conditioning and source-specific particles as modifiers of the effect of PM_{10} on hospital admissions for heart and lung disease. *Environmental Health Perspectives*, **110**, 43–49.

Michael Jerrett, Richard T. Burnett, Renjun Ma, C. Arden Pope III, Daniel Krewski, K. Bruce Newbold, et al. (2005). Spatial Analysis of Air Pollution and Mortality in Los Angeles. *Epidemiology*, **16**, 727–736.

Kinney, P. L., Aggarwal, M., Northridge, M. E., Janssen, N. A. H., and Shepard, P. (2000). Airborne concentrations of (PM2.5) and diesel exhaust particles on Harlem side-walks: A community-based pilogt study. *Environmental Health Perspectives*, **108**, 213–218.

Kioumourtzoglou, M. A., Spiegelman, D., Szpiro, A. A., Sheppard, L., Kaufman, J. D., Yanosky, J. D., et al. (2014). Exposure measurement error in $PM_{2.5}$ health effects studies: A pooled analysis of eight personal exposure validation studies. *Environmental Health*, **13**, 2. doi: 10.1186/1476-069X-13-2

Koutrakis, P., Briggs, S. L. K., and Leaderer, B. P. (1992). Source apportionment of indoor aerosols in Suffolk and Onondaga Counties, New York. *Environmental Science and Technology*, **26**, 521–527.

Kramer, U., Koch, T., Ranft, U., Ring, J., and Behrendt, H. (2000). Traffic related air pollution is associated with atopy in children living in urban areas. *Epidemiology*, **11**, 64–70.

Laden, F., Neas, L. M., Dockery, D. W., and Schwartz, J. (2000). Association of fine particulate matter from different sources with daily mortality in six US cities. *Environmental Health Perspectives*, **108**, 941–947.

Larson, T., Gould, T., Simpson, C., Liu, L. J. S., Claiborn, C., and Lewtas, J. (2004). Source apportionment of indoor, outdoor, and personal PM2.5 in Seattle, Washington, using positive matrix factorization. *Journal of Air Waste Management*, **54**, 1175–1187.

Levy, J. I., Houseman, E. A., Spengler, J. D., Loh, P., and Ryan, L. (2001). Fine particulate matter and polycyclic aromatic hydrocarbon concentration patterns in Roxbury, Massachusetts: A community-based GIS analysis. *Environmental Health Perspectives*, **109**, 341–347.

Levy, J. I., Chemerynski, S. M., and Sarnat, J. A. (2005). Ozone exposure and mortality: an empiric Bayes metaregression analysis. *Epidemiology*, **16**, 458–468.

Lin, S., Munsie, J. P., Hwang, S. A., Fitzgerald, E., and Cayo, M. R. (2002). Childhood asthma hospitalization and residential exposure to state route traffic. *Environmental Research*, **88**, 73–81.

Liu, Y., Paciorek, C. J., and Koutrakis. P. (2009). Estimating regional spatial and temporal variability of pm concentrations using satellite data, meteorology, and land use information. *Environmental Health Perspectives*, **117**, 886–892.

Long, CM, Suh HH, Catalano PJ, Koutrakis P. (2001) Using Time- and Size-Resolved Particulate Data to Quantify Indoor Penetration and Deposition Behavior. *Environmental Science Technology*, **35**, 2089–2099.

National Research Council. (1998). *Research priorities for airborne particulate matter. 1. Immediate priorities and a long-range research portfolio*. Washington, DC: National Academy Press.

Nitta, H., Sato, T., Nakai, S., Maeda, K., Aoki, S., and Ono, M. (1993). Respiratory health associated with exposure to automobile exhaust. I: Results of cross-sectional studies in 1979, 1982, and 1983. *Archives of Environmental Health*, **48**, 53–58.

Ntziachristos, L., Ning, Z., Geller, M. D., Sheesley, R. J., Schauer, J. J., and Sioutas, C. (2007). Fine, ultrafine and nanoparticle trace element compositions near a major freeway with a high heavy-duty diesel fraction. *Atmospheric Environment*, **41**, 5684–5696.

O'Neill, M. S., Zanobetti, A., Schwartz, J. (2005). Disparities by race in heat-related mortality in four US cities: the role of air conditioning prevalence. *Journal of Urban Health*, **82**, 191–197.

Paciorek, C. J., Yanosky, J. D., Pruett, R. C., Laden, F., and Suh, H. H. (2009). Practical large-scale spatio-temporal modeling of particulate matter concentrations. Harvard University Biostatistics Working Paper 76. *Annals of Applied Statistics*, **3**, 369–396.

Pinto, J. P., Lefohn, A. S., and Shadwick, D. S. (2004). Spatial variability of PM2.5 in urban areas in the United States. *Journal of Air Waste Management Association*, **54**, 440–449. doi : 10.1080/10473289.2004.10470919

Pope, C. A. (2000). Review: epidemiological basis for particulate air pollution health standards. *Aerosol Science Technology*, **32**, 4–14.

Puett, R., Hart, J. E., Yanosky, J., Paciorek, C. J., Schwartz, J., Suh, H., et al. (2009). Chronic fine and coarse particulate exposure, mortality and coronary heart disease in the nurses' health study. *Environmental Health Perspectives*, **117**, 1697–1701. doi:10.1289/ehp/.0900572

Puett, R., Schwartz, J., Hart, J. E., Yanosky, J. D., Speizer, F. E., Suh, H., et al. (2008). Chronic particulate exposure, mortality and coronary heart disease in the nurses' health study. *American Journal of Epidemiology*, **168**, 1161–1168. doi: 10.1093/aje/kwn232.

Quintana, P. J. E., Samimi, B. S., Kleinman, M. T., Liu, L. J., Soto, K., Warner, G. Y., et al. (2000). Evaluation of a real-time passive personal particle monitor in fixed site residential indoor and ambient measurements. *Journal of Exposure Analysis and Environmental Epidemiology*, **10**, 437–445.

Rojas-Bracho, L., Suh, H., and Koutrakis, P. (2000). Relationship among personal, indoor, and outdoor fine and coarse particulate concentrations for individuals with COPD. *Journal of Exposure Analysis and Environmental Epidemiology*, **10**, 294–306.

Rojas-Bracho, L., Suh, H. H., Oyola, P., and Koutrakis, P. (2002). Measurements of children's exposures to particles and nitrogen dioxide in Santiago, Chile. *Science of Total Environment*, **287**, 249–264.

Roorda-Knape, M. C., Janssen, N. A., de Hartog, J., Van Vliet, P. H., Harssema, H., and Brunekreef, B. (1998). Air pollution from traffic in city districts near motorways. *Atmopheric Environment*, **32**, 1921–1930.

Salmon, L. G., Cass, G. R., Pederen, D. U., Durant, J. L., Gibb, R., Lunts, A., and Utell, M. (1997). Determination of fine particle concentration and chemical composition in the Northeastern United States, 1995. Report to NESCAUM.

Samet, J. M., Dominici, F., Curriero, F. C., Coursac, I., and Zeger, S. L. (2000). Fine particulate air pollution and mortality in 20 U.S. cities, 1987-1994. *New England Journal of Medicine*, **343**, 1742–1749.

Santos-Burgoa, C., Rojas-Bracho, L., Rosas-Perez, I., Ramierez-Sanchez, A., Sanchez-Rico, G., and Mejia-Hernandez, S. (1998). Particle exposure modeling in the general population and risk or respiratory disease. *Gaceta Médica de México*, **134**, 407–417.

Sarnat, J., Koutrakis, P., and Suh, H. H. (2000). Assessing the relationship between personal particulate and gaseous exposures of senior citizens living in Baltimore, MD. *Journal of Air Waste Management Association*, **50**, 1184–1198.

Sarnat, J.A., Koutrakis, P., Long, C. M., Coull, B., Schwart, J., and Suh, H. H. (2002). Using sulfur as a tracer for outdoor fine particulate matter. *Environmental Science Technology*, **36**, 5305–5314.

Sarnat, J. A., Schwartz, J., Catalano, P. J., Suh, H. H. (2001). Gaseous pollutants in particulate matter epidemiology: Confounders or surrogates? *Environmental Health Perspectives*, **109**, 1053–1061.

Sarnat, S. E., Coull, B. A., Schwartz, J., Gold, D. R., and Suh, H. H. (2006). Factors affecting the association between ambient concentrations and personal exposures to particles and gases: Implications for air pollution epidemiology. *Environmental Health Perspectives*, **114**, 649–654.

Suh, H. H., Nishioka, Y., Koutrakis, P., and Burton, R. M. (1997). The Metropolitan Acid Aerosol Characterization Study: Results from Washington, DC. *Environmental Health Perspectives*, **105**, 826–834.

Suh, H. H., and Zanobetti, A. (2010). Exposure error masks the relation between traffic pollution and heart rate variability. *Journal of Occupational and Environmental Medicine*, **52**, 685–692.

Tamura, J. K., Ando, M., Sagai, M., and Matsumoto, Y. (1996). Estimation of levels of personal exposures to suspended particulate matter and nitrogen dioxide in Tokyo. *Environmental Science (Japan)*, **4**, 37–51.

Thomas, D., Stram, D., Dwyer, J. (1993). Exposure measurement error: Influence on exposure-disease relationships and methods of correction. *Annual Review of Public Health*, **14**, 69–93.

Tolocka, M. P, Solomon, P. A., Mitchell, W., Norris, G. A., Gemmill, D. B., Wiener, R. W., et al. (2001). East versus west in the US: Chemical characteristics of $PM_{2.5}$ during the winter of 1999. *Aerosol Science and Technology*, **34**, 88–96.

U.S. Environmental Protection Agency. (2002). Third external review draft of air quality criteria for particulate matter. Office of Research and Development, Washington DC.

World Health Organization. (2007). The world health report 2007—A safer future: Global public health security in the 21st century.

Williams, R., Creason, J., Zweidinger, R., Watts, R., Sheldon, L., and Shy, C. (2000). Indoor, outdoor, and personal exposure monitoring of particulate air pollution: the Baltimore elderly epidemiology-exposure pilot study. *Atmospheric Environment*, **34**, 4193–4204.

Yanosky, J., Paciorek, C., Schwartz, J., Laden, F., Puett, R., and Suh, H. (2008). Spatio-temporal modeling of chronic PM_{10} exposure for the Nurses' Health Study. *Atmospheric Environment*, **42**, 4047–4062.

Yanosky, J. D., Paciorek, C. J., Suh, H. H. (2009). Predicting chronic fine and coarse particulate exposures using spatio-temporal models for the northeastern and midwestern US. *Environmental Health Perspectives*, **117**, 522–529 doi: 10.1289/ehp.11692.

Zeger, S. L., Thomas, D., Dominici, F., Samet, J. M., Schwartz, J., Dockery, D., Cohen, A. (2000). Exposure measurement error in time-series studies of air pollution: concepts and consequences. *Environmental Health Perspectives*, **108**, 419–426.

Zhu, Y., Hinds, W. C., Kim, S., Shen, S., and Sioutas, C. (2002). Study of ultrafine particles near a major highway with heavy-duty diesel traffic. *Atmospheric Environment*, **36**, 4323–4335.

13

LAND USE REGRESSION MODELS
FOR OUTDOOR AIR POLLUTION

Gerard Hoek, Rob Beelen, and Bert Brunekreef

13.1 INTRODUCTION

Exposure assessment for epidemiological studies of long-term exposure to ambient air pollution remains a difficult challenge. The cohort studies published in the mid-1990s have compared mortality between cities, with exposure characterized by the average concentration measured at a central site within each city (Dockery et al. 1993; Pope et al. 2002). Various studies have documented significant variation of outdoor air pollution at a small scale within urban areas for important pollutants such as nitrogen dioxide (NO_2), black carbon and ultrafine particles (Zhu et al. 2002; Eeftens et al. 2012; HEI 2013). The within-city spatial contrast may be larger than the between-city contrast (Eeftens 2012). Epidemiological studies need to take these intra-urban contrasts into account. Monitoring of long-term average air pollution exposures will generally not be feasible, as the study population of epidemiological studies generally comprises several hundreds to thousands of subjects, living or working at different places.

Current approaches that have been developed to meet the challenge of assessing intra-urban air pollution contrasts include the use of exposure indicator variables (e.g., traffic intensity at the residential address or distance to a major road), interpolation methods (e.g., kriging, inverse distance weighing), dispersion models, and land-use regression models (Jerrett 2005). All these methods have been extensively applied in epidemiological studies. Although land use regression models have mostly been applied in epidemiological studies of long-term exposure, increasingly spatiotemporal models are developed that allow modeling of spatially resolved short-term exposures.

13.2 THE LAND USE REGRESSION METHOD

Land use regression (LUR) combines monitoring of air pollution at a limited number of locations, collection of variables usually through geographic information systems (GIS), which can potentially predict the measured spatial variation, and development of regression models. The regression model is then applied to a large number of locations in the study area where no measurements are available, for

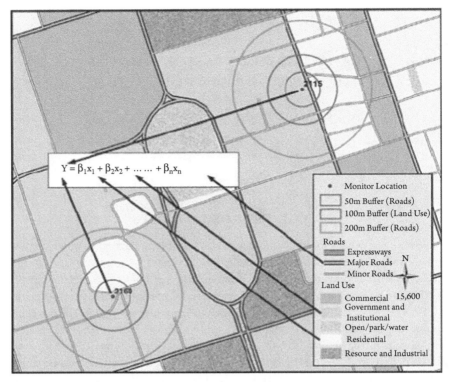

$$Y = \beta_1 x_1 + \beta_2 x_2 + \ldots \ldots + \beta_n x_n$$

Figure 13.1 Circular buffers of predictor variables for land use regression. *Source:* Jerrett et al., 2005.

example, the residential, school, or work addresses of subjects in an epidemiological study. Land use regression modeling uses as predictor variables various traffic representations, population/address density, land use, and variables such as altitude. Predictor variables are often calculated for specific circles around the sampling points, called buffers, as illustrated in Figure 13.1. Figures 13.2 and 13.3 further illustrate the land use regression method based on a study in Rome (Cesaroni 2012). Measurements were made at 67 locations in 1995–1996 and 78 locations in 2007 spread over the city (see Figure 13.2). After LUR models were developed for the 2 years, maps were generated for the entire city (see Figure 13.3). An interesting feature of the Rome study was the repetition of measurements and modeling after 12 years. Strong stability of measured and modeled spatial patterns was observed.

Land use regression is an empirical approach, in contrast with dispersion models, which are based upon physical principles and emission data. Epidemiologists have applied land use regression extensively because of the direct link with measured air pollution data, the relative ease of applying the method, the lower demand on input data compared with dispersion models, and the typically good performance of the models. Developments in GIS have contributed to the popularity of LUR methods. Epidemiologists prefer to use land use regression compared with interpolation methods because in urban areas spatial variability is characterized more by local

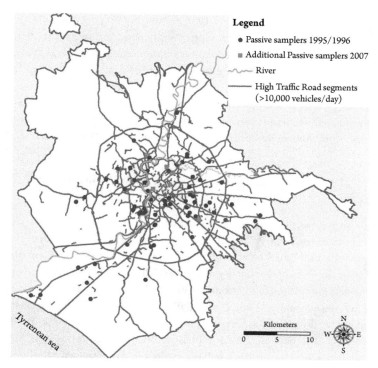

Figure 13.2 Map of monitoring locations for a LUR study in Rome. *Source:* Cesaroni, 2012.

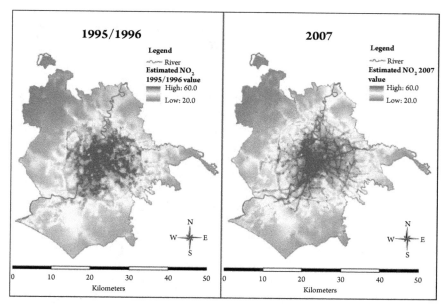

Figure 13.3 Map of modeled NO$_2$ concentrations from LUR model in Rome. *Source:* Cesaroni, 2012.

sources, such as traffic on major roads, than a smoothly varying concentration field, as assumed in spatial interpolation. Consistently, land use regression performed substantially better than simple spatial interpolation methods (Briggs et al. 2000).

After illustrating the method by introducing the first application of land use regression, a more systematic discussion of the key components of land use regression modeling follows. The key components are the monitoring data, GIS predictor data, model development, model validation, and model application. The chapter builds upon a previous review of LUR model studies up to 2008 (Hoek et al. 2008).

13.2.1 An Example: The Small Area Variations in Air Quality and Health Study

The land use regression approach was introduced in the Small Area Variations in Air Quality and Health (SAVIAH) study (Briggs et al. 1997). The aim of the study was to generate individual-level long-term average exposure to ambient air pollution to assess the risks of respiratory disease of children. Because the study population involved several thousand children, monitoring ambient air pollution at their home addresses was not feasible. Instead, in each of the three cities (Amsterdam, Huddersfield, and Prague), a purpose-designed monitoring network of 80 monitoring sites was established. At each site, the NO_2 concentration was measured for 14 days in each season with passive samplers. Measurements at all sites were performed simultaneously to avoid bias due to differences in weather conditions. The average concentration of the four seasons was used to develop linear regression models. Variables potentially related to contrasts in air pollution, including measures of traffic, population density, land use, and altitude, were compiled in a GIS. Linear regression was used to develop a model that explained the largest fraction of observed variability in annual average NO_2 concentration. The final prediction models explained between 61% and 72% of the observed variability in concentrations between sites (Briggs et al. 1997).

After the successful pioneering work in SAVIAH, LUR methods have been increasingly used in epidemiological studies (Hoek 2008). Although in 2008 it was still possible to provide an exhaustive review of LUR studies, the application of LUR in epidemiological studies has increased exponentially since then. The scope of land use regression modeling has widened, in terms of pollutants modeled, study areas covered, and temporal resolution. The methodology has been developed substantially. In 2008 most applications were limited to nitrogen dioxide (NO_2), largely because of the ease of monitoring of this pollutant with simple passive samplers. Only few studies had developed models for particulate matter ($PM_{2.5}$), the elemental carbon content of particulate matter (EC), and volatile organic compounds (VOCs), including benzene and toluene. Currently, a sizable number of studies have assessed particulate matter, including PM2.5 and the elemental carbon content of PM (Eeftens 2012). A few studies have also modeled the composition of particulate matter, including elemental composition (de Hoogh 2013), the organic carbon (OC) and PAH content of PM (Jedynska et al. 2014), and the oxidative potential of PM (Yanosky 2012). In 2008 the majority of studies were from Europe, but nowadays a sizable number of LUR models have been developed for North America and some Asian countries. Furthermore, there is a tendency toward national scale models that still provide the fine-scale spatial variation needed within urban areas, compared with studies that were performed mostly in a large urban area. Spatiotemporal models have been developed that provide spatially resolved models for daily variation of air pollutants.

13.3 KEY COMPONENTS OF LAND USE REGRESSION

The success of land use regression modeling depends on the quality of monitoring data, predictor data, and the model development method.

13.3.1 Monitoring Data

To obtain good quality land use regression models the monitoring sites need to cover the relevant variation of air pollution sources in the study area. The monitoring domain should be representative for the locations to which the model will be applied. In most urban areas, this implies that a reasonable number of sites need to be located in or near major streets. Depending on the area, other sources, such as major ports, industrial areas, or areas with significant wood burning may need to be covered. A detailed example of a site selection procedure can be found in the study manual of the European Study of Cohorts for Air Pollution Effects (ESCAPE) study (Eeftens 2012; http://www.escapeproject.eu). The ESCAPE study was a large European project using standardized monitoring of NO_2 and particulate matter across Europe and standardized development of LUR models. The monitoring base for land use regression modeling studies has been derived from existing routine monitoring and from purpose designed monitoring campaigns.

13.3.1.1 Routine Monitoring Data

National or supra-national studies have often been based upon routine monitoring networks (Stedman et al. 1997; Beelen et al. 2009; Gulliver 2013; Hystad 2011; Beckerman 2013b; Vienneau 2013). Land use regression models for particulate matter are also often based upon routine monitoring data because of the significantly higher cost of particle monitoring compared with monitoring of NO_2 (Moore et al. 2007; Ross et al. 2007). Advantages of routine monitoring data include low costs, the typically high temporal coverage of the measurements (continuous, especially for gaseous pollutants), and the availability of data for multiple years. Routine data may be the only choice when historic exposure assessment is needed. When routine monitoring data are used, however, careful attention must be paid to the site type because routine monitoring networks are often designed to monitor compliance with regulatory standards rather than to assess human exposures. Siting of monitors may differ substantially between countries. For example, in Southern Europe routine monitors are often located in hotspots, whereas in North America monitors tend to be located away from major roads. The siting strategy strongly affects the possibility to address specific sources. In a Canadian study, the authors noted that the network design did not allow assessment of fine-scale variation related to traffic because of the paucity of monitoring near major roads (Hystad 2011). Furthermore, few routine monitoring networks are sufficiently dense to characterize intra-urban variation well. Finally, the use of routine monitoring data limits the study to pollutants that are routinely measured, typically those that are regulated. This is one explanation for the limited amount of models for the (unregulated) ultrafine particles.

13.3.1.2 Purpose Designed Campaigns

Many studies have undertaken monitoring specifically for the purpose of model development. The networks that are operated for a limited time are typically spatially denser within urban areas than routine networks. A further advantage of purpose designed monitoring is that the distribution of site types (e.g., traffic, background) and pollutants can be optimized for the study objective. Disadvantages of purpose designed monitoring include the additional cost and the limited temporal coverage of the measurements. The typical purpose designed monitoring campaign consists of 7 to 14 days' sampling campaigns that are repeated one to four times. This method has been applied to the gaseous components NO_2, NO_x, and VOCs. Measurements are generally performed with passive samplers such as the Palmes tube (Briggs et al. 1997; Lewne et al. 2004) and the Ogawa badge (Gilbert et al. 2005; Henderson et al. 2007; Beelen et al. 2013). Because investigators typically have access to large numbers of passive samplers due to their low cost, monitoring campaigns are usually conducted simultaneously at all sites. Because of the cost of equipment, campaigns for particulate matter typically involve designs with simultaneous measurements at a subset of sites. Examples include the ESCAPE and the US National Particle Components Toxicity (NPACT) study (Eeftens 2012; Vedal 2013). In the Dutch study area of ESCAPE, including 40 sites with PM measurements, PM measurements were performed simultaneously at 10 sites because of available equipment. The comparison of concentrations between sites in non-simultaneous designs may include spatial and temporal variation. These designs therefore require one or more reference sites in the study area with continuous measurements to adjust for potential temporal bias in the comparison between sites. Adjustments can be made in the calculation of average concentrations (Eeftens 2012) or by specifying spatiotemporal models as in NPACT (Vedal 2013). The reference site should be a background location that represents temporal concentration variation in the wider surroundings of the site.

13.3.1.3 Short-Term or Mobile Measuring Campaigns

Short-term or mobile measuring campaigns have recently been carried out to develop models for especially ultrafine particles (UFP) and black carbon (Larson et al. 2009; Padró-Martínez et al. 2012; Rivera et al. 2012; Abernethy et al. 2013). The instruments available to measure ultrafine particle or total particle number concentrations are either too expensive or require too much operator supervision to be used in the monitoring campaigns based upon fixed sites where instruments are left unattended for 1 to 2 weeks. The mobile campaigns are typically conducted with one instrument for mobile sampling. In this design the potential for temporal bias is even larger than in the previously discussed design with fixed sites. One or more reference sites are typically used to adjust for temporal variation. The campaigns have short sampling periods per location (15–60 min) and a small number of repeats at each site. On-road mobile monitoring has also been used with typically even shorter sampling periods in a specific street but more repeats. The strength of the design is the large number of sites that can be measured, for example, over 600 sites in a study in Girona, Spain (Rivera et al. 2012). Because of the short sampling period, temporal fluctuations have more impact on results of measurements than in studies using longer sampling times. Therefore, these short-term sampling campaigns are likely less precise in determining spatial variation of long-term average concentrations, which could affect the development of robust land use regression models based upon the monitored average concentrations. Land use regression models based upon mobile campaigns typically have moderate explained variation of LUR models~50% or less, compared to LUR models for NO_2 and Black carbon based on larger averaging times which typically have explained variances above 70%.

13.3.1.4 Number of Monitoring Locations

Although there is no rigorous methodology to determine the required number of monitoring locations for a given study, progress has been made in assessing the robustness of LUR models in relation to the number of sites (Basagana 2012; Wang 2012). The ability of models to predict variability of measured concentrations at independent sites not used for modeling especially increased between 20 and about 80 sites in two studies conducted in the city of Girona, Spain (Basagana 2012) and the Netherlands (Wang 2012). Most published studies included between 20 and 100 sites, with the lower range representing those studies that modeled PM. Probably 40 to 80 sites is a desirable number to choose for study-specific monitoring, but the size of the population and city should be taken into account to determine the actual number.

There are several ways in which the selected number of monitoring sites can be distributed over the study area. Most studies have used informal methods to maximize the contrast in variables hypothesized to be potentially important predictors for spatial variation, taking into account the distribution of locations to which the model will be applied. An example can be found in the study manual of the ESCAPE study (Eeftens 2012). In each study area a total of 40 monitoring sites was available. In each area urban and regional background locations and traffic locations needed to be represented. Traffic sites were over-represented based upon the expectation that in all cities motorized traffic was an important source of spatial variation. The monitoring sites had to represent the anticipated range of predictor variables within the study area. Traffic locations were required to have a variety of (high) traffic intensities and street configurations.

Kanaroglou et al. (2005) developed a systematic methodology for selecting monitoring sites that uses the anticipated spatial variation in air pollution as well as the distribution of addresses over the study area, to assign monitoring locations. The network density is increased in locations where concentration variability is higher and more people live. The method specifies a continuous demand (for monitoring) surface over the area. An algorithm from the general family of location allocation problems is then used to select the optimal locations from a fixed number of monitoring sites. The demand surface incorporates an initial concentration surface, determined from monitoring data in a wider area than the study area, for example. The demand surface is then adapted by incorporating weights that reflect for example population density.

13.3.2 Predictor Data

Land use regression studies typically offer a large number of potential predictor variables to model variation of monitored concentrations. Frequently used predictor data include: traffic variables, population or address density, land use, altitude and topography, and indicators of location (Table 13.1). As an example, a study by Henderson et al. (2007) included 55 potential predictors, and a study by Moore et al. (2007) examined 140 predictors. The large number of predictors is especially due to the definition of multiple buffer sizes to represent predictor variables. In the ESCAPE study, for the land use variables five buffer sizes (radius 100, 300, 500, 1000, and 5000 m) were offered (Eeftens 2012). Often the number of potential predictor variables exceeds the number of sites significantly. Most predictor variables represent source strength such as traffic density or distance to a source.

Geographic information system predictor variables may be affected by the general problems associated with geographic data, such as completeness, precision, and availability for the period of interest (Vine et al. 1997; Nuckols et al. 2004). Traffic intensity data, especially those for municipal roads, are not always available for the investigators, despite the fact that most traffic data have been obtained with public funds. In many cities, traffic counts are only available for a small number of typically major roads. Therefore, assumptions about the traffic intensity of other roads must be made. The quality of traffic intensity data may also be limited, especially if traffic counts are derived from traffic models. In the absence of traffic data, several LUR studies have successfully used the length of specific road types without traffic intensity data (Brauer et al. 2003; Henderson et al. 2007). In Vancouver, the R^2 of

Table 13.1 Overview of often used predictor variables in LUR studies

Variable	Representation	Comment
Traffic		
Traffic intensity	Traffic intensity on nearest street or nearest major street	Nearest may be redefined if a minor and major road are parallel and represented as two separate roads. Best used in conjunction with distance to this road
Road length	Length of roads in buffers of typically 25–1000 m	More specific if road type is included, e.g., road length of freeways
Traffic load	Traffic intensity * road length in buffers of typically 25–1000 m	Accounts for intensity and distance
Distance major road	Non-linear, e.g., inverse distance	Exponential decay with distance to road
Intensity/ distance	Intensity divided by distance or distance squared	Accounts for interaction (close to a low traffic street leads to low concentrations), but needs high geographical precision for distances
Distance to intersection	Intersection density also used	Higher emissions for stop and go traffic
Population	In buffers of 100–10,000 m	Often not precise for small buffers
Land use	Industry Commercial Port Residential land Impervious surface Agricultural Natural land Water	Type of industry should be included. Major sources best as point sources. Proximity to water may reduce or increase concentrations depending on shipping emissions.
Physical geography	Altitude Distance to coast Distance to border crossing	Non-linear functions likely. Altitude often offered as square root.
Emission	Source-specific emission in grids of e.g. 1 km^2	Often scale too crude and data imprecise for the smallest (1*1 km) scales
Satellite NO$_2$ or AOD		
Coordinates	Study-area specific functions or regional indicators	Recommended only if other GIS variables do not represent trends well
Street con-figuration	Canyon or more continuous factors such as aspect ratio or sky view factor	May have a major influence, standard in dispersion models

the models based on traffic intensity did not differ from the models using only road length of highways and major roads for the evaluated pollutants (Henderson et al. 2007). In the ESCAPE study, models developed with traffic intensity predicted the spatial variation of NO_2 better than models developed with road length variables (Beelen 2013). The national models developed within North America were all based upon road length of major roads to represent road traffic (Novotny, 2011; Hystad, 2011).

Predictor variables in LUR models are usually computed for circular zones around each monitoring site, using buffer functions in the GIS. The selection of buffer size is crucial for the performance and the spatial resolution of the model. Ideally, buffer sizes should be selected to take account of known dispersion patterns. Various monitoring studies have shown that the impact of a major road on concentrations of traffic-related air pollutants declines exponentially with distance to the road (Zhu 2002). Beyond about 100 meters from a major urban road or 500 meters from a major freeway, the influence of emissions from that road is limited. In inner-city areas, buildings may limit the influence zone of roads. Air pollution concentrations fall virtually to background levels behind a row of uninterrupted buildings. Especially in the compact European urban areas, much of the variation in traffic-related air pollution is therefore extremely local. To represent the influence of freeways with higher traffic intensity and often located in more open terrain, larger buffers sizes can be used (300–500 m). Investigators have offered traffic intensity (or road length) in larger buffers (e.g., 1000 m). These buffers do not represent a single road, but rather the totality of traffic in a certain area, such as city center versus suburb.

The large spatial variability that occurs within tens of meters from major roads is potentially challenging given the geographic precision of monitoring sites, addresses, and roads (Briggs et al. 1997). In a Dutch study, it was found that direct observations of traffic by a technician at the monitoring sites improved the prediction models for soot and PM2.5 over the GIS variables (Brauer et al. 2003). In Amsterdam, a model based upon technician observations of distance and GIS variables explained 67% of the spatial variability in measured UFP concentrations, whereas a model with only GIS variables explained 44% of the UFP variability (Hoek et al. 2011). In epidemiology studies with a moderate population size (several hundreds), therefore, it may be useful to include direct traffic observations at the home address. This is especially attractive if home visits have been planned to collect specific additional data for the epidemiological study of interest (e.g., collect house dust in a birth cohort study). Another conclusion is that buffer sizes should not be too small. Within the ESCAPE study, it was observed that the smallest buffer for traffic variables (25 m) was only rarely selected in the LUR models, likely due to geographic imprecision.

Land use regression models have largely ignored vertical gradients. Geographical coordinates define the position using X- and Y-coordinates, but often do not have the height attached. In high-rise apartment buildings this may be an important issue, as several monitoring studies have suggested important differences in air pollution related to height for homes located in major streets (Vakeva et al. 1999; Janhall et al. 2003). A Korean study showed that VOC concentrations were up to 70% higher outside low-floor (first or second) apartments compared to high-floor (10th–15th floor) apartments in the same building located within 30 to 100 meters of a major road (Jo and Ky 2002). There is very limited vertical gradient at urban background locations. This suggests that applying LUR models in study areas where a large fraction of the population lives in high rise apartment buildings may misclassify exposure. A recent study from Taiwan showed that floor of the building was a significant predictor in a LUR model developed based upon monitoring at sites at low and high floors across the city (Wu 2014).

Methodological work has shown that the typical setting of LUR studies with a large number of correlated predictor variables and a limited number of monitoring sites may lead to overfitting (Johnson 2010; Basagana 2012; Wang 2012). Models may be developed that predict the monitoring data well, but do not predict independent measurements equally well. The main lesson from these studies for the definition of predictor variables is to be restrictive with respect to the number of predictors and use subject matter knowledge to offer only specific variables. Based upon monitoring studies, it is well known that the decay of pollution with distance from roads follows an exponential decay. Based on this knowledge, LUR studies should offer only distance to road variables that reflect these patterns, for example, inverse distance rather than offering various options for distance functions (e.g., linear, inverse distance, logarithmic). Some predictor variables only have non-zero values for a small fraction of sites. Examples may be industry or port in buffers of 100 meters. Models with these variables may not be robust and therefore one should limit offering variables with many zeros. Investigators have used as a cut point 10% of the sites for non-zero values, but probably a stricter cut point of, for example, 50% would be better. The issue with low variability in a predictor variable is not limited to zero values—percentage urban land in small buffers may be 100% for many sites within an urban study area.

Although many land use regression studies have focused on traffic, the method is by no means limited to modeling traffic-related air pollution. Population and household density representing multiple sources have been included as predictors in models. Industrial sources and distance to ports have been included, particularly if location of point sources and type of industry was available. The key is whether robust indicators of source strength or proximity to sources can be defined. Land use regression models with moderate explained variance have been developed to model pollution from wood smoke in studies in Vancouver and Seattle (Larson 2007; Su 2008). The monitoring campaign and collection of predictor variables were designed specifically to model wood smoke emissions. In these studies, night-time mobile monitoring of $PM_{2.5}$ was performed and careful consideration of direction of air flows at nighttime affecting the monitoring sites instead of simple circular buffers was used to obtain predictor variables (Larson 2007).

A very interesting development is the use of satellite observations in developing LUR models. Satellite observations of NO_2 and aerosol optical density (AOD) are publicly available and have been shown to correlate moderately well with surface measurements of NO_2 and fine particles (Martin 2008). It has recently been suggested in studies within North America and Europe that satellite observations of air pollutants may be useful in providing particularly the regional scale component of ambient air pollution in land use regression models (Hystad 2011; Novotny 2011; Vienneau 2013). Satellite AOD observations have been used to develop global models of fine particles (Brauer 2012). The major advantage of satellite observations is that data are available globally, in contrast to surface monitoring data that are available in a more limited number of countries and often concentrated in urban areas in those countries with sufficient monitoring. In international studies, the consistency of monitoring is another advantage of satellite data. Concentration contrasts between countries derived from surface monitoring may be affected by differences in monitoring methods and selection of monitoring sites. Because satellite data are available on a daily basis, spatio-temporal LUR models combining daily satellite observations, land use, and surface monitoring have been developed successfully in a series of North American studies (Kloog 2012, 2014; Lee 2014). These studies provided daily pollution estimates for the 1*1 km scale. The method provides spatially varying temporal trends, relaxing the assumption of a single temporal trend often applied in time series studies based on surface monitors. Because of the current spatial scale of the observations (at best 1*1, but often 10*10 km), satellite data cannot represent the fine-scale variation related to local traffic emissions, for example. Satellites may further provide important information about land use predictor variables, such as greenness.

13.3.3 Model Development

Methods for developing models based upon monitoring and GIS predictor data have been improved over the past decade. Studies have used linear regression to develop a parsimonious model from a large set of predictor variables that maximizes the percentage explained variability (R^2) or the cross-validation R^2. Based upon the observation that models may overfit the data (Basagana, 2012; Wang 2012), we recommend not to use fully automated procedures without constraints such as forward or backward selection. One constraint that investigators have specified in order to increase the applicability of the model beyond the monitoring sites is an a priori definition of the sign of regression slopes for specific variables (e.g., positive for traffic intensity) (Briggs 1997; Brauer et al. 2003; Henderson et al. 2007; Eeftens 2012). Standard diagnostic tests for ordinary least squares regression should be applied, such as checks on the normality of residuals, heteroscedasticity, and influential observations measured by Cook's D. Because linear regression assumes independence of the residuals, most studies do check whether the residuals of the model exhibit spatial autocorrelation using a variety of techniques including kriging and Moran's I (Ross et al. 2007). Moran's I is a statistic between −1 and +1, with 0 indicating no correlation of nearby sampling points. Most studies observed that, although significant spatial autocorrelation is present in the measured concentrations, the residuals of land use regression models are independent, indicating that ordinary least squares regression can be used. In large study areas, significant spatial autocorrelation may remain in the data related to regional variation of concentrations resulting for example from slow pollution formation processes. Universal kriging may then be used to extend LUR models (Beelen 2009; Sampson 2013).

Studies have used a structured approach in which different predictors were used for different spatial scales (Beelen et al. 2007, 2009). These were studies applying LUR models to larger geographical areas than most studies that model large metropolitan areas. Spatial variation was assumed to comprise a regional, urban, and local component for which a different set of monitoring locations and predictor variables was used. A model was first developed for the regional and next for the urban and local scale. The approach incorporates more theoretical knowledge about processes governing spatial variation, possibly increasing the applicability of the developed model elsewhere. The structured approach may increase the likelihood that the model predicts well for background and traffic locations. Models developed for all sites may be dominated by the most important predictors, as observed in a LUR study in Amsterdam, which predicted well for traffic locations but much less for urban background locations (Hoek 2011).

Different methods have been applied to develop LUR models, including the ADDRESS and Deletion-Substitution Algorithm (DSA) (Su 2009; Beckerman 2013a). The DSA is a machine-learning algorithm that uses a covariate search algorithm to fit a generalized linear model, minimizing the cross-validation mean squared error (Beckerman 2013a). The DSA has optimal properties in selecting the subset of variables that best explains variability. However, the method is less transparent than the simpler methods discussed previously. ADDRESS (A Distance Decay REgression Selection Strategy) is a technique to select optimal buffer sizes and optimize model performance (Su 2009), using the correlation of measured concentrations and the predictor variable in a large number of buffer sizes. Few comparisons have been made between the performance of different variable selection methods. In a study in Girona, Spain, performance measured by hold-out validation statistics did not differ substantially between DSA and the supervised stepwise method used in the ESCAPE study (Basagana 2012). In the US NPACT study, spatiotemporal models were developed that accounted for the common unbalanced spatiotemporal data structure by incorporating spatial and temporal predictors in one model (Sampson 2011; Vedal 2013). The model can account for continuous temporal data from a few sites and spatial data at many sites but at a few time points, which differ per site. The model allows specification of spatially varying temporal trends. Modeling can be performed with the R package SpatioTemporal.

Model R^2 of published LUR models are often high. In the ESCAPE study, many models had R^2 exceeding 80% (Eeftens 2012; Beelen 2013). The models were developed based upon monitoring at 20 to 80 locations. Three studies recently documented that the model R^2 values are a substantial overestimate of the predictive ability of the models at independent sites (Johnson 2010;

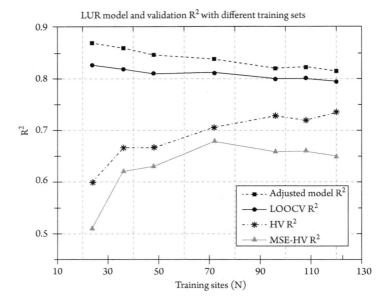

Figure 13.4 Difference in model explained variance and validation explained variance. *Source:* Wang, 2012.

Basagana 2012; Wang 2012). The gap was attributed to overfitting. The difference between model and hold-out validation R^2 decreased with increasing number of monitoring sites in the dataset to develop the models. Figure 13.4 illustrates this for a study based upon 144 monitoring locations across the Netherlands. Note that although the hold-out validation R^2 was much lower than the model R^2, the absolute value of the hold-out validation R^2 was still reasonably high, even for the smaller number of sites. An important lesson from these studies is that maximizing explained variance should not be too empirical. Restricting the number of offered predictors and the shape of the offered predictor variables by incorporating theoretical knowledge likely leads to more robust models. If good traffic intensity data are available, it may be better to a priori choose one or a few local traffic representations (e.g., traffic load in a 50 m buffer, traffic intensity/distance to nearest road) rather than multiple buffers and various road length buffers.

Few studies have attempted to model the spatial variation of particle composition. In a large European study, LUR models for eight key elements of PM10 and PM2.5 were developed (de Hoogh 2013). Elements for which the main source was motorized traffic (Cu, Fe, markers of nonexhaust traffic emissions) were well modeled. The models for components with major nontraffic predictors had lower performance, related to the lack of specific predictor variables for sources such as wood burning in commonly available geographic databases. A similar observation was made in North American studies of wood smoke (Larson 2007; Su 2008).

13.3.4 Model Validation

Model validation is an essential part of developing LUR models. One often used approach is leave-one-out cross-validation (LOOCV), in which a model is developed for n-1 sites and the predicted concentrations are compared with the actually measured concentrations at the left-out site. This procedure is repeated *n* times and the agreement between the predicted and observed concentrations calculated. Usually the structure of the model is based on the model developed for the full dataset and remains constant for each model. Methodological work has documented that LOOCV does not sufficiently address the overestimate of the predictive ability of regression models, especially for smaller number of sites (Johnson 2010; Basagana 2012; Wang 2012). Figure 13.4 illustrates that LOOCV R^2, although lower than model R^2, substantially exceeds the hold-out validation R^2 in a study in the Netherlands. The main reason is likely that no new model is developed in each of the *n* steps. Adaptation of the procedure by relaxing the requirement to have the same model structure may result in better performance. Leave-one-out cross-validation has been applied especially in studies with a small number of monitoring locations, which does not allow the separation of the dataset in a training set for model development and a test set for model validation.

A better approach is to subdivide the monitoring sites into a training dataset for model development and a smaller group of sites for model validation (Briggs et al. 1997; Beelen 2009; Vienneau 2013). This approach has been applied especially in studies with a large number of monitoring sites. A disadvantage is that the a priori division of sites, distributions of predictors, and concentrations measured at the training and validation sites may differ. Recent LUR studies have used tenfold cross-validation, in which the monitoring sites are divided into training sets of 90% of the sites and test sets of 10% of the sites. The division is repeated 10 times using a different group for validation such that all sites are used in model development and validation (Vedal 2013). Predicted and measured concentrations are then compared.

13.3.5 Model Application

Little attention has been given to issues related to applying the developed LUR models to the residential addresses of an epidemiological study population, for example. The most important issue is that the monitoring domain should be representative for the locations to which the model is applied. Because LUR models are empirical models, extrapolation beyond the range of predictor variables for which the model was developed may not be valid. Within the ESCAPE project, a strict interpretation of this principle was applied by truncating the minimum and maximum of predictor variables at the residential addresses to the minimum and maximum at the monitoring sites. Note that prediction of higher concentrations than measured is still possible if an address has high values for multiple predictors. Truncation was shown to improve hold-out validation (Wang 2012). Prevention of unrealistic predictions due to errors in GIS variables is one rationale for truncation; for example, distances of 10 cm to major roads from coordinates may occur and these may lead to extreme predictions if inverse distance is one of the predictors. Extreme predictions can also be prevented by assigning a realistic minimum distance of say, 2 meters as the smallest distance.

Often the period of interest for exposure assessment does not coincide with the monitoring period of the LUR study. Monitoring may for example may be more recent than the recruitment period of the epidemiological studies, such as in the large ESCAPE study, in which monitoring occurred mostly in 2009–2010 and recruitment went back to the mid-1990s in some cohorts. Four recent studies in the Netherlands (Eeftens et al. 2011), Great Britain (Gulliver et al. 2013), Rome (Cesaroni et al. 2012), and Vancouver (Wang et al. 2013) have shown that for periods up to 10 years spatial air pollution contrasts of NO_2 often remained the same. Moreover, LUR models based on current NO_2 data were able to predict historical exposure well. Even if the spatial ranking of study areas remains the same accounting for temporal trends by back-extrapolating using long-term trends from routine monitoring networks may still be needed, for example, if one wants to document associations with health at air pollution levels below current air quality guidelines. Stability of spatial patterns will not apply universally. In rapidly developing areas, spatial patterns may change substantially, as observed in a cohort study conducted in China in which the ranking of pollution of study areas changed during follow-up (Zhang 2011).

13.4 CRITICISM OF LAND USE REGRESSION MODELS

Land use regression models have received various criticisms. First, LUR models have been judged to be too empirical and inferior in predictive abilities to dispersion models that attempt to model spatial variation based upon physical principles. However, there is little empirical support for this claim (Hoek 2008). A recent comparison between predictions of LUR models and dispersion models showed good agreement for NO_2 and moderate agreement for $PM_{2.5}$ (de Hoogh 2014). The LUR models may outperform dispersion models if the input data from the dispersion model are imprecise and if in complex urban areas the physical model does not adequately reflect reality.

As most predictor variables for LUR models reflect source strength and do not describe atmospheric formation processes, LUR models may be less applicable for secondary pollutants, including ozone and sulfate. Incorporation of the typically large-scale chemical transport models in the land use regression framework could be useful for more secondary pollutants, however.

Some of the predictors used for developing air pollution exposures with LUR could introduce *confounding* when applied in epidemiological studies. Land use regression models, including population density, may be problematic because population density may also be associated with other risk factors such as low socio-economic status or poor housing stock, which could influence the disease of interest (e.g., asthma prevalence). One solution to this potential problem is the inclusion of area-level confounders that are more closely related to the disease of interest (e.g., percentage of low-income families in a neighborhood) than the variable used in predicting air pollution (number of addresses in a 300-m buffer).

Although land use regression models provide individual estimates of exposure at usually the residential address, the estimates may not relate well to actual long-term average *personal exposure.* This issue applies equally to other modeling methods focusing on outdoor air, such as dispersion models and interpolation methods, such as kriging. The predictor variables do not take account of factors (e.g., air exchange rate) related to infiltration of outdoor air in the home where people spend a large fraction of their time. Time activity patterns such as the fraction of time spent at home, the work or school location, and mode of and time in transport are likely important determinants of personal exposure (Dons 2012; de Nazelle 2013). In a group of 62 pregnant women personal exposure of especially NO was moderately correlated with ambient NO assessed by LUR (Nethery et al. 2008). Little association was found between LUR modeled and personal exposure of soot. In a Canadian study, 72-hour personal exposure of 33 elderly adults measured in three seasons were not associated with NO_2 concentrations predicted by LUR models (Sahsuvaroglu 2009). The LUR models, which predict long-term average concentrations, were compared with short-term personal exposure measurements, which could have limited the agreement. The difficulty of obtaining long-term average personal exposure with current monitoring technology is a serious limitation of all validation studies published to date. Soot LUR models explained 39%, 44%, and 20% of personal exposure variability (R^2) in Helsinki, Utrecht, and Barcelona in a study of 45 volunteers with repeated personal exposure monitoring (Montagne 2013). In Utrecht and Helsinki, but not Barcelona, NO_2 LUR models significantly predicted personal exposure; $PM_{2.5}$ models were not correlated with personal $PM_{2.5}$ in any of the cities. However, $PM_{2.5}$ and NO_2 model predictions were correlated with personal soot. Soot is the pollutant that is least affected by indoor sources, illustrating the major problem indoor sources pose in validation studies of ambient pollution models. Land use regression modeled and measured personal exposure and were highly correlated for all pollutants when data from the three cities were pooled (Montagne 2013), supporting studies using between city contrasts in exposure. A few studies showed that some of the traffic variables used in land use regression models were associated with small but significant contrasts in personal exposure of soot (Wichmann et al. 2005; Van Roosbroeck et al. 2006, 2007).

13.5 HYBRID MODELS

Recognizing the limitations of LUR models, dispersion models, and interpolation methods, studies have started to develop hybrid models incorporating multiple methods in one framework. A study in Catalonia developed a modeling framework based on the Bayesian Maximum Entropy (BME) method that integrated NO_2 monitoring data and outputs from LUR and chemical transport models (Akita 2014). The model performed better than the individual model components. A hybrid model predicted $PM_{2.5}$ across the United States better than LUR only (Beckerman 2013b). The hybrid model was developed by combining a land use regression model (including remote sensing PM2.5) and Bayesian Maximum Entropy interpolation of the LUR spatio-temporal residuals. Remote sensing was a strong predictor of ground-level concentrations (Beckerman 2013b). A hybrid model incorporating monitoring data and a LUR model also performed well to predict ozone concentrations in Quebec, Canada (Adam-Poupart 2014). A North American study documented slightly better prediction of NO_2 concentrations when the CALINE-3 dispersion model was combined with LUR modeling compared with the individual models (Wilton 2010).

13.6 CONCLUSION

Land use regression models have been successfully developed and applied for a variety of pollutants and study areas. The scope has expanded from the pollutants NO_2, $PM_{2.5}$, and the black carbon content of particulate matter to new pollutants, including ultrafine particles, composition of particles (elements, PAH), and ozone. Ultrafine particle models have become possible, by designing short-term and mobile monitoring campaigns. The short-term monitoring design requires more evaluation and development before being applied with confidence in epidemiological studies. Land use regression models have been applied now in Europe, North America, and Asia. Increasingly, national and supra-national scale models have been developed that include fine-scale variation, for example, by combining satellite and local traffic information. Land use regression models are increasingly applied as an important exposure assessment method in epidemiological studies characterizing small-scale spatial variation. The method has evolved significantly in the past decade, improving the performance of the method. New developments included development of spatiotemporal models allowing more detailed temporal resolution compared with spatial models for typically the annual average. New insights were obtained in the validity of LUR models in relation to the number of sampling locations, the number of predictor variables offered, and the statistics used to characterize validity. The model R^2 may be a substantial overestimate of the true predictive ability of the models. More systematic identification of models has been developed, including regression models maximizing R^2 or cross-validation R^2 incorporating a priori selection of direction of effect for predictor variables, the deletion substitution algorithm, ADDRESS, and spatiotemporal methods. The development of hybrid models, including dispersion models, satellite observations of NO_2, and fine particles as predictors in LUR models, often using Bayesian methods is another promising trend. Finally, LUR models may be an important tool to assess fine-scale spatial variation of outdoor pollution, but the moderate agreement with personal exposure suggests that accounting for time activity patterns and infiltration of ambient pollution in buildings needs to be developed as well. Use of new technology, including GPS, smartphones, and smaller pollution sensors, may offer new possibilities.

REFERENCES

Abernethy, R. C., Allen, R. W., McKendry, I. G., and Brauer, M. (2013). A land use regression model for ultrafine particles in Vancouver, Canada. *Environmental Science & Technology*, **47**, 5217–5225.

Adam-Poupart, A., Brand, A., Fournier, M., Jerrett, M., and Smargiassi, A. (2014). Spatiotemporal modeling of ozone levels in Quebec (Canada): A comparison of kriging, land-use regression (LUR), and combined Bayesian maximum entropy-LUR approaches. *Environmental Health Perspectives*, **122**, 970–976.

Akita, Y., Baldasano, J. M., Beelen, R., Cirach, M., de Hoogh, K., Hoek, G., et al. (2014). A large scale air pollution estimation method combining land use regression and chemical transport modeling in a geostatistical framework. *Environmental Science & Technology*, **48**, 4452–4459.

Basagaña, X., Rivera, M., Aguilera, I., Agis, D., Bouso, L., Elosua, R., et al. (2012). Effect of the number of measurement sites on land use regression models in estimating local air pollution. *Atmospheric Environment*, **54**, 634–642.

Beckerman, B. S., Jerrett, M., Martin, R. V., van Donkelaar, A., Ross, Z., and Burnett, R. T. (2013a). Application of the deletion/substitution/addition algorithm to selecting land use regression models for interpolating air pollution measurements in California. *Atmospheric Environment*, **77**, 172–177.

Beckerman, B. S., Jerrett, M., Serre, M., Martin, R. V., Lee, S. J., van Donkelaar, A., et al. (2013b). A hybrid approach to estimating national scale spatiotemporal variability of PM2.5 in the contiguous United States. *Environmental Science & Technology*, **47**, 7233–7241.

Beelen, R., Hoek, G., Fischer, P., van den Brandt, P. A., and Brunekreef, B. (2007). Estimated long-term outdoor air pollution concentrations in a cohort study. *Atmospheric Environment*, **41**, 1343–1358.

Beelen, R., Hoek, G., Pebesma, E., Vienneau, D., de Hoogh, K., and Briggs, D. J. (2009). Mapping of background air pollution at a fine spatial scale across the European Union. *Science of the Total Environment*, **407**, 1852–1867.

Beelen, R., Hoek, G., Vienneau, D., Eeftens, M., Dimakopoulou, K., Pedeli, X., et al. (2013). Development of NO2 and NOx land use regression models for estimating air pollution exposure in 36 study areas in Europe—The ESCAPE project. *Atmospheric Environment*, **72**, 10–23.

Brauer, M., Amann, M., Burnett, R. T., Cohen, A., Dentener, F., Ezzati, M., et al. (2012). Exposure assessment for estimation of the global burden of disease attributable to outdoor air pollution. *Environmental Science & Technology*, **46**, 652–660.

Brauer, M., Hoek, G., van Vliet, P., Meliefste, K., Fischer, P., Gehring, U., et al. (2003). Estimating long-term average particulate air pollution concentrations: application of traffic indicators and geographic information systems. *Epidemiology*, **14**, 228–239.

Briggs, D., Collins, S., Elliot, P., Fischer, P., Kingham, S., Lebret, E., Pryl, K., et al. (1997). Mapping urban air pollution using GIS: A regression-based approach. *International Journal of Geographical Information Science*, **11**, 699–718.

Briggs, D. J., de Hoogh, C., Gulliver, J., Wills, J., Elliott, P., Kingham, S., and Smallbone K. (2000). A regression-based method for mapping traffic-related air pollution: Application and testing in four contrasting urban environments. *Science of the Total Environment*, **253**, 151–167.

Cesaroni, G., Porta, D., Badaloni, C., Stafoggia, M., Eeftens, M., Meliefste, K., et al. (2012). Nitrogen dioxide levels estimated from land use regression models several years apart and association with mortality in a large cohort study. *Environmental Health*, **11**, 48.

de Hoogh, K., Korek, M., Vienneau., D., Keuken, M., Kukkonen, J., Nieuwenhuijsen, M. J., et al. (2014). Comparing land use regression and dispersion modelling to assess residential exposure to ambient air pollution for epidemiological studies. *Environment International*, **73**, 382–392.

de Hoogh, K., Wang, M., Adam, M., Badaloni, C., Beelen, R., Birk, M., et al. (2013). Development of land use regression models for particle composition in twenty study areas in Europe. *Environmental Science & Technology*, **47**, 5778–5786.

de Nazelle, A., Seto, E., Donaire-Gonzalez, D., Mendez, M., Matamala, J., Nieuwenhuijsen, M. J., and Jerrett, M. (2013). Improving estimates of air pollution exposure through ubiquitous sensing technologies. *Environmental Pollution*, **176**, 92–99.

Dockery, D. W., Pope, C. A. III., Xu, X., Spengler, J. D., Ware, J. H., Fay, M. E., et al. (1993). An association between air pollution and mortality in six U.S. cities. *New England Journal of Medicine*, **329**, 1753–1759.

Dons, E., Int Panis, L., Van Poppel, M., Theunis, J., and Wets, G. (2012). Personal exposure to black carbon in transport microenvironments. *Atmospheric Environment*, **55**, 392–398.

Eeftens, M., Beelen, R., de Hoogh, K., Bellander, T., Cesaroni, G., Cirach, M., et al. (2012). Development of Land Use Regression models for PM(2.5), PM(2.5) absorbance, PM(10) and PM(coarse) in 20 European study areas: Results of the ESCAPE project. *Environmental Science & Technology*, **46**, 11195–11205.

Eeftens, M., Beelen, R., Fischer, P., Brunekreef, B., Meliefste, K., and Hoek, G. (2011). Stability of measured and modelled spatial contrasts in NO2 over time. *Occupational & Environmental Medicine*, **68**, 765–770.

Gilbert, N. L., Goldberg, M. S., Beckerman, B., Brook, J. R., and Jerrett, M. (2005). Assessing spatial variability of ambient nitrogen dioxide in Montreal, Canada, with a land-use regression model. *Journal of the Air & Waste Management Association*, **55**, 1059–1063.

Gulliver, J., de Hoogh, K., Hansell, A., and Vienneau, D. (2013). Development and back-extrapolation of NO2 land use regression models for historic exposure assessment in Great Britain. *Environmental Science & Technology*, **47**, 7804–7811.

HEI Review Panel. (2013). *Understanding the health effects of Ambient Ultrafine Particles Report*. Health Effects Institute, London.

Henderson, S., Beckerman, B., Jerrett, M., and Brauer, M. (2007). Application of land use regression to estimate long-term concentrations of traffic-related nitrogen oxides and fine particulate matter. *Environmental Science & Technology*, **41**, 2422–2428.

Hoek, G., Beelen, R., de Hoogh, K., et al. (2008). A review of land-use regression models to assess spatial variation of outdoor air pollution. *Atmospheric Environment*, **42**, 7561–7578.

Hoek, G., Beelen, R., Kos, G., Dijkema, M., van der Zee, S. C., Fischer, P. H., and Brunekreef, B. (2011). Land use regression model for ultrafine particles in Amsterdam. *Environmental Science & Technology*, **45**, 622–628.

Hystad, P., Setton, E., Cervantes, A., Poplawski, K., Deschenes, S., Brauer, M., et al. (2011). Creating national air pollution models for population exposure assessment in Canada. *Environmental Health Perspectives*, **119**, 1123–1129.

Janhall, S., Molnar, P., and Molnar, H. (2003). Vertical distribution of air pollutants at the Gustavii Cathedral in Goteborg, Sweden. *Atmospheric Environment*, **37**, 209–217.

Jedynska, A., Gerard, H., Marloes, E., Josef, C., Menno, K., Christophe, A., et al. (2014). Spatial variations of PAH, hopanes/steranes and EC/OC concentrations within and between European study areas. *Atmospheric Environment*, **87**, 239–248.

Jerrett, M., Arain, A., Kanaroglou, P., Beckerman, B., Potoglou, D., Sahsuvaroglu, T., et al. (2005). A review and evaluation of intraurban air pollution exposure models. *Journal of Exposure Analysis and Environmental Epidemiology*, **15**, 185–204.

Jo, W. K., and Ky, K. (2002). Vertical variability of volatile organic compound (VOC) levels in ambient air of high-rise apartment buildings with and without occurrence of surface inversion. *Atmospheric Environment*, **36**, 5645–5652.

Johnson, M., Isakov, V., Touma, J. S., Mukerjee, S., and Ozkaynak, H. (2010). Evaluation of land-use regression models used to predict air quality concentrations in an urban area. *Atmospheric Environment*, **44**, 3660–3668.

Kanaroglou, P. S., Jerrett, M., Morrison, J., Beckerman, B., Altaf, A. M., Gilbert, N. L., and Brook, J. R. (2005). Establishing an air pollution monitoring network for intra-urban population exposure assessment: A location-allocation approach. *Atmospheric Environment*, **39**, 2399–2409.

Kloog, I., Nordio, F., Coull, B. A., and Schwartz, J. (2012). Incorporating local land use regression and satellite aerosol optical depth in a hybrid model of spatiotemporal PM2. 5 exposures in the Mid-Atlantic states. *Environmental Science & Technology 2012*, **46**, 11913–11921.

Kloog, I., Nordio, F., Coull, B. A., and Schwartz, J. (2014). Predicting spatiotemporal mean air temperature using MODIS satellite surface temperature measurements across the Northeastern USA. *Remote Sensing of Environment*, **150**, 132–139.

Larson, T., Henderson, S., and Brauer, M. (2009). Mobile monitoring of particle light absorption coefficient in an urban area as a basis for land use regression. *Environmental Science & Technology*, **43**, 4672–4678.

Larson, T., Su, J., Baribeau, A., Buzzelli, M., Setton, E., and Brauer, M. (2007). A spatial model of urban winter woodsmoke concentrations. *Environmental Science & Technology*, **41**, 2429–2436.

Lee, H. J., and Koutrakis, P. (2014). Daily ambient NO2 concentration predictions using satellite ozone monitoring instrument NO2 data and land use regression. *Environmental Science and Technology*, **48**, 2305–2311.

Lewne, M., Cyrys, J., Meliefste, K., Hoek, G., Brauer, M., Fischer, P., et al. (2004). Spatial variation in nitrogen dioxide in three European areas. *Science of the Total Environment*, **332**, 217–230.

Martin, R. V. (2008). Satellite remote sensing of surface air quality. *Atmospheric Environment*, **42**, 7823–7843.

Monn, C. (2001). Exposure assessment of air pollutants: A review on spatial heterogeneity and indoor/outdoor/personal exposure to suspended particulate matter, nitrogen dioxide and ozone. *Atmospheric Environment*, **35**, 1–32.

Montagne, D., Hoek, G., Nieuwenhuijsen, M., Lanki, T., Pennanen, A., Portella, M., et al. (2013). Agreement of land use regression models with personal exposure measurements of particulate matter and nitrogen oxides air pollution. *Environmental Science & Technology*, **47**, 8523–8531.

Moore, D. K., Jerrett, M., Mack, W. J., and Kunzli, N. (2007). A land use regression model for predicting ambient fine particulate matter across Los Angeles, CA. *Journal of Environmental Monitoring*, **9**, 246–252.

Nethery, E., Leckie, S. E., Teschke, K., and Brauer, M. (2008). From measures to models: an evaluation of air pollution exposure assessment for epidemiological studies of pregnant women. *Occupational & Environmental Medicine*, **65**, 579–586.

Novotny, E.V., Bechle, M. J., Millet, D. B., and Marshall, J. D. (2011). National satellite-based land-use regression: NO2 in the United States. *Environmental Science & Technology*, **45**, 4407–4414.

Nuckols, J. R., Ward, M. H., and Jarup, L. (2004). Using geographic information systems for exposure assessment in environmental epidemiology studies. *Environmental Health Perspectives*, **112**, 1007–1015.

Padró-Martínez, L. T., Patton, A. P., Trull, J. B., Zamore, W., Brugge, D., Durant, J. L. (2012). Mobile monitoring of particle number concentration and other traffic-related air pollutants in a near-highway neighborhood over the course of a year. *Atmospheric Environment*, **61**, 253–264.

Pope, C. A. 3rd., Burnett, R. T., Thun, M. J., Calle, E. E., Krewski, D., Ito, K., and Thurston, G. D. (2002). Lung cancer, cardiopulmonary mortality, and long-term exposure to fine particulate air pollution. *Journal of the American Medical Association*, **287**, 1132–1141.

Rivera, M., Basagaña, X., Aguilera, I., Agis, D., Bouso, L., Foraster, M., et al. (2012). Spatial distribution of ultrafine particles in urban settings: A land use regression model. *Atmospheric Environment*, **54**, 657–666.

Ross, Z., Jerrett, M., Ito, K., Tempalski, B., and Thurston, G. D. (2007). A land use regression for predicting fine particulate matter concentrations in the New York City region. *Atmospheric Environment*, **41**, 2255–2269.

Sahsuvaroglu, T., Su, J. G., Brook, J., Burnett, R., Loeb, M., and Jerrett, M. (2009). Predicting personal nitrogen dioxide exposure in an elderly population: Integrating residential indoor and outdoor measurements, fixed-site ambient pollution concentrations, modeled pollutant levels, and time-activity patterns. *Journal of Toxicology and Environmental Health Part A: Current Issues*, **72**, 1520–1533.

Sampson, P. D., Szpiro, A. A., Sheppard, L., Lindström, J., and Kaufman, J. D. (2011). Pragmatic estimation of a spatio-temporal air quality model with irregular monitoring data. *Atmospheric Environment*, **45**, 6593–6606.

Sampson, P. D., Richards, M., Szpiro, A. A., Bergen, S., Sheppard, L., Larson, T. V., and Kaufman, J. D. (2013). A regionalized national universal kriging model using Partial Least Squares regression for estimating annual PM2.5 concentrations in epidemiology. *Atmospheric Environment*, **75**, 383–392.

Stedman, J., Vincent, K., Campbell, G., Goodwin, J., and Downing, C. (1997). New high resolution maps of estimated background ambient NOx and NO2 concentrations in the U.K. *Atmospheric Environment*, **31**, 3591–3602.

Su, J. G., Buzzelli, M., Brauer, M., Gould, T., and Larson, T. V. (2008). Modeling spatial variability of airborne levoglucosan in Seattle, Washington. *Atmospheric Environment*, **42**, 5519–5525.

Su, J. G., Jerrett, M., Beckerman, B., Wilhelm, M., Ghosh, J. K., and Ritz, B. (2009). Predicting traffic-related air pollution in Los Angeles using a distance decay regression selection strategy. *Environmental Research*, **109**(6), 657–670.

Vakeva, M., Hameri, K., Kulmala, M., Ruuskanen, J., and Laitinen, T. (1999). Street level versus rooftop concentrations of submicron aerosol particles and gaseous pollutants in an urban street canyon. *Atmospheric Environment*, **33**, 1385–1397.

Van Roosbroeck, S., Jacobs, J., Janssen, N., Oldenwening, M., Hoek, G., and Brunekreef, B. (2007). Long-term personal exposure to PM2.5, soot and NOx in children attending schools located near busy roads: A validation study. *Atmospheric Environment*, **41**, 3381–3394.

Van Roosbroeck, S., Wichmann, J., Janssen, N. A., Hoek, G., van Wijnen, J. H., Lebret, E., and Brunekreef, B. (2006). Long-term personal exposure to traffic-related air pollution among school children: A validation study. *Science of the Total Environment*, **368**(2-3), 565–573.

Vedal, S., Campen, M. J., McDonald, J. D., Larson, T. V., Sampson, P. D., Sheppard, L., et al. (2013). National Particle Component Toxicity (NPACT) initiative report on cardiovascular effects. *Research Report of the Health Effects Institute*, **178**, 5–8.

Vienneau, D., de Hoogh, K., Bechle, M. J., Beelen, R., van Donkelaar, A., Martin, R. V., et al. (2013). Western European land use regression incorporating satellite- and ground-based measurements of NO2 and PM10. *Environmental Science & Technology*, **47**, 13555–13564.

Vine, M. F., Degnan, D., and Hanchette, C. (1997). Geographic information systems: Their use in environmental epidemiologic research. *Environmental Health Perspectives*, **105**, 598–605.

Wang, M., Beelen, R., Eeftens, M., Meliefste, K., Hoek, G., and Brunekreef, B. (2012). Systematic evaluation of land use regression models for NO2. *Environmental Science & Technology*, **46**, 4481–4489.

Wang, R. R., Henderson, S. B., Sbihi, H., Allen, R. W., and Brauer, M. (2013). Temporal stability of land use regression models for traffic-related air pollution. *Atmospheric Environment*, **64**, 312–319.

Wichmann, J., Janssen, N., van der Zee, S., and Brunekreef, B. (2005). Traffic-related differences in indoor and personal absorbation coefficient measurements in Amsterdam, the Netherlands. *Atmospheric Environment*, **39**, 7384–7392.

Wilton, D., Szpiro, A., Gould, T., and Larson, T. (2010). Improving spatial concentration estimates for nitrogen oxides using a hybrid meteorological dispersion/land use regression model in Los Angeles, CA and Seattle, WA. *Science of the Total Environment*, **408**, 1120–1130.

Wu, C. F., Lin, H. I., Ho, C. C., Yang, T. H., Chen, C. C., and Chan, C. C. (2014). Modeling horizontal and vertical variation in intraurban exposure to PM2.5 concentrations and compositions. *Environmental Research*, **133**, 96–102

Yanosky, J. D., Tonne, C. C., Beevers, S. D., Wilkinson, P., and Kelly, F. J. (2012). Modeling exposures to the oxidative potential of PM10. *Environmental Science & Technology*, **46**, 7612–7620.

Zhang, P., Dong, G., Sun, B., Zhang, L., Chen, X., Ma, N., et al. (2011). Long-term exposure to ambient air pollution and mortality due to cardiovascular disease and cerebrovascular disease in Shenyang, China. *PLoS One*, **6**, e20827.

Zhu, Y., Hinds, W., Kim, S., Shen, S., and Sioutas, C. (2002). Study of ultrafine particles near a major highway with heavy-duty diesel traffic. *Atmospheric Environment*, **36**, 4233–4335.

14

THE EXPOSOME—CONCEPT AND
IMPLEMENTATION IN BIRTH COHORTS

Martine Vrijheid

14.1 INTRODUCTION

The "exposome" was first proposed by Wild (2005) to encompass the totality of human environmental (meaning all non-genetic) exposures from conception onward, complementing the genome. The concept was proposed primarily to draw attention to the need for better and more complete environmental exposure data, in order to balance the investment, tools, and knowledge in genetics. Many associations between environmental factors and health remain poorly characterized, giving rise to uncertain health risk and impact assessments, and uncertain directions for prevention. This is due to the many uncertainties in assessment of environmental exposures, which are traditionally measured through questionnaires and geographical mapping, and to the lack of studies that tackle multiple exposures; the environmental component in disease etiology has thus far largely been studied using a "one-exposure-one-health-effect" approach. We have not been able to measure environmental factors with the same degree of accuracy and comprehensiveness as the genome. Wild (2012) further defined three overlapping domains within the exposome: 1) a general external environment to include factors such as the urban environment, climate factors, social capital, and stress; 2) a specific external environment with specific contaminants, diet, physical activity, tobacco, infections, etc., and 3) an internal environment to include internal biological factors such as metabolic factors, gut microflora, inflammation, and oxidative stress (Figure 14.1; reprinted from Vrijheid 2014). Measurement of these three domains of the exposome requires the employment of a range of diverse methods and tools that can capture many exposures in a single measurement; a "one-agent-at-a-time" approach will not be able to do this, nor is it likely that one single tool can be developed for this purpose.

14.1.1 Tools to Measure the External Exposome

In the exposome concept, the traditional challenge of accurate estimation of exposure (reduction of misclassification) is multiplied because it requires obtaining exposure data for many different exposures. Within the external exposome, a

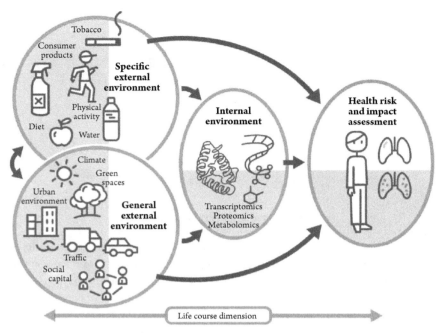

Figure 14.1 Three domains of the exposome. (Reprinted from Vrijheid, M. (2014). The exposome: A new paradigm to study the impact of environment on health. *Thorax*, **69**(9), 876–878.)

distinction can be made between exposures in the specific external environment, including environmental tobacco smoke (ETS), water contaminants, persistent organic pollutants (POPs), pesticides, and metals, which are traditionally assessed at the *individual level* through questionnaires and/or biomonitoring, and exposures in the general external environment, such as outdoor air pollutants, noise, and green space, which are mainly assessed at the *community level* through geographical mapping methods (see Figure 14.1).

For *individually assessed exposures*, improvement in exposure assessment can be achieved by improving conventional methods and introducing new imaging, sensor, and computer technologies. As an example of the former, more frequent measurement of biomarkers combined with better modeling of exposure will improve assessments. Individually assessed exposures can vary on an hourly, daily, or yearly basis. Temporal variability is particularly high for exposures with a short biological half-life and little constancy in the underlying exposure behavior (e.g., bisphenol A [BPA], phthalates, organophosphorus pesticides; Preau et al. 2010; Braun et al. 2011; Bradman et al. 2013; Philippat et al. 2013). For such exposures, intra- compared with inter-individual variability is known to be high and only many repeat measurements, or measurement of a pool of many samples, over time may give improved exposure estimates. For more persistent exposures, biomarkers give more long-term exposure estimates that are influenced by changes in diet or behavior, for example, by breastfeeding patterns. Here, modeling the toxico-kinetics of the chemical using physiologically based pharmacokinetics (PBPK) may help the interpretation of the measured biomarker data. Physiologically based pharmicokinetic models describe the fate of chemicals in the body using individual-specific information about the physiology (age, gender, weight) and the biochemistry (enzyme content) of the individual as well as information on the individual's behavior (breastfeeding, physical activity, diet) (Beaudouin et al. 2010). In the context of population (epidemiological) studies, PBPK models can be used to simulate exposure during critical time periods between biomarker measurement points. To be relevant, this approach requires detailed input data on individual characteristics and behaviors to minimize assumptions and uncertainties (refer to chapter 8). New smartphone-linked diaries and imaging are also promising tools for more accurate and complete exposure assessment, for example, of diet and use of consumer products.

For *community-level exposures* that are traditionally assessed on the basis of residential location, major improvements in exposure assessment and reduction in measurement error can be achieved by collecting information on where people are, how they move through their environment, and, in case of air pollution, how much air they inhale. New geographic information system (GIS)–based exposure assessments (Beelen et al. 2013), remote sensing (Dadvand et al. 2012), and smartphone technologies (Nieuwenhuijsen et al. 2014) have made it easier to assess outdoor exposures, and to integrate personal mobility and physical activity data. Knowledge about the inhalation rate, for example, may be integrated with personal air pollution measurements to estimate inhalation dose. For this, information about physical activity is needed and this can be collected through readily available accelerometers or sensors in smartphones. Further, people tend to move around in micro-environments: for example, near busy roads where exposures such as air pollutants or noise can be considerable higher compared with the rest of the time, or in parks where exposure to green space is higher and exposure to air pollution and noise is lower. Smartphone applications that integrate global positioning systems (GPS) location data with physical activity information and pollution measurements are now being developed to better characterize the external exposome (Nieuwenhuijsen et al. 2014).

14.1.2 Tools to Measure the Internal Exposome

High-throughput molecular "omics" techniques can analyze complete sets of biological molecules, including smaller molecules (metabolomics), larger molecules (proteome), gene expression profiles (transcriptomics and epigenomics), and reactive electrophiles (adductomics). Recent years have seen the rapid development of omics applications in animal and in vitro experimental studies; for example, there are now numerous reports of epigenetic (methylation and miRNA) modifications arising from exposure to environmental toxicants. In human studies, applications have been extremely limited, but promising new results relate to their use to predict exposure-related health risks and individual susceptibilities, for example, methylation profiles in relation to air pollution and cigarette smoking, metabolomic profiles to diet, and protein profiling in relation to benzene, arsenic, and lead (Holmes et al. 2008; Bollati and Baccarelli 2010; Vlaanderen et al. 2010; Hou et al. 2012). In the development of the exposome concept, the contribution of omics techniques is likely to lie mainly in their potential to measure profiles (or signatures) of the biological response to complex exposure mixtures or a cumulative exposure experience. In particular, the hope is to find a unique matrix that could play an equivalent role to the DNA sequence in genome-wide association studies (GWAS), and allow the characterization of the exposome without characterizing each exposure separately (Wild 2012). This is exactly the point where classical, single, exposure biomarkers have reached their limits: The measurement of numerous single analytes has limits both in cost and available sample quantity. A "blood exposome" has now been proposed to encompass all endogenous and exogenous chemicals in the blood (Rappaport et al. 2014). It is expected that the untargeted nature of omics data will capture biological responses to exposure in a more holistic way, providing clues about thus far unidentified risk factors. Further, omics data are likely to provide extra information on the molecular mechanisms underlying exposure-related health effects. Specifically, using omics tools we may be able to identify how diverse exposures act on common pathways to cause common disease outcomes. Further evaluation of omics tools for use in environmental health research requires careful attention to be paid to challenges relating to study design, validation, replication, temporal variance, and meta-data analysis (Vlaanderen et al. 2010). For example, for these techniques to be useful in larger studies, it has to be shown that intra-individual variability in the molecular profiles measured in systemic body fluids that can be collected in population studies (blood, urine) is less important than inter-individual variability. Profiles of RNA transcripts, proteins, and metabolites are highly variable over time; teasing out variations due to exposure changes remains a major challenge.

14.1.3 The Dynamic Exposome

The exposome is dynamic, as opposed to the static genome. Exposures vary on an hourly to yearly basis both in the external and internal environments and this is reflected in the high degree of variation in their measurements (Figure 14.2).

For example, spatial models for the outdoor exposures are constructed for a specific year and can then be extrapolated to relevant time periods (days, weeks, months, or years) backward or forward in time using available monitoring stations data. For persistent pollutants we may assume that biomarkers give estimates over a relatively long time period, whereas for non-persistent pollutants biomarkers will reflect only very recent exposures; in some cases we may assume a fairly constant

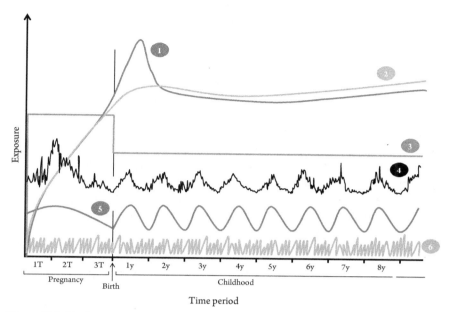

Figure 14.2 The dynamic exposome—six different hypothetical exposure scenarios during early life. 1. Persistent organic pollutants, including organochlorines, brominated and perfluorinataed compounds (breastfeeding exposure). 2. Metals, including Hg and Pb (cumulative during pregnancy). 3. Environmental Tobacco Smoke. 4. Air pollution, noise, and green space with daily and seasonal variations. 5. UV radiation, pesticides, benzophenone-3 with mainly seasonal variation. 6. Non-persistent pollutants, including phthalates, phenols, and triclosan.

exposure pattern depending on the habits underlying the exposure (e.g., cosmetics use, dietary patterns), whereas in other cases exposure variations may be largely seasonal (e.g., sunscreens, pesticides). Moreover, a given exposure or dose will not have the same effect during various developmental periods that are critical to health and disease. For example, neurodevelopment, growth and obesity, and asthma and allergies, are each driven by extremely complex multistage developmental processes that take place prenatally and during the first years of postnatal life. Measurement of the exposome (internal or external) at one given point in time would not be sufficient to characterize all health impacts of the environment, but there are currently no prospective study populations that would allow lifelong repeated characterization. One way forward would be to start developing the exposome at certain key points in exposure experience or disease development (Wild 2012). For example, it is well recognized that the periods of organ development during prenatal life and infancy are especially vulnerable to the effects of environmental risk factors, which may manifest themselves throughout the lifetime in adult diseases. Early life is thus a key point for defining the exposome. Another option is to apply the exposome concept to several cohorts that span the life course.

14.2 IMPLEMENTATION OF THE EARLY LIFE EXPOSOME

Here, we aim to illustrate how the exposome concept may be implemented in an epidemiological study design, using the Human Early Life Exposome (HELIX) project as an example (full study design described in Vrijheid et al. 2014). The HELIX project has as its general aim to implement novel tools and methods (biomarkers, omics-based approaches, remote sensing and GIS-based spatial methods, personal exposure devices, statistical tools for combined exposures, and burden of disease methodologies), to characterize early-life exposure to a wide range of chemical and physical environmental factors and associate these with data on major child health outcomes (e.g., growth and obesity, neurodevelopment, respiratory health). The project takes pregnancy and childhood periods (early life) as the starting point for putting the exposome into practice.

14.2.1 The Human Early Life Exposome Study Design

The HELIX will develop the early-life exposome approach and database in three overlapping steps. A first step will measure the external exposome—exposure estimates for a broad range of chemical and physical exposures; a second step will measure the internal exposome (molecular signatures) and integrate the multiple dimensions of the exposome—multiple exposures, multiple time points, individual variability—and a third step will develop the tools and methods to evaluate the exposome's impact on child health. Six existing longitudinal population-based birth cohort studies in Europe form the basis of the project: BiB (UK), EDEN (France), INMA (Spain), KANC (Lithuania), MoBa (Norway), and RHEA (Greece). The cohorts were selected because 1) they each have a large amount of existing longitudinal data from early pregnancy through childhood; 2) they can implement new follow-up examinations of the children at similar ages (6–9 y), old enough for accurate measurement of the phenotypes of interest for HELIX; and 3) they can integrate new questionnaires, biosampling, and clinical examinations in their new follow-ups using common protocols. The selection of cohorts followed a strategy to obtain data in different regions of Europe. In general, exposure estimates can be obtained in cohort studies for very large numbers of subjects by exposure models and questionnaires, whereas exposure and omics biomarkers can, for cost reasons, only be obtained in smaller numbers of subjects. Assessment of individual exposure variability and validation of exposure models require very intensive data collection that is only feasible in an even smaller number of subjects. Therefore, to construct the exposome, HELIX uses a multilevel study design, drawing on nested study populations for different levels of data collection. Exposure assessment methods used in the HELIX project are summarized in Table 14.1 and further described in Vrijheid et al. (2014).

Table 14.1 Exposure groups and assessment methods included in HELIX

Exposure group	Assessment method
POPS: PCB-153, DDE, HCB, PBDE-47	Biomarkers: in stored pregnancy blood samples* and in newly collected child blood samples.
PFAS: PFOS, PFOA, PFBS, PFHxS, PFNA	Biomarkers: in stored pregnancy blood samples* and in newly collected child blood samples. PBPK models for pregnancy and childhood.
Metals: Hg, Pb, and TMS	Biomarkers: in stored pregnancy samples* and in newly collected child samples: blood (Pb), urine (TMS), and hair (Hg).
Phthalates: 13 metabolites	Biomarkers: in stored pregnancy urine samples[b] and in newly collected child urine samples (last night and first morning void) in subcohort; In daily repeat urine samples in panel studies. Daily data on diet, cosmetics. PBPK model for DEHP.
Phenols: BPA, parabens, TCS, BP3	Biomarkers: in stored pregnancy urine samples** and in newly collected child urine samples (last night and first morning void) in subcohort. In daily repeat urine samples in panel studies. Daily data on diet, cosmetics.
OP pesticides	Biomarkers: in stored pregnancy urine samples* and in newly collected child urine samples (last night and first morning void) in subcohort. In daily repeat urine samples in two seasons in panel studies. Daily data on diet and repellent use in panel studies.
Water DBPs	Estimates available from previous HiWATE project during and after pregnancy. New questionnaire in subcohort children on water consumption and swimming combined with water company data. Water consumption diaries in panel studies
Indoor air: BTEX, NO_2, $PM_{2.5}$	Existing questionnaire data on indoor sources during and after pregnancy. New questionnaire in subcohort children on cooking, heating, cleaning, and ventilation. Passive BTEX and NO_2 sampling in the home in panel studies. Active $PM_{2.5}$ sampling in panel studies.
ETS	Existing questionnaire and cotinine data during and after pregnancy. New questionnaire in subcohort children. Biomarkers: cotinine measurement in newly collected child urine and/or hair samples.
Ambient air pollutants	LUR model for NO_2, $PM_{2.5}$. PM_{10}, PM_{coarse} $PM_{2.5}$ aborbance, PM elemental analyses. Routine monitoring and OMI satellite data for temporal variability. Panel studies: Inhalation rates and mobility (GPS) data from smartphones. Personal monitoring (24 hours) of $PM_{2.5}$ (BGI-400-4 with cyclone pump) and black carbon MicroAthelometer (AE51).

(continued)

Table 14.1 Continued

Exposure group	Assessment method
Noise	Existing municipal noise maps to obtain spatial estimates. Address-based modeling of noise at the most and least exposed facade. New questionnaires in subcohort children on bedroom position, noise perception, etc. Noise estimates based on maps and questions. Time-activity and mobility (GPS) data from smartphones in panel studies.
UV	Remote sensing (satellite) UV radiation maps. New questionnaires in subcohort children on traveling, use of sunscreens, clothes, skin color. UV radiation estimates based on maps and questions. Panel studies: Time-activity and mobility (GPS) data from smartphones and questionnaires. Personal monitoring using electronic UV dosimeters.
Temperature	Remote sensing (satellite) temperature maps (from thermal infrared band) and data from local meteorological stations. New questionnaires in subcohort children on heating and air conditioning. Temperature estimates based on maps and questions. Panel studies: Time-activity and mobility (GPS) data from smartphones and questionnaires. Personal monitoring of temperature using electronic dosimeters.
Built environment/ green spaces	Normalized Difference Vegetation Index from satellite. Building density, walkability score, accessibility, bike lanes, etc. derived from GIS data. New questionnaires in subcohort children on use of green spaces, public spaces, active transportation. Panel studies: Time-activity and mobility (GPS) data from smartphones and questionnaires.

BP3: benzophenone-3; BPA: bisphenol A; BETX: benzene, toluene, ethylbenzene, xylene; DBPs: disinfection by-products; DDE: dichlorodiphenyldichloroethylene; DEHP: bis(2-ethylhexyl) phthalate (di-2-ethylhexyl phthalate; ETS: environmental tobacco smoke; HCB: hexachlorobenzene; Hg: mercury; NO_2: nitrogen dioxide; OP: organophospate pesticides; Pb: lead; PBDE-47: polybrominated diphenyl ethers-47; PCB-153:polychlorinated biphenyl-153; PFAS: perfluoroalkyl substances; PFBS: perfluorobutanesulfonic acid; PFHxS: perfluorohexane sulfonic acid; PFNA: perfluorononanoic acid; PFOA: perfluorooctanoic acid; PFOS: perfluorooctane sulfonic acid; TCS: triclosan; TMS: total metal spectrum. LUR: land use regression, NO_2: nitrogen dioxide, NO_x: nitrous oxides, $PM_{2.5}$: mass concentration of particles less than 2.5 μm in size, PM_{10}: mass concentration of particles less than 10 μm in size, PM2.5 absorbance: measurement of the blackness of $PM_{2.5}$ filters; a proxy for elemental carbon, which is the dominant light absorbing substance, PM_{coarse}: mass concentration of particles between 2.5 and 10 μm in size, GPS: global positioning system.

* Where measurements are available from previous studies these will be used.

** Pooling of 2 or more urine samples when available.

14.2.2 Measurement of the External Exposome

The "Outdoor Exposome" in the Entire Six Cohorts of 32,000 Mother–Child Pairs

Risk estimates for the effects of combined outdoor exposures (the "outdoor exposome") on child health will be obtained in the entire study population of the six cohorts combined. Outcomes will include birth outcomes, postnatal growth and body mass index (BMI), wheezing and asthma, lung function, and neurodevelopmental constructs, including general cognition, language development, and motor abilities, across different age groupings. The cohorts will provide existing exposure data such as on tobacco use, air pollution land-use regression model estimates, and existing confounder and outcome data. Further, a GIS environment will be constructed for the six study areas, and exposure will be estimated for air pollutants, noise, UV radiation, temperature, built environment/green spaces, during pregnancy and childhood (see Table 14.1). Data from existing regulatory monitors and remote sensing data will be used to inform ambient spatial exposure models. The aim is to obtain average exposure estimates for the pregnancy period, and during childhood for different time periods, including 1 day, 1 week, 1 month, and 1 year before outcome assessment.

The "Total Exposome" in a HELIX Subcohort of 1200 Mother–Child Pairs

A subcohort of 1200 mother–child pairs will be fully characterized for the external and internal exposome, including exposure biomarkers during pregnancy and childhood, and omics biomarkers during childhood. The impact of the total early-life exposome on child health will be characterized in these subjects. The 1200 mother–child pairs will be nested within the entire cohorts by selecting 200 pairs from each cohort. The nested design means that for the subcohort subjects, the outdoor exposome will have been characterized following the methods outlined in the preceding. During the subcohort follow-up examination, new biological samples are collected suitable for all planned biomarker (see Table 14.1) and omics analyses. Questionnaires will collect information on water consumption habits, which will be combined with information on concentrations of DBPs in drinking water from water companies to obtain estimates of exposure to DBPs. Questionnaires will also collect information on sources of indoor air pollution, including ETS, cooking and heating appliances, and ventilation (see Table 14.1). The collection of two urine samples (one before bedtime and one first morning void) will better capture short-lived biomarker metabolites and provide more stable metabolome coverage than would be achieved with one spot urine sample. During the follow-up examination, trained nurses will carry out health examinations of the children. The subcohort children will be examined by trained nurses to measure weight, height, waist circumference, skin folds, blood pressure, and lung function. Interviews with the mothers will collect information on exposures, physical activity, time activity, diet, social factors, stress, and asthma and allergy. Neurodevelopmental outcomes will be assessed through a battery of internationally standardized, non-linguistic, and culturally blind computer tests. Parents will complete the Conner's and Child Behaviour Checklist (CBCL) questionnaire to assess child behavioral problems.

"Exposome Variability" Panel Studies

Panel studies will collect data on short-term temporal variability in exposure bio-markers and omics biomarkers, individual behaviors (physical activity, mobility, time activity), and personal and indoor exposures. A *children panel study* will include children from the HELIX subcohort ($n = 150$). A *pregnant women panel* will include 150 pregnant women from outside the cohorts; mothers from the cohorts cannot be used for this purpose because their pregnancies were several years ago. Subjects in the children and pregnant women panel study will be followed for 1 week in two seasons. From these subjects we will collect daily urine samples and at the end of each monitoring week, blood samples will be collected following the same proce-dures as for the subcohort. The daily urine samples will be used to measure repeat biomarkers of the non-persistent chemicals (phthalates, phenols, organophos-phate pesticides) (see Table 14.1); these data will be used to characterize inter- and intra-individual variability in these urine biomarkers, and where possible, correct for the uncertainties in the larger cohort. Smartphones will be worn by the partic-ipants in the panel studies to provide geolocation data, the metabolic equivalent of tasks (METs) derived from the in-built accelerometer and GPS and integrated on the specially developed ExpoApp. We will then translate these data into activ-ity type (resting, cycling, car travel) and derive inhalation rates. The panel study subjects will also wear electronic wristband UV dosimeters, $PM_{2.5}$ active samplers, and MicroAthelometers for continuous black carbon monitoring (see Table 14.1). Personal exposure estimates will be used to characterize uncertainties in the spatial exposure models. Indoor air pollution will be measured to characterize errors when using exposure information from questionnaires and models. This will be done using passive samplers for nitrogen dioxide (NO_2) and BTEX (benzene, toluene, ethylene, and xylene), and active $PM_{2.5}$ Cyclone pumps, installed in the home.

The HELIX project will also evaluate the use of PBPK modeling to interpret bio-markers of exposure to perfluorinated alkyl substances (perfluorooctane sulfonate [PFOS], perfluorooctanoic acid [PFOA], and di-2-ethyl hexyl phthalate [DEHP]). For the PFAS, the biomarker measurement in the subcohort children will be related to that in the mothers during pregnancy using an exposure scenario that integrates maternal–fetal transfers during pregnancy, transfers via breast milk, and diet dur-ing childhood. For DEHP, repeat biomarkers in the panel studies and information on exposure-related behaviors and urination times will be used to evaluate the pre-dictable value of different numbers of biomarker measurements.

Once individual and outdoor exposures have been estimated, analysis-of-variance techniques, incorporating data from both the HELIX subcohort and the panel studies, will be used to understand the variance components for each key exposure (for instance, arising from diet, physical activity, or time of sampling) and describe the uncertainties in each of the exposure estimates. Statistical techniques such as factor analysis and latent class analysis will be used to create a reduced set of continuous exposure indices based on commonly occurring exposures, whereas individuals who share similar exposure profiles or "exposomes" will be defined. We will then determine the influence of variables such as diet, socioeconomic status, study region, and seasonality on these exposure indices or profiles. Specific attention will be given to the detection of cohort-specific exposure patterns.

14.2.3 Measurement of the Internal Exposome

The HELIX will determine molecular signatures associated with environmental exposures through the measurement of endogenous and xenobiotic metabolite profiles in blood and urine, proteins in plasma, and coding and small non-coding RNAs (including miRNAs) and DNA methylation in whole blood. Omics tools will be employed mainly in the subcohort of 1200 children with newly collected biosamples at age 6 to 9 years and in the two repeat panel study periods; the use of new samples ensures comparability between techniques and cohorts. The use of a similar time point for all omics techniques also allows integration of the different techniques during data analysis. The omics work will be implemented in three general stages:

Stage 1. Study design optimization: Biological samples collected in the panel studies (daily urine samples, two blood samples) will be used to assess detectability of omics markers and the likely sources of variability within and between individuals, using small numbers of subjects. These results will inform the design and interpretation of stages 2 and 3.

Stage 2. Omics-exposure associations in the biological samples newly collected in the subcohort ($n = 1200$): Primary analyses will evaluate three a priori defined exposures for which long-term pre and post natal exposure estimates can be obtained (ETS, total POP concentration, and air pollution). Secondary analyses will examine other exposures. Panel study data will evaluate short-term exposure-omics associations for a range of exposures for which detailed data are collected in the panels: air pollution, noise, UV, and non-persistent chemicals.

Stage 3. Biologically meaningful omics "hits" will be then linked to our main child health endpoints, similar to the "meet-in-the middle" approach to biomarker discovery (Chadeau-Hyam et al. 2011). The child health outcomes will be largely continuous outcome scores (BMI z-score, cognitive score, lung function). If relevant, reverse causality potential may be evaluated in blood and urine samples available in some of the cohorts at earlier time points.

In order to analyze, integrate, and interpret the large amounts of data generated by individual omics techniques, HELIX will apply a pathway analysis approach.

The biomarkers obtained from the association analysis, in combination with available libraries of biological pathways (GO, KEGG, Reactome, Comparative Toxicogenomics Database), will be used to identify biological pathways affected by the exposures. Identification and representation of biological-toxicological pathways will be done using software such as Ingenuity Pathway Analysis, Cytoscape, and Impala (Kamburov et al. 2011).

14.2.4 Associating the Exposome with Child Health

One of the greatest challenges of the exposome concept lies in the assessment of its association with health outcomes: How can we integrate multi-dimensional exposome data to draw meaningful conclusions about (child) health impacts? In general, environmental health studies have considered single exposures or single families of exposure (e.g., atmospheric pollutants, drinking water pollutants). Issues of co-linearity when investigating multiple exposures that may be highly correlated due to common sources or temporality will require new statistical frameworks (Sun et al. 2013). In developing statistical tools for the analysis of many exposure factors, important lessons should be drawn from the achievements but also the limitations (Shi and Weinberg 2011) of the parallel genome-wide association studies (GWAS) field, particularly regarding the probably weak efficiency of purely agnostic approaches, the very large sample sizes required, and the need to use complementary approaches (e.g., pathway analysis) making use of a priori information. It is apparent that different statistical approaches will be needed for the different objectives of exposome analyses, which can include identifying the most important individual exposures (crucial for regulatory policy), describing exposure mixtures or exposome patterns (as most normally encountered in reality), and indentifying synergistic or interactive effects, which mainly due to issues of power has been relatively unexplored in the epidemiological literature. The HELIX will develop a multistep statistical analysis approach that is based on several tools and methods (reviewed by Billionnet et al. 2012; Chadeau-Hyam et al. 2013; Sun et al. 2014), including an agnostic environment-wide association study (EWAS) approach, reduction dimension and variable selection techniques, and clustering techniques such as Bayesian Profile Regression. The latter aims to identify groups of individuals sharing a similar exposome that at the same time show marked differences according to the health outcome variable of study (Molitor et al. 2010; Papathomas et al. 2011).

Finally, HELIX will estimate the burden of common childhood diseases that may be attributed to multiple environmental exposures in Europe. It will construct scenarios for the health impact assessment, working from traditional one-exposure-one-outcome assessments (e.g., traffic-related air pollution and asthma, mercury, and neurodevelopment) to more complex benefit–harm scenarios. For example, given increasing obesity rates, children are encouraged to walk or cycle to school, which may lead to increased energy expenditure and possible reduction in weight and improvement in mental health. However, at the same time, longer duration of exposure to air pollutants, noise, and UV may lead to adverse health effects and higher risks of accidents (Rojas-Rueda et al. 2012). Do the overall benefits outweigh these risks and what should policymakers do to improve these conditions of active transportation? This work will integrate exposure, uncertainty, and biomarker data obtained in HELIX, risk estimates obtained in HELIX, exposure–response data from the literature, exposure data from other existing birth and child cohorts (Vrijheid et al. 2012), and Europe-wide surveys, and prevalence data from existing health registries/surveys in Europe.

14.3 CONCLUSION

Among much debate on the definition and application of the exposome (Rappaport and Smith 2010; Rappaport 2011; Peters et al. 2012; Buck-Louis et al. 2013; Miller and Jones 2014), we should bear in mind that complementing (not replacing) the "one-exposure-one-health-effect" approach of current etiological studies with a more holistic approach is essential to improve our understanding of the predictors, risk factors, and protective factors of complex, multifactorial, chronic pathologies. The exposome offers a framework for improvement and integration of currently scattered and uncertain data on the environment over the life course. Clearly, there are large challenges in developing this framework into a workable approach: A complete exposome would have to integrate many external and internal exposures from different sources continuously over the life course; we may have to accept that we will never be able to measure a truly "complete" exposome. The management, analysis, and interpretation of these multi-dimensional exposome data also pose new challenges for population studies. Practical applications to measure partial exposomes are underway (Patel et al. 2010; Exposomics 2014; Golding et al. 2014; Lenters et al. 2014; Vrijheid et al. 2014), making the time ripe now to evaluate the exposome challenges in carefully designed epidemiological projects.

REFERENCES

Beaudouin, R., Micallef, S., and Brochot, C. (2010). A stochastic whole-body physiologically based pharmacokinetic model to assess the impact of inter-individual variability on tissue dosimetry over the human lifespan. *Regulatory Toxicology and Pharmacology*, **57**(1), 103–116.

Beelen, R., Hoek, G., Vienneau, D., Eeftens, M., Dimakopoulou, K., Pedeli, X., et al. (2013). Development of NO2 and NOx land use regression models for estimating air pollution exposure in 36 study areas in Europe—The ESCAPE project. *Atmospheric Environment*, **72**, 10–23.

Billionnet, C., Sherrill, D., and Annesi-Maesano I. (2012). Estimating the health effects of exposure to multi-pollutant mixture. *Annals of Epidemiology*, **22**, 126–141.

Bollati, V., and Baccarelli, A. (2010). Environmental epigenetics. *Heredity* (Edinburgh), **105**, 105–112.

Bradman, A., Kogut, K., Eisen, E. A., Jewell, N. P., Quiros-Alcala, L., Castorina, R., et al. (2013). Variability of organophosphorous pesticide metabolite levels in spot and 24-hr urine samples collected from young children during 1 week. *Environmental Health Perspectives*, **121**(1), 118–124.

Braun, J. M., Kalkbrenner, A. E., Calafat, A. M., Bernert, J. T., Ye, X., Silva, M. J., et al. (2011). Variability and predictors of urinary bisphenol A concentrations during pregnancy. *Environmental Health Perspectives*, **119**(1), 131–137.

Buck Louis, G. M., Yeung, E., Sundaram, R., Laughon, S. K., and Zhang, C. (2013). The exposome—exciting opportunities for discoveries in reproductive and perinatal epidemiology. *Paediatric and Perinatal Epidemiology*, **27**, 229–236.

Chadeau-Hyam, M., Athersuch, T. J., Keun, H. C., De Iorio, M., Ebbels, T. M., Jenab, M., et al. (2011). Meeting-in-the-middle using metabolic profiling—a strategy for the identification of intermediate biomarkers in cohort studies. *Biomarkers*, **16**(1), 83–88.

Chadeau-Hyam, M., Campanella, G., Jombart, T., Bottolo, L., Portengen, L., Vineis, P., et al. (2013). Deciphering the complex: Methodological overview of statistical models to derive OMICS-based biomarkers. *Environmental and Molecular Mutagenesis*, **54**(7), 542–557.

Dadvand, P., Sunyer, J., Basagana, X., Ballester, F., Lertxundi, A., Fernandez-Somoano, A., et al. (2012). Surrounding greenness and pregnancy outcomes in four Spanish birth cohorts. *Environmental Health Perspectives*, **120**(10), 1481–1487.

Exposomics. (2014). Cited November 3, 2014. http://www.exposomicsproject.eu/

Golding, J., Gregory, S., Iles-Caven, Y., Lingam, R., Davis, J. M., Emmett, P., et al. (2014). Parental, prenatal, and neonatal associations with ball skills at age 8 using an Exposome approach. *Journal of Child Neurology*, **29**(10), 1390–1398.

Holmes, E., Loo, R. L., Stamler, J., Bictash, M., Yap, I. K., Chan, Q., et al. (2008). Human metabolic phenotype diversity and its association with diet and blood pressure. *Nature*, **453**(7193), 396–400.

Hou, L., Zhang, X., Wang, D., and Baccarelli, A. (2012). Environmental chemical exposures and human epigenetics. *International Journal of Epidemiology*, **41**(1), 79–105.

Kamburov, A., Cavill, R., Ebbels, T. M., Herwig, R., and Keun, H. C. (2011). Integrated pathway-level analysis of transcriptomics and metabolomics data with IMPaLA. *Bioinformatics*, **27**(20), 2917–2918.

Lenters, V., Portengen, L., Smit, L. A., Jonsson, B. A., Giwercman, A., Rylander, L., et al. (2014). Phthalates, perfluoroalkyl acids, metals and organochlorines and reproductive function: A multipollutant assessment in Greenlandic, Polish and Ukrainian men. Occupational and Environmental Health. doi: 10.1136/oemed-2014-102264. [Epub ahead of print]

Miller, G. W., and Jones, D. P. (2014). The nature of nurture: Refining the definition of the exposome. *Toxicological Sciences*, **137**, 1–2.

Molitor, J., Papathomas, M., Jerrett, M., and Richardson, S. (2010). Bayesian profile regression with an application to the National Survey of Children's Health. *Biostatistics*, **11**(3), 484–498.

Nieuwenhuijsen, M. J., Donaire-Gonzalez, D., Foraster, M., Martinez, D., and Cisneros, A. (2014). Using personal sensors to assess the exposome and acute health effects. *International Journal of Environmental Research and Public Health*, **11**(8), 7805–7819.

Patel, C. J., Bhattacharya, J., and Butte, A. J. (2010). An Environment-Wide Association Study (EWAS) on type 2 diabetes mellitus. *PLoS One*, **5**, e10746.

Papathomas, M., Molitor, J., Richardson, S., Riboli, E., and Vineis, P. (2011). Examining the joint effect of multiple risk factors using exposure risk profiles: Lung cancer in nonsmokers. *Environmental Health Perspectives*, **119**(1), 84–91.

Peters, A., Hoek, G., and Katsouyanni, K. (2012). Understanding the link between environmental exposures and health: Does the exposome promise too much? *Journal of Epidemiological and Community Health*, **66**, 103–105.

Philippat, C., Wolff, M. S., Calafat, A. M., Ye, X., Bausell, R., Meadows, M., et al. (2013). Prenatal exposure to environmental phenols: Concentrations in amniotic fluid and variability in urinary concentrations during pregnancy. *Environmental Health Perspectives*, **121**(10), 1225–1231.

Preau, J. L. Jr., Wong, L. Y., Silva, M. J., Needham, L. L., and Calafat, A. M. (2010). Variability over 1 week in the urinary concentrations of metabolites of diethyl phthalate and di(2-ethylhexyl) phthalate among eight adults: An observational study. *Environmental Health Perspectives*, **118**(12), 1748–1754.

Rappaport, S. M. (2011). Implications of the exposome for exposure science. *Journal of Exposure Science and Environmental Epidemiology*, **21**(1), 5–9.

Rappaport, S. M., Barupal, D. K., Wishart, D., Vineis, P., and Scalbert, A. (2014). The blood exposome and its role in discovering causes of disease. *Environmental Health Perspectives*, **122**, 769–774.

Rappaport, S. M., and Smith, M. T. (2010). Epidemiology. Environment and disease risks. *Science*, **330**(6003), 460–461.

Rojas-Rueda, D., de Nazelle, A., Teixido, O., and Nieuwenhuijsen, M. J. (2012). Replacing car trips by increasing bike and public transport in the greater Barcelona metropolitan area: A health impact assessment study. *Environment International*, **49**, 100–109.

Shi, M., and Weinberg, C. R. (2011). How much are we missing in SNP-by-SNP analyses of genome-wide association studies? *Epidemiology*, **22**(6), 845–847.

Sun, Z., Tao, Y., Li, S., Ferguson, K. K., Meeker, J. D., Park, S. K., et al. (2013). Statistical strategies for constructing health risk models with multiple pollutants and their interactions: Possible choices and comparisons. *Environmental Health*, **12**, 85.

Vlaanderen, J., Moore, L. E., Smith, M. T., et al. (2010). Application of OMICS technologies in occupational and environmental health research: Current status and projections. *Occupational and Environmental Health*, **67**(2), 136–143.

Vrijheid, M., Casas, M., Bergstrom, A., Carmichael, A., Cordier, S., Eggesbo, M., et al. (2012). European birth cohorts for environmental health research. *Environmental Health Perspectives*, **120**(1), 29–37.

Vrijheid, M., Slama, R., Robinson, O., Chatzi, L., Coen, M., van den Hazel, P., et al. (2014). The human early-life exposome (HELIX): Project rationale and design. *Environmental Health Perspectives*, **122**, 535–544.

Vrijheid, M. (2014). The exposome: A new paradigm to study the impact of environment on health. *Thorax*, **69**(9), 876–878.

Wild, C. P. (2005). Complementing the genome with an "exposome": The outstanding challenge of environmental exposure measurement in molecular epidemiology. *Cancer Epidemiology, Biomarkers & Prevention*, **14**, 1847–1850.

Wild, C. P. (2012). The exposome: From concept to utility. *International Journal of Epidemiology*, **41**, 24–32.

15

REMOTE SENSING

Payam Dadvand

15.1 INTRODUCTION

Remote sensing can be defined as gathering information on a phenomenon or an object from a distance using optic, acoustical, or microwave signals (Schowengerdt 2007). This broad definition includes a wide range of fields, from medical imaging to video surveillance, sonar, traffic and aviation radars, and astronomy (RAdio Detection And Ranging) (Schott 2007). Accordingly, remote sensing instruments can be installed on or in a number of mobile or stationary platforms, such as medical instruments, vehicles, ships, aircrafts, satellites, or observatories (Ostfeld et al. 2005). For our purpose, we restrict this definition to measuring or characterizing phenomena or objects on earth or in the atmosphere applying data on optical (i.e., electromagnetic) signals obtained by sensors on-board satellites or aircraft (Schott 2007; Schowengerdt 2007).

Remote sensing has been used for environmental monitoring (e.g., deforestation, land use and land cover dynamics, sea and land surface temperature, temporal changes in glaciers, impacts of natural disasters) since the second half the twentieth century. Over recent years there has been a growing interest in applying remote sensing data in environmental epidemiological studies, either to develop new methods for assessing exposure or to improve the estimates of available exposure assessment methods. This increasing interest has been partly because of the increasing tendency for more refined exposure assessments, especially across large study areas, and partly because of better availability and quality of remote sensing data together with recent advances in computational power, retrieval algorithms, and geographical information systems (GIS). Nowadays, freely available satellite data provide repeated measurements of environmental factors over a long period of time and large areas, which offer a credible tool to explore trends in these environmental factors in an objective and standardized way for a large part of the world.

This chapter describes methods applied to acquire remote sensing data and provides some examples of the application of remote sensing data in assessing exposure to air pollution, heat, greenness, and ultraviolet radiation.

15.2 REMOTE SENSING DATA

Remote sensing instruments generally record data on electromagnetic radiation with wavelengths ranging from 260 nm (ultraviolet radiation) to 0.1–10 cm (radar) (Hoff and Christopher 2009). Remote sensing instruments can be classified as active or passive (Figure 15.1). Passive instruments, such as radiometers and spectrometers, collect electromagnetic signals that are naturally emitted (e.g., thermal infrared) or reflected (mostly solar backscatter) by the target, whereas active instruments record the electromagnetic signal that was first emitted by the instrument itself and then reflected by the target. Radar (RAdio Detection And Ranging) and Lidar (Light Detection and Ranging) are examples of active instruments. To date, environmental epidemiologists have mostly used data generated by passive remote sensing instruments; however, there are increasing numbers of studies applying active remote sensing data.

Remote sensing data are characterized according to their spatial, temporal, spectral, and radiometric resolutions. Spatial resolution is the size of pixels constituting the image captured by remote sensing sensors. It is often expressed as ground sample distance (GSD), which is the distance between centers of image pixels on the ground. Based on their spatial resolution, remote sensing data available for civilian use are classified as high-resolution (0.5–1.8 m), mid-resolution (2.0–36 m), and low-resolution (>36 m) (Ostfeld et al. 2005). Intuitively, higher resolution data would offer higher classification accuracy but, at the same time, they are less likely to be freely available, often cover smaller areas in a single image, and are more computationally heavy to process (Ostfeld et al. 2005). Therefore, the choice of proper spatial resolution is a trade-off between required classification accuracy and available resources.

Temporal resolution indicates the frequency of revisiting and collecting data of the target by satellite or aircraft. In the case of satellite remote sensing, the temporal resolution is a function of satellite orbit characteristics (e.g., altitude, inclination,

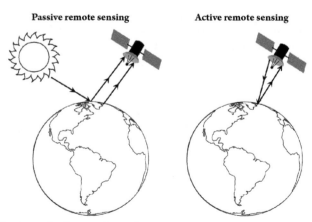

Figure 15.1 Passive and active remote sensing.

and eccentricity), technical specifications (e.g., swath width and overlap), and meteorological conditions (e.g., clear vs. cloudy sky), and often is a matter of days (Martin 2008). Temporal resolution is important for studies concerned with short- or long-term temporal trends (e.g., daily, seasonal, or year-to-year variations) in environmental factors.

Spectral resolution indicates the range of wavelengths (bandwidth) recorded by each spectral band of the sensor, which is a function of total bandwidth covered by the sensor and the number of bands. For a given sensor, a narrower bandwidth in each band and larger number of bands can be translated to higher spectral resolution. For example, hyperspectral sensors collect data on a large number of narrow and contiguous bands that cover a large part of the electromagnetic spectrum (Ostfeld et al. 2005). Radiometric resolution reflects the ability of a sensor to classify the intensity of radiation it has received. It is presented as the number of data bits that can be recorded for each spectral band. For example, an 8-bit sensor is able to store 256 ($2\times2\times2\times2\times2\times2\times2\times2$) levels of radiation intensity for each spectral band.

There are two different approaches in using remote sensing data: image-centered and data-centered (Schowengerdt 2007). In the image-centered approach, the principal interest lays in the spatial relationship among objects with an ultimate goal of developing a map. In the data-centered approach, instead, the prime interest is the data dimension rather than the spatial relation between the objects. Likewise, remote sensing data can be analyzed in two different ways: *image interpretation* by a skilled human analyst based on viewing spatial patterns in an image, and *quantitative analysis* by computer-based algorithms based on quantitative measures of radiance levels and spectral characteristics (Schott 2007). To date, environmental epidemiologists have mostly adapted a data-centered approach for exposure assessment purposes. Use of satellite data on atmospheric pollution or land surface temperate for assessing exposure to air pollution and heat, respectively, are examples of a data-centered approach.

15.3 AIR POLLUTION

During the past few decades, remote sensing has been applied in monitoring levels and trends of surface air pollutants, forecasting air quality, assessing emission activities of sources (anthropogenic and natural sources such as forest fires and volcanic activities), enforcing air quality standards, detecting long-range transport of pollutants (e.g., dust storms), and characterizing visibility impairment (Martin 2008; Hoff and Christopher 2009). Of relevance to epidemiological studies, remote-sensing retrievals have been used to assess the levels of particulate air pollutants, including particulate matter with aerodynamic diameter ≤ 2.5 μm ($PM_{2.5}$) and ≤ 10 μm (PM_{10}), as well as gaseous air pollutants, including ozone, nitrogen dioxide (NO_2), sulfur dioxide (SO_2), carbon monoxide (CO), methane (CH_4), and formaldehyde (CH_2O).

To date, a limited number of epidemiological studies have relied on remote-sensing retrievals in assessing exposure to air pollution (mostly $PM_{2.5}$); however, there is an increasing tendency to apply such data as a way to assess the exposure to air pollution or as an input to available modeling techniques to improve their efficacy. Remote sensing retrievals are increasingly seen as an alternative way to assess exposure to air pollution in rural areas or developing countries, where ground monitoring stations are scarce or non-existent. They can also provide a standardized way of assessing exposure to air pollution across large areas for studies that deal with health outcomes at a global or intercontinental level (e.g. assessing the global burden of disease attributable to ambient air pollution). MODerate resolution Imaging Spectroradiometer (MODIS) on-board Terra and Auqa satellites, Scanning Imaging Absorption spectrometer for Atmospheric Cartography (SCIAMACHY) on-board ENVISAT, Global Ozone Monitoring Experiment (GOME) on-board ERS-2, Measurements Of Pollution In The Troposphere (MOPITT) on-board Terra, Tropospheric Emission Spectrometer (TES) on-board Aura, and Cloud-Aerosol LIdar with Orthogonal Polarization (CALIOP) on-board Cloud-Aerosol Lidar, and Infrared Pathfinder Satellite Observations (CALIPSO) are among the sensors that have been widely used to retrieve levels of surface air pollutants (Martin 2008) (Table 15.1).

Surface air pollutant levels are not directly measured by remote-sensing instruments. Instead, algorithms are required to retrieve such levels from recorded atmospheric radiative transfer in different wavelengths. These algorithms, based on the Beer–Lambert law, try to optimize mixing ratio or levels of surface pollutants that can explain the observed abatement in the intensity, spectral difference in absorbed and emitted radiation, and changes in reflectance (Martin 2008; Hoff and Christopher 2009). For gaseous pollutants, different algorithms have been developed to process data generated by thermal infrared and visible light remote sensing. For thermal infrared, algorithms generally apply the spectral difference in emitted and absorbed radiation to estimate levels of gaseous pollutants, whereas for visible light remote sensing, the algorithms rely on the characterization of the abatement of the intensity of solar reflectance while passing through the atmosphere (Martin 2008).

Aerosol optical depth (AOD) has been used extensively to retrieve particulate air pollution (mainly $PM_{2.5}$) from data generated by visible light remote sensing. Aerosol optical depth is a unitless indicator of the attenuation of the light due to absorption or scattering by atmospheric particulate matter (Boys et al. 2014). The association between surface $PM_{2.5}$ levels and AOD can be formulized as $PM_{2.5} = \eta \times AOD$ (Boys et al. 2014). η Can be abstracted using atmospheric chemical transport models. Brauer et al. (2012), for example, applied the global chemical transport model *GEOS-Chem* to abstract η in order to estimate global levels of surface $PM_{2.5}$ levels at $0.1° \times 0.1°$ spatial resolution for the period 1990–2005 (Figure 15.2) (Brauer et al. 2012). Another way of estimating η is to use measured $PM_{2.5}$ levels by ground monitoring stations as a training dataset to quantify the association between PM2.5 and AOD (Boys et al. 2014). In this approach, for those areas with available

Table 15.1 More commonly used sensors and platforms for the remote sensing of air pollution, surface temperature, greenness, and ultraviolet radiation

Sensor	Platform
Air pollution	
MODerate resolution Imaging Spectroradiometer (MODIS)	Terra and Auqa satellites
Measurements Of Pollution In The Troposphere (MOPITT)	Terra sattelite
Scanning Imaging Absorption spectrometer for Atmospheric Cartography (SCIAMACHY)	ENVISAT
Tropospheric Emission Spectrometer (TES)	Aura satellite
Global Ozone Monitoring Experiment (GOME)	ERS-2
Cloud-Aerosol LIdar with Orthogonal Polarization (CALIOP)	CALIPSO
Surface temperature	
Thematic Mapper (TM)	Landsat 4 and 5
Enhanced Thematic Mapper (ETM+)	Landsat 7
Thermal Infrared Sensor (TIRS)	Landsat 8
MODIS	Terra and Auqa satellites
Advanced Very High Resolution Radiometer (AVHRR)	NOAA satellites
Advanced Spaceborne Thermal Emission and Reflection Radiometer (ASTER)	Terra satellite
Greenness	
TM	Landsat 4 and 5
ETM+	Landsat 7
Operational Land Imager (OLI)	Landsat 8
MODIS	Terra and Auqa satellites
ASTER	Terras satellite
Ultraviolet radiation	
Total Ozone Mapping Spectrometer (TOMS)	Nimbus 7 satellite
Ozone Monitoring Instrument (OMI)	Aura satellite
GOME	ERS-2
GOME-2	METOP-A satellite
SCIAMACHY	ENVISAT

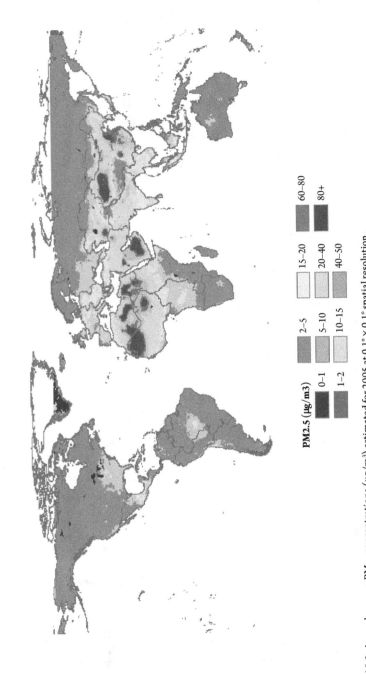

Figure 15.2 Annual average PM$_{2.5}$ concentrations (μg/m³) estimated for 2005 at 0.1° × 0.1° spatial resolution.
Source: Brauer, M., Amann, M., Burnett, R. T., Cohen, A., Dentener, F., Ezzati, M., et al. (2012). Exposure assessment for estimation of the global burden of disease attributable to outdoor air pollution. *Environmental Science & Technology, 46,* 652–660.

measures of $PM_{2.5}$ (from ground stations) and AOD (from satellites), η is estimated and will be applied to predict $PM_{2.5}$ levels from AOD for those places without available ground monitoring data. More elaborate approaches have been developed to improve estimations of particulate pollution levels by including other predictors, such as the height of the planetary boundary layer, or meteorological and surface information, such as land surface temperature, relative humidity, and albedo in addition to AOD in a regression modeling framework (Hoff and Christopher 2009). Further details on methods to estimate air pollutant levels are presented in reviews by Hoff and Christopher (2009) and Martin (2008).

Surface air pollutant levels retrieved from remote-sensing data require validation using ground monitoring stations. Ground-based Dobson O_3 spectrophotometer and more recently Brewer spectrophotometer are examples of ground monitoring stations that have been used to validate remote sensing retrievals for O_3, SO_2, and AOD. For AOD, however, ground-based sunphotometer is considered the gold standard instrument for validation purposes (Hoff and Christopher 2009). For particulate pollutants, there is also a need to validate the AOD to $PM_{2.5}$ conversion. Such validations are necessary because retrieval of AOD is prone to misclassification as a result of erroneous sampling, inaccurate assumptions of particulate matter and land surface characteristics, cloud effects, and erroneous sensor calibration (Boys et al. 2014). Furthermore, the relationship between AOD and particulate matter levels can change through the seasons and years as well as between regions as a result of variations in particulate matter characteristics (e.g., composition, size distribution, number of particles per unit space, reflective properties, and hygroscopicity), ground surface albedo (e.g., presence of ice and snow), meteorological factors (e.g., cloud cover, temperature, and relative humidity), and the height of the planetary boundary layer (Martin 2008; Hoff and Christopher 2009; Boys et al. 2014). Such seasonal and year-to-year variations in the AOD–particulate matter relationship can have important implications on assessing temporal trends in particulate pollution (e.g., time-series analyses) (Hoff and Christopher 2009; Boys et al. 2014). Furthermore, the regional variations in the AOD–particulate matter relationship needs to be considered when extrapolating predictions of particulate pollution levels from one region to another or when predicting pollution levels at very large (e.g., continental or intercontinental) scales (Hoff and Christopher 2009).

Environmental epidemiological studies generally require air pollution levels at fine spatial and temporal resolution. To date, the finest spatial resolution of the available air pollution data based on remote sensing retrievals ranges between 4 and 10 km, which are often not sufficient for studies at the intra-urban level (Martin 2008; Hoff and Christopher 2009). This has led a number of studies to use remote sensing retrievals to improve predictions of air pollution levels by already-available modeling approaches (e.g., land use regression models) instead of directly using them to assess exposure. Covering large areas, the air pollution levels based on remote sensing retrievals can provide context to air pollution estimates by regional models and are used as a predictor together with other predictors in these models (e.g., Kloog et al. 2011; Lee and Koutrakis 2014). Recently, some methods have also been developed to enhance the spatial resolution of remote sensing retrievals of air pollution levels, including use of Bayesian modeling approaches (e.g., Wang et al. 2013). Moreover, future hyperspectral satellite instruments are expected to be able to better characterize the pollutant properties, including composition and size distribution of particulate pollutants and mixing ratio of gaseous pollutants (Hoff and Christopher 2009).

15.4 SURFACE TEMPERATURE

Since the late 1960s, satellite retrievals of land and sea surface temperatures have been used for meteorological and climatological studies (Tomlinson et al. 2011). For example, time-series of land and sea surface temperatures based on satellite retrievals have been instrumental in documenting global warming. Land surface temperature (LST), defined as the skin temperature of the ground (Kloog et al. 2014), has also been applied for monitoring wildfires, volcanic activities, and heat waves (Leblon 2001; Dousset et al. 2011), investigating spatiotemporal dynamics of urban land use, including vegetation cover (Jenerette et al. 2007; Weng 2009), evaluating land surface moisture (Petropoulos et al. 2009) and evapotranspiration (Kalma et al. 2008), and surveillance of vector-based diseases such as malaria (Garske et al. 2013) and leishmaniasis (Ntais et al. 2013). Furthermore, LST has been extensively applied to investigate urban heat island effect, a phenomenon characterized by higher-temperature in urban areas compared with their surroundings (White-Newsome et al. 2013).

About half of the world's population is currently living in cities, and it is projected that by 2030 three of every five persons will live in urban areas worldwide (Smith and Guarnizo 2009). There is an increase in the proportion of old population who are among the most vulnerable groups to extreme climatic conditions. At the same time, the future climate is predicted to have more intense, longer, and/or more frequent extreme heat conditions (Meehl and Tebaldi 2004). All these together have resulted in an increasing tendency to study the adverse health effects of these conditions or to identify vulnerable neighborhoods/population subgroups to such effects in urban areas (Kestens et al. 2011; White-Newsome et al. 2013; Kloog et al. 2014). To date, most of the epidemiological studies on the adverse health effects of exposure to heat have relied on routinely collected measurements of *air temperature* (normally measured at 1.5–2 m height) by meteorological monitoring networks. These networks are often spatially sparse, especially in nonurban areas. Thus, although data generated by them can be applied to characterize the temporal variation in temperature to be used, for example, in time-series analyses, they do not properly address the spatial variation in temperature, particularly in urban areas. Spatial variation in temperature in urban areas has been well documented, and land cover type (e.g., vegetation cover, concrete, or asphalt surfaces), surface imperviousness, elevation, and topography have been suggested to contribute to this variation (Kestens et al. 2011). Therefore, the inability of routinely collected data by meteorological monitoring networks to properly address the within-city variation in temperature can result in exposure measurement error. Accordingly, there is a growing interest in developing methods capable of better characterization of within-city variation in heat and determining the temperature hot spots (referred to as *micro-urban heat islands*) across urban areas (Kestens et al. 2011). Land surface temperature together with geostatistical interpolation techniques (e.g., kriging; Zhang et al. 2011) and land use regression models (e.g., Kestens et al. 2011) are among methods used to better characterize the spatial variation in temperature in urban areas.

Land surface temperature can be retrieved from thermal infrared radiation or passive microwave data recorded by sensors on-board satellites as well as aircraft (Tomlinson et al. 2011). Land surface temperature retrieved from passive microwave data often have coarse spatial resolutions that are not sufficient for epidemiological studies. The data generated by aircraft sensors often provides better spatial and thermal resolutions, but they usually cover small areas and are costly, making them less suitable for epidemiological studies (Tomlinson et al. 2011). Consequently, almost all epidemiological studies of the health effects of heat have used satellite-based remote sensing data on thermal infrared radiation. Thematic Mapper (TM) on-board Landsat 4 and 5, Enhanced Thematic Mapper (ETM+) on-board Landsat 7, Thermal Infrared Sensor (TIRS) on-board Landsat 8, MODIS on-board Aqua and Terra satellites, Advanced Very High Resolution Radiometer (AVHRR) sensor on-board National Oceanic and Atmospheric Administration (NOAA) satellites, and the Advanced Spaceborne Thermal Emission and Reflection Radiometer (ASTER) on-board Terra satellite are among the sensors recording thermal infrared data that can be used to retrieve LST (Tomlinson et al. 2011) (Table 15.1).

Radiative transfer equation and generalized split window are two main approaches to convert thermal infrared data to LST (Tomlinson et al. 2011). The accuracy of retrieved LST depends on several factors, including sensor characteristics, land surface properties (spectral emissivity), atmospheric attenuation (absorption, reflection or refraction, and scattering), and angular effects (satellite–sun geometry and surface geometry) (Tomlinson et al. 2011; Li et al. 2013; Kloog et al. 2014). Spectral emissivity itself can be influenced by surface cover, vegetation cover, and soil moisture, which can vary considerably over time and space, especially if the study area is large or the study period is long (Tomlinson et al. 2011). Therefore, LST retrievals need to be validated. Temperature-based methods, radiance-based methods, and cross-validation are the three main approaches to validate LST retrievals (Li et al. 2013). Briefly, temperature-based methods rely on in situ measures of temperature by ground-based temperature monitors, the radiance-based methods make use of land surface spectral emissivity and atmospheric profile, and the cross-validations compare the LST retrievals of one sensor with those of a gold standard sensor to validate LST retrievals. More details on the theoretical basis and applied algorithms to retrieve and validate LST can be found in a number of reviews (Tomlinson et al. 2011; Li et al. 2013).

Land surface temperature has been used as the surrogate of exposure to heat in a number of epidemiological studies (Smargiassi et al. 2009; Harlan et al. 2013; Dadvand et al. 2014). However, the association between LST and air temperature is complex. It has been suggested that although LST could be an acceptable surrogate for heat exposures over longer periods, it has less capability to characterize shorter-term exposure to air temperature, which can be of interest in studies of short-term effects of extreme heat conditions such as heat waves (Tomlinson et al. 2011; White-Newsome et al. 2013). Recently some methods have been developed to predict spatiotemporal variations air temperature based on LST together with a number of other predictors (e.g., Kloog et al. 2014), which can be promising for future epidemiological studies of such effects.

15.5 GREENNESS

Remote sensing has been widely used to classify land cover/land use, mostly to monitor the changes in forestland, croplands, and urbanized landscapes over time (Hansen and Loveland 2012). Since the 1980s, remote sensing data have been applied to classify vegetation species, characterize vegetation traits and canopy properties (e.g., plant height, leaf phenology, and leaf chlorophyll, water and elemental content), monitor vegetation growth and photosynthetic activity, estimate crop yield, evaluate vegetation flammability properties, surveil vegetation stress and diseases, and evaluate impacts of drought and deforestations (Xie et al. 2008; Homolová et al. 2013). Compared with traditional methods like field surveys, remote sensing has the advantage of covering large areas, providing an opportunity to evaluate temporal trends in vegetation cover in a standardized way, and being less costly and time and resource consuming for the end users, considering the increasing number of freely available remote sensing datasets relevant to vegetation cover (Xie et al. 2008).

Recently there has been a growing interest in applying remote sensing data on vegetation in epidemiological studies of the effects of green spaces on human health. Characterizing the vegetation density surrounding living environments (e.g., Dadvand et al. 2012), quantifying tree canopies around residential addresses (e.g., Donovan et al. 2011), and assessing the road-adjacent tree coverage (e.g., Dadvand et al. 2014) are examples of the application of remote sensing data in epidemiological studies of the health effects of green spaces. Furthermore, remote sensing data on vegetation cover have been used as an input in models to assess exposure to air pollution (e.g., Su et al. 2010) and heat (e.g., Kestens et al. 2011) in epidemiological studies.

NASA's Airborne Visible InfraRed Imaging Spectrometer (AVIRIS) and the US National Ecological Observatory Network (NEON)'s Airborne Observation Platform (AOP) are examples of aircraft-based remote sensing that have been used to monitor vegetation cover over parts of the United States, Canada, and Europe. Aircraft-based data on vegetation have the advantage of high spatial resolution, but they generally offer low temporal resolution because of the cost and logistical limitations.

TM (Landsat 4 and 5), ETM+ (Landsat 7), Operational Land Imager (Landsat 8), MODIS (Aqua and Terra), AVHRR (NOAA), and ASTER (Terra), and also sensors on-board commercial satellites IKONOS, RapidEye, and QuickBird are among the sensors that produce data usable to characterize vegetation cover (Table 15.1). Satellite-based data on vegetation usually undergo preprocessing to reduce the noise/errors and improve the interpretability of data (Xie et al. 2008). Retrieval of vegetation data is based on characterization of unique spectral properties of vegetations. A number of algorithms have been developed to convert satellite-recorded spectral data into different vegetation indices in order to quantify the fraction of the photosynthetically active radiation absorbed by vegetations (some example of these methods can be found in reviews by Xie et al. [2008] and Homolová et al. [2013]). These algorithms mostly rely on the difference between reflectance of visible light (wavelength of 0.4–0.7 μm), which is strongly absorbed by chlorophyll content of leaves and near-infrared light (wavelength of 0.7–1.1 μm), which is reflected by the cell structure of the leaves (Weier and Herring 2011). Here we focus on those indices that have been applied or have a potential to be applied by epidemiological studies.

To date, the most widely used vegetation index in epidemiological studies is the normalized difference vegetation index (NDVI), which was developed in the late 1970s mainly to monitor drought and crop yields. The NDVI is calculated as

(reflected near infrared – reflected visible light) / (reflected near infrared
   + reflected visible light)

It ranges between –1 and +1 with higher numbers indicating more density of photosynthetically active vegetation (e.g., Figure 15.3). Measurement of NDVI can be affected by distortion of light by atmospheric particles and land cover below the vegetation. It can also become saturated over regions with large amounts of chlorophyll such as rainforests. The enhanced vegetation index (EVI) has been developed to overcome these limitations using data on atmospherically corrected near-infrared, red, and blue reflectance, canopy background, and atmospheric particle resistance terms (Weier and Herring 2011). However, both NDVI and EVI can both be affected by cloud cover, which can be a major limitation, especially in regions or seasons with frequent cloudy skies. Furthermore, neither NDVI nor EVI distinguish between different types of vegetation. The vegetation type can be relevant to some of the proposed underlying mechanisms for the health benefits of green spaces. For example, the ability of green space in reducing air pollutants is reported to be type dependent, with trees being the most effective and grasses being the least effective (Givoni 1991). The Vegetation Continuous Fields (VCF) is another satellite-based vegetation index that provides proportional estimates for vegetation types, including woody vegetation (i.e., trees), herbaceous vegetation (i.e., non-tree vegetation), and bare ground (Townshend et al. 2001). In contrast with traditional classification approaches, in which vegetation types are distinctly concentrated, VCF offers

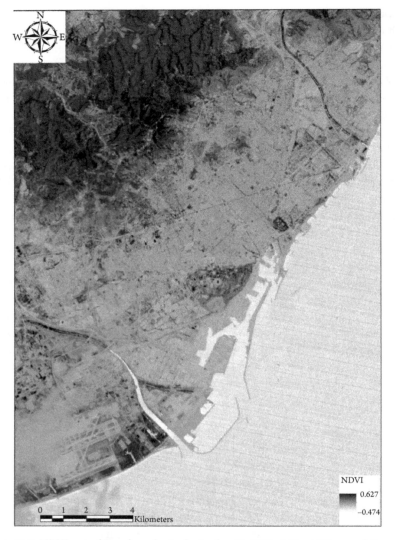

Figure 15.3 NDVI map of Barcelona, Spain, September 12, 2009, at 30 m × 30 m resolution. Source: Landsat 5 TM, NASA.

a continuous classification of vegetation type over the space (Townshend et al. 2001). Like NDVI and EVI, the retrieval of VCF can be affected by cloud cover and requires clear sky to achieve the best results. Furthermore, VCF is not capable of separating species within each vegetation type, which can be of interest, for example, for epidemiological studies of the allergic reactions to certain species. Separating vegetation species based on remote sensing data is still in its first steps; however, there are growing efforts to develop algorithms capable of separating vegetation species using data generated by hyperspectral sensors (Pettorelli et al. 2014), which ultimately can be used in future epidemiological studies. Methods have also been developed to integrate aforementioned passive remote sensing data with data generated by active remote sensing sensors such as Lidars in order to better classify vegetation types (Homolová et al. 2013).

Lidars have been used to estimate, among others, vegetation height, canopy density, leaf morphology, and more recently three-dimensional mapping of vegetation in ecological studies. Radars are other active remote sensing techniques used to estimate vegetation height and biomass density (Homolová et al. 2013). Active remote sensing techniques appear to be effective in characterizing exposure to green spaces in epidemiological studies and are being used by increasing numbers of epidemiological studies.

The available evidence on the validity of satellite-based measures of greenness in epidemiological studies is still limited. However, measures of residential surrounding greenness based on NDVI has been shown to strongly correlate with the perception of the greenness of corresponding residential areas (Rhew et al. 2011). Characterization of the quality of green spaces has remained as a major limitation of remote sensing techniques. Characteristics such as aesthetics, biodiversity, walkability, presence of sport/play facilities, and organized social events have been suggested to affect the use of green spaces (McCormack, Rock, Toohey, and Hignell 2010) and therefore are important for epidemiological studies of the health effects of such spaces. Recently, there has been a limited effort to use remote-sensing images (e.g., Google Earth Pro; Taylor et al. 2011) to assess the quality characteristics of green spaces like walkability, and the presence of sport facilities, water features, lighting, and birdlife, which showed a strong correlation with the assessments made by in-person surveys. Such use of remote sensing, if proved to be valid, can result in a considerable reduction in the cost and time required to assess the quality of green spaces in future epidemiological studies.

15.6 ULTRAVIOLET RADIATION

Ultraviolet (UV) radiation is a non-ionizing part of the electromagnetic spectrum. The sun is the main source of UV, but substantial exposure can occur from occupational as well as artificial sources, such as sunbeds. Based on wavelength, solar UV is classified as UV-A (400–320 nm), which passes through the atmosphere with little change; UV-B (320–290 nm), of which 70% to 90% is absorbed by the stratospheric ozone; and UV-C (290–200 nm), which is totally absorbed by stratospheric ozone (Lucas et al. 2006). Exposure to UV is associated with both beneficial (e.g., vitamin D production) and harmful (e.g., skin cancers and cataract) health effects, with UV-B being the main agent responsible for such effects.

Since the 1980s, a network of ground-based UV monitoring stations started to develop, mostly as a reaction to the concerns over the depletion of the stratospheric ozone layer. This monitoring network has generated reliable measures of UV irradiance at different parts of the globe, which have been instrumental in our understanding of the impacts of stratospheric ozone depletion. However, this monitoring network is spatially sparse, especially in the developing world, and provides point estimates of surface UV irradiance that may not be generalizable to regional or con-tinental levels. Moreover, most of these monitoring sites have been active for only 15 to 20 years, restricting the ability to evaluate long-term trends in UV irradiance. To overcome these limitations, remote-sensing data have been applied that can pro-vide standardized measures of surface UV irradiance over large areas with decades of available historical data. Total Ozone Mapping Spectrometer (TOMS) on-board NASA's Nimbus 7 satellite, Ozone Monitoring Instrument (OMI) on-board Aura, Global Ozone Monitoring Experiments (GOME on-board ERS-2 and GOME-2 on-board METOP-A), and SCIAMACHY on-board Envisat are among the sen-sors that have been extensively used to estimate surface UV irradiance (Torres et al. 2007) (Table 15.1).

Surface UV irradiance varies by solar altitude (zenith angle), total column ozone, aerosols and trace gases, cloud cover, altitude, and surface albedo. Solar alti-tude itself is a function of latitude, season, and time of day (Torres et al. 2007). In other words, the surface UV irradiance is a function of the incident UV radiation on the top of the atmosphere and the transmission of UV through the atmosphere. Because the top of the atmosphere incident UV radiation is rather constant, the surface UV irradiance is mainly determined by UV atmospheric transmission. Therefore, algorithms developed to retrieve surface UV irradiance are mainly based on characterization of UV transmission in atmosphere using radiative trans-fer equations with satellite-observed total column ozone as an input (Torres et al. 2007; Gadhavi et al. 2008). To improve estimations of surface UV irradiance, other satellite-observed characteristics, such as cloud cover, levels of aerosol and trace gases, climatological surface albedo, elevation, temperature profiles, and solar zenith angle and latitude, have also been used, together with total column ozone as input for the radiative transfer models (Tanskanen et al. 2007). Cloud cover is a major determinant of atmospheric UV transmission and has a substan-tial impact on the accuracy of the satellite retrievals of surface UV irradiance. Different indicators like *cloud optical depth* or *cloud water thickness* based on data generated by the sensors on-board the same satellite or on-board other satellites have been used to address the impact of cloud cover on retrievals of surface UV irradiance (Janjai et al. 2010).

Satellite retrievals of surface UV irradiance have been extensively validated using measurements made by ground-based UV monitors. Generally, although results of these validation studies generally suggest an overestimation of surface UV irradiance by satellite retrievals, especially in cloudy conditions or regions with high surface albedo, the satellite estimations have been reported to have a strong temporal correlation with measurements by ground-based monitors (Gao et al. 2010; Janjai et al. 2010). Such strong temporal correlation, if established by more studies in different settings, make satellite retrievals of surface UV irradi-ance a valuable source of data to assess exposure to UV (either as a surrogate of UV exposure or as an input for models predicting individual UV exposure levels as a function of ambient UV levels and personal behavior) in epidemiologi-cal studies of the health effects of UV. However, the use of satellite retrieval of surface UV irradiance in epidemiological studies faces some challenges. The spatial resolution of the most of available satellite-based surface UV irradiance maps is relatively coarse and there are reports showing a considerable within-pixel variation in surface UV irradiance (Weihs et al. 2008). Furthermore, these maps mostly provide daily levels of surface UV irradiance without characterization of within-day variation in UV levels, which can be important for some studies. To date, epidemiological studies of the long-term effects of UVR exposure have mainly relied on measures of surface UV irradiation or its surrogates (latitude of the city of residence), and, to a lesser extent, aspects of personal behavior (e.g., questionnaire-based data on time spent outdoors or habits in relation to sun exposure). Among those few studies using measures of surface UV irradiance, almost all have used measured surface irradiance by ground-based monitors, and only a handful of studies (e.g., Grant 2002; Grant et al. 2005) have applied satellite-retrievals of surface UV irradiance to assess exposure to UV.

REFERENCES

Boys, B. L., Martin, R. V., van Donkelaar, A., MacDonell, R. J., Hsu, N. C., Cooper, M. J., et al. (2014). Fifteen-year global time series of satellite-derived fine particulate matter. *Environmental Science & Technology*, 48, 11109–11118.

Brauer, M., Amann, M., Burnett, R. T., Cohen, A., Dentener, F., Ezzati, M., et al. (2012). Exposure assessment for estimation of the global burden of disease attributable to outdoor air pollution. *Environmental Science & Technology*, 46, 652–660.

Dadvand, P., Ostro, B., Figueras, F., Foraster, M., Basagaña, X., Valentín, A., et al. (2014). Residential proximity to major roads and term low birth weight: The roles of air pollution, heat, noise, and road-adjacent trees. *Epidemiology*, 25, 518–525.

Dadvand, P., Sunyer, J., Basagaña, X., Ballester, F., Lertxundi, A., Fernández-Somoano, A., et al. (2012). Surrounding greenness and pregnancy outcomes in four Spanish birth cohorts. *Environmental Health Perspectives*, 120, 1481–1487.

Donovan, G. H., Michael, Y. L., Butry, D. T., Sullivan, A. D., and Chase, J. M. (2011). Urban trees and the risk of poor birth outcomes. *Health Place*, 17, 390–393.

Dousset, B., Gourmelon, F., Laaidi, K., Zeghnoun, A., Giraudet, E., Bretin, P., et al. (2011). Satellite monitoring of summer heat waves in the Paris metropolitan area. *International Journal of Climatology*, 31, 313–323.

Gadhavi, H., Pinker, R. T., and Laszlo, I. (2008). Estimates of surface ultraviolet radiation over North America using Geostationary Operational Environmental Satellites observations. *Journal of Geophysical Research: Atmospheres*, 113, D21205.

Gao, Z., Gao, W., and Chang, N.-B. (2010). Comparative analyses of the ultraviolet-B flux over the continental United States based on the NASA total ozone mapping spectrometer data and USDA ground-based measurements. *Journal of Applied Remote Sensing*, 4, 043547.

Garske, T., Ferguson, N. M., and Ghani, A. C. (2013). Estimating air temperature and its influence on malaria transmission across Africa. *PloS One*, 8, e56487.

Givoni, B. (1991). Impact of planted areas on urban environmental quality: A review. *Atmospheric Environment Part B Urban Atmosphere*, 25, 289–299.

Grant, W. B. (2002). An estimate of premature cancer mortality in the U.S. due to inadequate doses of solar ultraviolet-B radiation. *Cancer*, **94**, 1867–1875.

Grant, W. B., Garland, C. F., and Holick, M. F. (2005). Comparisons of estimated economic burdens due to insufficient solar ultraviolet irradiance and vitamin D and excess solar UV irradiance for the United States. *Journal of Photochemistry and Photobiology*, **81**, 1276–1286.

Hansen, M. C., and Loveland, T. R. (2012). A review of large area monitoring of land cover change using Landsat data. *Remote Sensing of Environment*, **122**, 66–74.

Harlan, S. L., Declet-Barreto, J. H., Stefanov, W. L., and Petitti, D. B. (2013). Neighborhood effects on heat deaths: Social and environmental predictors of vulnerability in Maricopa County, Arizona. *Environmental Health Perspectives*, **121**, 197–204.

Hoff, R. M., and Christopher, S. A. (2009). Remote sensing of particulate pollution from space: Have we reached the promised land? *Journal of the Air & Waste Management Association*, **59**, 645–675.

Homolová, L., Malenovský, Z., Clevers, J. G. P. W., García-Santos, G., and Schaepman, M. E. (2013). Review of optical-based remote sensing for plant trait mapping. *Ecological Complexity*, **15**, 1–16.

Janjai, S., Buntung, S., Wattan, R., and Masiri, I. (2010). Mapping solar ultraviolet radiation from satellite data in a tropical environment. *Remote Sensing of Environment*, **114**, 682–691.

Jenerette, G. D., Harlan, S. L., Brazel, A., Jones, N., Larsen, L., and Stefanov, W. L. (2007). Regional relationships between surface temperature, vegetation, and human settlement in a rapidly urbanizing ecosystem. *Landscape Ecology*, **22**, 353–365.

Kalma, J. D., McVicar, T. R., and McCabe, M. F. (2008). Estimating land surface evaporation: A review of methods using remotely sensed surface temperature data. *Surveys in Geophysics*, **29**, 421–469.

Kestens, Y., Brand, A., Fournier, M., Goudreau, S., Kosatsky, T., Maloley, M., et al. (2011). Modelling the variation of land surface temperature as determinant of risk of heat-related health events. *International Journal of Health Geographics*, **10**, 1–9.

Kloog, I., Koutrakis, P., Coull, B. A., Lee, H. J., and Schwartz, J. (2011). Assessing temporally and spatially resolved PM2.5 exposures for epidemiological studies using satellite aerosol optical depth measurements. *Atmospheric Environment*, **45**, 6267–6275.

Kloog, I., Nordio, F., Coull, B. A., and Schwartz, J. (2014). Predicting spatiotemporal mean air temperature using MODIS satellite surface temperature measurements across the Northeastern USA. *Remote Sensing of Environment*, **150**, 132–139.

Leblon, B. (2001). Forest wildfire hazard monitoring using remote sensing: A review. *Remote Sensing Reviews*, **20**, 1–43.

Lee, H. J., and Koutrakis, P. (2014). Daily ambient NO_2 concentration predictions using satellite ozone monitoring instrument NO_2 data and land use regression. *Environmental Science & Technology*, **48**, 2305–2311.

Li, Z.-L., Tang, B.-H., Wu, H., Ren, H., Yan, G., Wan, Z., et al. (2013). Satellite-derived land surface temperature: Current status and perspectives. *Remote Sensing of Environment*, **131**, 14–37.

Lucas, R., McMichael, T., Smith, W., and Armstrong, B. (2006). *Solar ultraviolet radiation.* (Assessing the environmental burden of disease at national and local levels Environmental Burden of Disease Series). World Health Organization, Geneva.

Martin, R. V. (2008). Satellite remote sensing of surface air quality. *Atmospheric Environment*, **42**, 7823–7843.

McCormack, G. R., Rock, M., Toohey, A. M., and Hignell, D. (2010). Characteristics of urban parks associated with park use and physical activity: A review of qualitative research. *Health Place*, **16**(4), 712–726.

Meehl, G. A., and Tebaldi, C. (2004). More intense, more frequent, and longer lasting heat waves in the 21st century. *Science*, **305**, 994–997.

Ntais, P., Sifaki-Pistola, D., Christodoulou, V., Messaritakis, I., Pratlong, F., Poupalos, G., et al. (2013). Leishmaniases in Greece. *American Journal of Tropical Medicine and Hygiene*, **89**, 906–915.

Ostfeld, R. S., Glass, G. E., and Keesing, F. (2005). Spatial epidemiology: An emerging (or re-emerging) discipline. *Trends in Ecology & Evolution*, **20**, 328–336.

Petropoulos, G., Carlson, T. N., Wooster, M. J., and Islam, S. (2009). A review of Ts/VI remote sensing based methods for the retrieval of land surface energy fluxes and soil surface moisture. *Progress in Physical Geography*, **33**, 224–250.

Pettorelli, N., Laurance, W. F., O'Brien, T. G., Wegmann, M., Nagendra, H., and Turner, W. (2014). Satellite remote sensing for applied ecologists: Opportunities and challenges. *Journal of Applied Ecology*, **51**, 839–848.

Rhew, I. C., Vander Stoep, A., Kearney, A., Smith, N. L., and Dunbar, M. D. (2011). Validation of the Normalized Difference Vegetation Index as a measure of neighborhood greenness. *Annals of Epidemiology*, **21**, 946–952.

Schott, J. R. (2007). *Remote sensing: The image chain approach.* Oxford University Press, New York.

Schowengerdt, R. A. (2007). *Remote sensing: Models and methods for image processing.* Academic Press, Burlington, MA.

Smargiassi, A., Goldberg, M. S., Plante, C., Fournier, M., Baudouin, Y., Kosatsky, T. (2009). Variation of daily warm season mortality as a function of micro-urban heat islands. *Journal of Epidemiology and Community Health*, **63**, 659–664.

Smith, M. P., and Guarnizo, L. E. (2009). Global mobility, shifting borders and urban citizenship. *Tijdschrift Voor Economische en Sociale Geografie*, **100**, 610–622.

Su, J., Jerrett, M., Beckerman, B., Verma, D., Arain, M. A., Kanaroglou, P., et al. (2010). A land use regression model for predicting ambient volatile organic compound concentrations in Toronto, Canada. *Atmospheric Environment*, **44**, 3529–3537.

Tanskanen, A., Lindfors, A., Määttä, A., Krotkov, N., Herman, J., Kaurola, J., et al. (2007). Validation of daily erythemal doses from Ozone Monitoring Instrument with ground-based UV measurement data. *Journal of Geophysical Research: Atmospheres*, **112**, D24S44.

Taylor, B. T., Fernando, P., Bauman, A. E., Williamson, A., Craig, J. C., and Redman, S. (2011). Measuring the quality of public open space using Google Earth. *American Journal of Preventive Medicine*, **40**, 105–112.

Tomlinson, C. J., Chapman, L., Thornes, J. E., and Baker, C. (2011). Remote sensing land surface temperature for meteorology and climatology: A review. *Meteorological Applications*, **18**, 296–306.

Torres, O., Tanskanen, A., Veihelmann, B., Ahn, C., Braak, R., Bhartia, P. K., et al. (2007). Aerosols and surface UV products from Ozone Monitoring Instrument observations: An overview. *Journal of Geophysical Research: Atmospheres*, **112**, D24S47.

Townshend, J. R. G., Carroll, M., Dimiceli, C., Sohlberg, R., Hansen, M., and DeFries, R. (2001). *Vegetation continuous fields MOD44B, 2002 percent tree cover, Collection 5.* Accessed January 15, 2013. https://lpdaac.usgs.gov/sites/default/files/public/modis/docs/VCF_C5_UserGuide_Dec2011.pdf

Wang, Y., Jiang, X., Yu, B., and Jiang, M. (2013). A hierarchical Bayesian approach for aerosol retrieval using MISR data. *Journal of the American Statistical Association,* **108,** 483–493.

Weier, J., and Herring, D. (2011). *Measuring vegetation (NDVI & EVI).* Accessed November 17, 2013. http://earthobservatory.nasa.gov/Features/MeasuringVegetation/

Weihs, P., Blumthaler, M., Rieder, H. E., Kreuter, A., Simic, S., Laube, W., et al. (2008). Measurements of UV irradiance within the area of one satellite pixel. *Atmospheric Chemistry and Physics,* **8,** 5615–5626.

Weng, Q. (2009). Thermal infrared remote sensing for urban climate and environmental studies: Methods, applications, and trends. *ISPRS Journal of Photogrammetry and Remote Sensing,* **64,** 335–344.

White-Newsome, J. L., Brines, S. J., Brown, D. G., Dvonch, J. T., Gronlund, C. J., Zhang, K., et al. (2013). Validating satellite-derived land surface temperature with in situ measurements: A public health perspective. *Environmental Health Perspectives,* **121,** 925–931.

Xie, Y., Sha, Z., and Yu, M. (2008). Remote sensing imagery in vegetation mapping: A review. *Journal of Plant Ecology,* **1,** 9–23.

Zhang, K., Oswald, E. M., Brown, D. G., Brines, S. J., Gronlund, C. J., White-Newsome, J. L., et al. (2011). Geostatistical exploration of spatial variation of summertime temperatures in the Detroit metropolitan region. *Environmental Research,* **111,** 1046–1053.

16

EXPOSURE ASSESSMENT
OF WATER CONTAMINANTS

Cristina M. Villanueva and Patrick Levallois

16.1 INTRODUCTION

Safe drinking water is essential for human life and well-being. Water is a limited natural resource under pressure by human activities, population growth, and climate change. The quality of drinking water may be compromised by the presence of microbes, chemicals, and eventually radionuclides. On a global scale, microbial contamination is the main stressor of drinking water quality, causing about 1/10 of the burden of disease worldwide. This is preventable by improving drinking water supply, sanitation, hygiene, and management of water resources (Prüss-Üstün 2008). Chemicals in drinking water are present worldwide and can be related to health effects (Thompson 2007). This chapter is devoted to the issue of exposure assessment of chemicals in drinking water and recreational water.

16.2 OCCURRENCE OF CONTAMINANTS
IN DRINKING WATER

16.2.1 Sources of Chemicals in Drinking Water

Chemicals may be present in drinking water as a consequence of natural geochemical processes. Such is the case for arsenic, fluoride, and hardness (calcium and magnesium salts). Arsenic is an element that occurs naturally in the earth's crust as a component of many minerals. Erosion of minerals or rocks containing arsenic leads to the release of arsenic, with the consequent contamination of water sources. Fluoride, although in some countries is added to drinking water at low concentrations to prevent dental caries, occurs naturally at high levels in certain parts of the world such as the Rift Valley in Africa (Malde 2011) and is associated with adverse health outcomes. The source of calcium and magnesium salts that confer water hardness is from the minerals through which water has circulated in the natural environment. Water hardness has been related to a protective effect on cardiovascular disease, although evidence is inconclusive. Other contaminants such as barium, manganese, and uranium can be released naturally by various types of rocks into groundwater and may become a risk for human health.

Human activities, for example, industry, agriculture, farming, water treatment, and wastewater from domestic use lead to the contamination of water bodies with a variety of chemicals. Domestic sources of chemicals are linked to ingredients of consumer products such as pharmaceuticals, personal care products, disinfectants, flame retardants used in electronic devices, food preservatives, food containers, and pesticides. For example, more than 100,000 chemicals are registered in the European Union (European Inventory of Existing Commercial Chemical Substances), and the contamination of water bodies with thousands of anthropogenic chemicals is an increasing environmental problem worldwide (Richardson and Ternes 2011). Although most of these chemicals when present are at low concentrations (e.g., ng/l range), there are toxicological concerns about them, especially because very few have been completely evaluated for toxicological effects and many of them are present as complex mixtures (Schwarzenbach 2006).

16.2.2 Role of Water Source, Treatment, and Distribution

The water source, treatment processes, and distribution determine the quality of drinking water. The type and characteristics of the raw water influence the choice of treatment. Common processes to treat water from surface sources include pre- or intermediate oxidation, coagulation, flocculation, sedimentation, filtration, and disinfection. Advanced (tertiary) treatment involves processes such as reverse osmosis or activated carbon filtration. Small community water supplies often receive minimal treatment and may be at greater risk and less able to control the problem of chemical contaminants. Private well water generally does not receive treatment. The water source quality and choice of treatment and disinfectant(s) dictates the resulting mixture of disinfection by-products (DBPs) in the final water. Switching from chlorination to chloramination may be effective to reduce the formation of regulated DBPs such as trihalomethanes, but increases the concentrations of nitrogen-containing DBPs such as nitrosamines (Bond 2011). The removal of chemicals such as pesticides, pharmaceutical residues, and endocrine-disrupting compounds may be less effective through traditional compared to advanced treatment processes (Templeton 2009). For example, conventional treatment processes with coagulation, filtration, and chlorination can remove about 50% of pharmaceuticals, whereas advanced treatment such as ozonation, advanced oxidation, activated carbon, and membrane processes (e.g., reverse osmosis, nanofiltration), can achieve higher removal rates for some contaminants (WHO 2012). Some chemicals derived from coagulants used during the coagulation process (aluminium, acrylamide) might also be of health concerns.

Several contaminants could be released from main pipe components, storage tanks, or domestic lines (e.g. asbestos, lead, copper, polycyclic aromatic hydrocarbons, polyvinyl chloride). Lead release is certainly the main issue that has been known for decades (Rabin 2008). However, other contaminants can be released and remain undetected from public authorities if they are not monitored appropriately (e.g., vinyl chloride found recently in French drinking water networks; http://www.actu-environnement.com/media/pdf/news-23485-avis-anses-eaux-chlorure-vynile.pdf, [consulted Feb 2015]).

16.2.3 Regulations and Emerging Substances

Drinking water quality is legislated in many countries, wherein regulated substances are routinely monitored. Legal limits reflect both the level that protects human health and the level that water systems can achieve using the best available technology, taking into account the cost of treatment and also the laboratory capacity of monitoring the water quality at that level. The World Health Organization produces guidelines that are used as the basis for regulation and standard setting in many countries. These guidelines require periodical review to be updated as new toxic chemicals are identified, and existing maximum contaminant levels need to be revised according to new knowledge. Examples of regulated substances include metals (e.g., lead), disinfection by-products (e.g., trihalomethanes), and pesticides (e.g., atrazine), among others.

Advances in analytical chemistry allow the identification of chemicals in water that previously had not been detected. These substances are generally known as emerging contaminants and mostly occur at very low concentrations, near the quantification limits (e.g., ng/l). Wastewater from human activities may contaminate downstream water supply sources with these emerging contaminants, which may be present in drinking water (Ternes 2007). The presence of these substances in wastewater, natural waters, and drinking water is of concern because the burden of human exposure and the consequences for human health and ecosystems is unknown. Examples of these emerging contaminants are pharmaceutical residues, nanoparticles, consumer products such as sunscreens, and nitrogenated and iodinated disinfection by-products (Richardson and Ternes 2011) (Table 16.1).

16.2.4 Recreational Bathing Water

Disinfection is necessary in swimming pools, hot tubs, and spa to avoid waterborne infections. The most widely used disinfectant is chlorine, which reacts with organic matter from bathers (urine, sweat, hair, cells, cosmetics, etc.) to generate disinfectant by-products such as haloacetic acids (HAAs), trihalomethanes (THMs), and chloral hydrate, among others (Zwiener 2007; Lee 2010), in a similar way as in drinking water treatment. The presence of nitrogen in the organic matter from bathers leads to the formation of nitrogenated by-products such as chloramines (mochloramine, dichloramine, trichloramine), haloacetonitriles (Weaver 2009), and nitrosamines (Walse 2008). The formation of disinfection by-products in swimming pools depends on several factors including the number of swimmers, water

Table 16.1 Emerging contaminants identified in water sources classified by the source

Source	Chemical group	Substance examples
Ingredients of consumer products or personal care products	Brominated flame retardants	Polybrominated diphenyl ethers (PBDEs)
	Benzotriazoles	Benzotriazole, tolytriazole
	Dioxane	(single chemical)
	Ionic liquids	Imidazolium, pyridinium
	Musks	Musk xylene, musk ketone
	Perfluorinated compounds	Perfluorooctanoic acid (PFOA)
	Siloxanes	Octamethylcyclotetrasiloxane (D4)
	Sunscreens/UV filters	Benzophenone-3 (BP3)
Pharmaceuticals, consumer or personal care products	Artificial sweeteners	Saccharine
	Illicit drugs	Amphetamine-like compounds
	Iodinated X ray contrast media (ICM)	Iohexol (IOX) and diatrizoate (DTZ)
	Pharmaceuticals	Antidepressants, antibiotics
Transformation products	Disinfection by-products	NDMA
	ICM transformation products	Iohexol TP599, iomeprol TP643
	Naphtenic acids	Trans-4-methyl-1-cyclohexane carboxylic acid (trans-4MCHCA)
	Pesticide transformation products	Alachlor ethanesulfonic acid (ESA)
Algal blooms	Cyanotoxins	Microcystin-LR
Heterogeneous sources	Nanomaterials	Nanotubes, quantum dots, TiO_2
	Perchlorate	(single chemical)

Adapted from Richardson, S. D., and Ternes, T. A. (2011). Water analysis: emerging contaminants and current issues. *Analytical Chemistry*, **83**, 4614–4648.

temperature, and total organic carbon (Chu and Nieuwenhuijsen 2002). Higher levels have been observed in winter compared with summer, suggesting that a low air exchange rate in winter leads to accumulation of pollutants (Bessonneau 2011). Outdoor compared with indoor pools tend to show higher THM levels in water (Font-Ribera 2010a), although there may be less inhalation exposure. Alternative disinfectants that are used in swimming pools include bromide-based substances, copper salts, ozone, ultraviolet radiation, etc. These are used in many cases in combination (e.g., ozonation + chlorination). Any disinfectants are highly reactive substance by definition, and produce chemical reactions leading to specific by-products (e.g., bromate as by-product of ozonation) (Lee 2010).

16.3 EXPOSURE ASSESSMENT

Accurate exposure assessment in human observational studies is essential to obtain valid results and constitutes a main methodological challenge. In the selection of methods to evaluate exposure we have to consider the study objectives and design, the specific outcome under study, and the substance of interest. Evaluation of exposure in individual-based studies requires much deeper personal and environmental information compared to ecological studies. The period of latency for the given exposure/outcome under study will dictate the exposure window to evaluate. Finally, the physicochemical characteristics of the substances of interest need to be well known and considered in order to evaluate all the relevant exposure pathways, such as inhalation for volatile substances, dermal absorption for skin-permeable substances, or incorporation though dietary items (e.g., in lypophilic substances).

16.3.1 Challenges of Exposure Assessment

16.3.1.1 Low Concentrations

Many substances, and particularly emerging contaminants, occur at low concentrations. However, even low concentrations may have important consequences across the entire population because the whole population is exposed to water. Difficulties in identifying and measuring contaminants in water supplies at very low concentrations hamper the evaluation of human exposure. Accuracy of analytical measurements in water is particularly important at the low range of exposure, as well as methods to minimize measurement error.

16.3.1.2 Lack of Suitable Monitoring Data

Monitoring data are collected on limited compounds, especially inorganics and a few organics. Available data are often not available at all, or is available but not suitable or enough for the purpose of exposure assessment for epidemiological studies. Data should be sufficient to evaluate temporal and geographical variation in the study areas for the time window of interest, and sometimes data are insufficient to properly evaluate real exposure in the population. This is particularly problematic for long-latency diseases such as cancer, because historical records are usually unavailable. In addition, monitoring data are limited to regulated substances, and research on emerging contaminants is hampered by the lack of historical records.

16.3.1.3 Mixtures

Chemical contamination of water supplies often constitutes mixtures of varying composition in time and space. The occurrence of substances as part of complex mixtures hampers the evaluation of human exposure and estimation of risks, requiring new methods in health risk analysis (Schwarzenbach 2006). Examples of substances occurring in mixtures include disinfection by-products (DBPs) and pharmaceutical residues. In the case of DBPs, the use of a few compounds (such as trihalomethanes) as surrogates of the mixture as a whole has been a way to address the complex nature of the mixture in epidemiological studies. However, the assumption that they correlate with other DBPs is not universally supported and correlations can vary in time and space (Villanueva 2012). In consequence, depending on the site of the study and the individual constituents of the mixture, chemical-by-chemical exposure assessment may not be feasible or could result in simplistic exposure estimates.

16.3.1.4 Multiple Exposure Routes

Exposure to water contaminants can occur through multiple routes, depending on the chemical characteristics of the substances. Volatile chemicals may be inhaled, and skin-permeable chemicals may be absorbed through the skin. This is the case for some disinfection by-products such as trihalomethanes, for which showering, bathing and dishwashing may substantially contribute to the exposure of these compounds, besides ingestion. In addition, most chemicals do not exclusively occur in drinking water and may be present in food, air, etc. For example, food is a main source of exposure to nitrosamines (such as NDMA) and nitrate, in addition to water (IARC 2010). When possible, exposure through all plausible routes and from all important sources should be assessed in order to produce accurate estimates of disease risk.

16.3.1.5 Lack of Validated Biomarkers of Exposure

Among the few available biomarkers specific for drinking water contaminants, many have short half-lives (e.g., urinary trichloroacetic acid) and are thus of limited value to associate with health outcomes with latency periods longer than the half-life of the biomarker compound (Savitz 2012). Sometimes, as for arsenic, other biological specimens such as nails can extend the exposure assessment to 12 to 18 months (Karagas 2004). However, limitations persist concerning exposure assessment for longer periods of time. Consequently, exposure assessment in most instances relies on assessment of personal behavior ascertained through questionnaires and measurement of environmental levels.

16.3.1.6 Long Latency Periods for Certain Outcomes

The evaluation of long exposure periods results in greater chances of exposure misclassification, and lack of historical data are frequent. The natural history of cancer may be long, and evaluation of the exposure should cover the initiation or promotion of the tumor, which constitutes a major challenge. This period varies between cancer sites or subtypes and specific exposures, but typically exposure should be assessed at least up to 40 years before diagnosis. Relevant information on levels and personal water use during this period should be collected.

16.3.2 Methods to Assess Exposure in Epidemiological Studies

16.3.2.1 Water Measurements and Other Environmental Data

Data on concentrations of the chemical(s) of interest in drinking water of study areas are essential to quantify the exposure. Data may be provided by routine monitoring records or by measurements designed and conducted by the researcher. Ideally, measurements should cover the relevant exposure period. Repeated measurements and distribution of sampling points covering different water zones are necessary to evaluate geographical and temporal variation during the relevant exposure period. In the case of cancer, historical data are necessary, and studies on cancer have mostly used routine monitoring data from regulatory agencies for contaminants with a long history of regulatory requirements. For instance, nitrate data from 396 communities between 1955 to 1988 was used to reconstruct exposure for a cohort of women in Iowa (Weyer 2001). The validity of regulatory monitoring data as a surrogate for levels at the tap of the consumers may be a concern when there is important variability within the distribution system or temporal variability, such as the case of disinfection by-products (Rodriguez 2004; Symanski 2004) and lead (Payne 2008). Regulatory measurements only apply to households connected to a distribution system because private wells are usually excluded from regulatory monitoring. This is problematic when the chemical occurs mainly in ground water and the study population is served by private wells in a large extent. For instance, 25% of participants supplied by private wells could not be evaluated in the study of Weyer et al. 2001. In these situations, historical levels could be modeled based on valid predictors (see section 16.3.2.4) or additional water sampling, which is costly and hardly feasible for retrospective studies but feasible for prospective studies. A summary of the environmental data to be collected for exposure assessment purposes is included in Table 16.2. Ideally, environmental data are combined with personal habits of water consumption gathered by questionnaires to derive individual exposure indices.

16.3.2.2 Questionnaires

Personal behavior involving exposure to water contaminants can be collected though questionnaires. The design of the questionnaire is a critical step in epidemiological studies and requires particular attention. Questionnaires may be self-administered or administered by a professional interviewer; in the second case, questionnaires may be conducted through face to face personal interviews or telephone interviews. Any modality of questionnaires has advantages and disadvantages, and the formulation of questions should consider the method of administration for proper data collection. For instance, personal interviews allow more complex questions compared with self-administered questionnaires. For the purpose of exposure assessment to water contaminants, in addition to ingestion, inhalation and dermal contact may be relevant exposure routes for volatile or skin-permeable chemicals. In consequence, activities involving different water uses at home (e.g., showering,

Table 16.2 Environmental data and other information to be collected for exposure assessment in epidemiologic studies on drinking water

Data	Details/comments	Index to derive
Environmental data		
Quality of water in the study areas	Concentration of the chemical of interest during the period of interest, from routine monitoring data or other sources	Depends on the outcome: e.g., annual average levels for cancer studies; monthly average for pregnancy outcomes
Predictors of the chemical of interest	Water source (ground/surface/other) Raw water parameters (based on the literature) Water treatment Land use During the period of interest (e.g., annual average values for cancer outcomes)	Models to estimate levels of the contaminant of interest, when data are limited
Other data		
Effect of home devices	E.g., filters, boiling. Effect based on the literature.	Estimate ingestion of chemicals
Toxicology data	Based on the literature. See Haddad et al. (2006) for details.	Combined with physiological data to estimate internal dose through physiologically based toxicokinetic model
Uptake factors	Based on the literature, for volatile or skin permeable chemicals: • Showering • Bathing • Swimming in pools	To be combined with water use and levels to estimate internal dose through different routes
Biomarkers		
	When valid biomarkers are available: • Define sample size and design according to the study objectives (exploratory/validity/etc.) • Define procedures to collect the relevant tissue, storage conditions, laboratory analysis and quality control	Estimate internal dose

bathing), in recreation (e.g., swimming in pools), and through occupations involving water contact should be considered. A summary of variables to be ascertained through questionnaires for exposure assessment purposes is included in Table 16.3.

16.3.2.2.1 Residential History and Source of Water

The address of the residences during the period of interest is needed to link with concentrations in the distribution systems. In North America, a complete postal code might be sufficient in urban areas, but less efficient in rural areas. In other countries, the full address may be needed for a precise location. The lack of information on the location of the residence or the geographical zone served by each distribution system may lead to exposure misclassification or exclusion of subjects. For instance, in a case-control study on disinfection by-products and leukemia in Canada, about 36% of cases and controls were discarded because this information was not available for the period under evaluation (Kasim 2006). The main source of water consumed (e.g., distribution system, private well) in each residence is important to gather, because subjects may use well water despite being served by a distribution network. Information on well depth might be important because it may indicate vulnerability to potential contaminants, as for instance increased nitrate concentration in shallow wells (Burow 2010). Changes may occur within a residence (e.g., shift from municipal to bottled water) and these should be collected, particularly when evaluating long-latency outcomes (e.g., cancer).

16.3.2.2.2 Water Consumption

Type (e.g., bottled, tap, private well) and quantity of water consumed at home during the relevant period should be collected, usually through consumption frequency questionnaires and validation diaries (Willet 1998; Riboli 2002). Because boiling and filtration may affect water composition (Levesque 2006; Weinberg 2006), information on water handling should be collected for different water-based fluids (e.g., food preparation, cold beverages, hot beverages) and eventually for different water sources (e.g., bottled water could be used only for a specific usage). This evaluation should be ideally repeated because consumption or water handling habits may change during the exposure window of interest. Few published questionnaires are available (Nieuwenhuijsen 2003) and few validation studies have been conducted. Most of them are conducted in studies on reproductive outcomes, with a time windows of exposure of a few months (Barbone 2002; Kaur 2004; Shimokura 1998). Water consumption outside home could be an important proportion of total water intake and should be taken into account (Levallois 1998; Shimokura 1998). However, because it is very difficult to get information on the water quality, it has not been done as detailed as for residential exposure, with some exceptions (Nuckols 2011). At least the amount of water consumed outside home could be gathered.

Table 16.3 Personal characteristics to be ascertained through questionnaires for exposure assessment in epidemiologic studies on drinking water contaminants

Data	Details	Index to derive
Personal characteristics	Age, Gender, Weight, Height	To be used in physiologically based toxicokinetic models
Type of water consumed	• Bottled/municipal/private well/other • At home and outside • Changes over time	
Amount of water ingested (l/day or glasses/day)	• Overall and by type of water or water-based fluids: Tap water, bottled water, water-based drinks (coffee, tea, herbal drinks, other), water-based food (soups, other) • At home and outside • Changes over time	Mean daily volume of water consumed
Use of filters	• Yes/no • Type of filter used (active carbon, reverse osmosis, other) • Date started using the device • Changes over time	To correct ingestion estimates
Home address and residential history	• Full address, currently • Lifetime residential history (for long-latency outcomes, e.g., cancer): • Complete address of residences above a certain duration (typically ≥1 year) • Year start, year stop living in each residence	Link with water supplier (by geocoding or other means) and quality data to assess the levels at the water supplied to the households
Water source serving the residence	• Community distribution/private well/other • For all residences	
Showering and bathing	• Frequency (times/day or week) • Duration (minutes)	For volatile or skin permeable chemicals, to estimate indices of inhalation and/or dermal exposure
Hand dishwashing	• Frequency (times/day or week) • Duration (minutes) • Use of gloves (always/usually/seldom/never)	
Swimming in pools	• Frequency (times/day or week) • Duration (minutes) • Type of pool (indoors/outdoors)	

16.3.2.2.3 Showering and Bathing

Frequency and duration of showering and bathing should be considered for volatile and skin-permeable chemicals. Based on experimental work on human exposure to chloroform and trichloroethylene in water, Weisel and Jo (Weisel 1996) estimated that inhalation and dermal exposure during a 10-minute shower equals the total internal dose from 2 liters of water ingestion. However, few studies have included such a component, few questionnaires are available, and there is a need for standardized and validated tools. From the US experience, individuals tend to overestimate the duration of a shower in a retrospective questionnaire (Wilkes 2005). Factors that influence exposure may be added to the questionnaire: ventilation, time spent in the bathroom after the shower, etc., although it will be difficult to analyze for quantifying exposure.

16.3.2.2.4 Swimming in Pools

For contaminants such as disinfection by-products, swimming pools could be a significant source of exposure via inhalation and dermal exposure (Levesque 1994; Nieuwenhuijsen 2000; Erdinger 2004; Font-Ribera 2010b). Data on frequency and duration of swimming in pools, by type of swimming pool (indoor or outdoor, type of disinfectant used), will be useful to evaluate exposure.

16.3.2.3 Biomarkers

Several exposure biomarkers have been used in water research but one limiting factor is the relative short half-life of waterborne contaminants in human tissues. Exposure biomarkers are a good choice to evaluate exposure in prospective studies, and even short-time half-life biomarkers could be used to validate other means of exposure assessment. For instance, using 24-hour urinary sampling, which is usually an indicator of recent exposure, authors were able to demonstrate the impact of low nitrate levels in water on the total exposure to nitrates of rural inhabitants of Quebec (Levallois 2000).

Urine trichloroacetic acid (TCAA) has been proposed as a valid exposure biomarker of ingested disinfection by-products, because the half-life (>2 days) is longer than consecutive exposure events and urine levels correlate with ingested levels through drinking water. However, this biomarker would only reflect exposure through ingestion, because haloacetic acids are not incorporated through inhalation and skin absorption. Urine trichloroacetic acid may also reflect exposure to chloral hydrate and trichloroethylene because these chemicals are metabolized to TCAA. Although the use of this biomarker is promising, it has only been used in a few epidemiological studies on reproductive outcomes (Xie 2011; Zhou 2012; Costet 2012; Smith 2013), and requires methodological development prior to generalized use in epidemiological studies (Savitz 2012). Trihalomethanes are highly volatile disinfection by-products, and short half-life hampers their use in epidemiological studies. Levels in exhaled air have been used in the evaluation of short-term effects, such as molecular changes after swimming in pools (Font-Ribera 2010c; Kogevinas 2010). Levels of trihalomethanes in blood can be measured and show a consistent correlation with levels in water (Rivera-Nunez 2012).

Arsenic can be measured in several body tissues. Urine levels reflect recent exposure, whereas levels in toenails would reflect a longer exposure period. For instance, Karagas et al. used toenail arsenic as a measure of cumulative exposure to arsenic in the past 12 to 18 months in a study on cancer (Karagas 2004). However, uncertainties concerning the validity to represent exposure during the relevant period limited the interpretation of results.

Before using a biomarker on a larger scale, it is important to conduct pilot studies to evaluate the sensitivity to the variation of exposure in the range of concern, within and between-person variability, as well as other practical requirements for good collection and storage (Savitz 2012). Other aspects to consider on biomarkers are indicated in Table 16.2. New biomarkers are promising but they cannot pass over systematic validation (Vineis and Perera 2007). The introduction of the "exposome" paradigm has renewed the interest to use biomarkers in exposure assessment through the evaluation of "omics" (Wild 2005); however, such new biomarkers have more challenges to overcome (Vineis 2013).

In summary, there are some but few validated biomarkers of exposure specific for contaminants of drinking water, and therefore exposure assessment in most epidemiological studies relies on personal habits ascertained through questionnaires and levels of contaminants in drinking water.

16.3.2.4 Statistical Modeling

When direct measurements are not sufficient for a valid assessment, modeling strategies based on predictors of the exposure of interest may be applied. Models used in the literature are multiple and in many instances make use of geographical information system. Models may be based on geographic distributions of contaminants (Toledano 2005), modeling of underground plumes, and hydraulic simulation of contaminants (Aral 2004; Nuckols 2004; Gallagher 2011), and/or surrogate parameters such as land use (Aschebrook-Kilfoy 2012). Several methods can be used in combination, tailored to the availability of data, such as in a study on the long-term exposure to arsenic and cancer (Nuckols 2011) that combines arsenic data from one's own measurements in water samples collected at the homes of participants, data from public water utilities, and historical data for aquifers. For chemicals generated by treatment (e.g., DBPs), models could be based on raw water and treatment characteristics (Singer 2001; Rodriguez 2004; Sadiq 2004). Given the important seasonal and temporal variability, such models need to be site specific and require validation. Finally, insufficient predictor data may lead to uncertainty and exposure misclassification, and this should be considered before undertaking any modeling in order to produce valid exposure estimates.

16.3.3 Estimation of Personal Exposure Indices

Once data collection is finished, several exposure indices can be estimated by combining concentration at the tap and water use habits. Time-weighted average concentrations are mean concentrations at the residence, weighted by duration, regardless of water use. Ingested dose is calculated by multiplying the water consumption (e.g., liters/day) times the concentration at the tap (e.g., mg/l) eventually corrected by factors accounting for the effect of water handling (e.g., filtering, boiling) (Savitz 2005; Levallois 2012). Internal dose after showering, bathing, and swimming in pools can be estimated, taking into consideration the frequency and duration, and using uptake factors derived from experimental studies (Savitz 2005; Hoffman 2008). A more precise value of the absorbed dose could be estimated using validated physiologically based toxicokinetic (PBTK) models based on physical properties of the substance (e.g., skin permeability, water-air ratio) and personal characteristics of participants (age, gender, body weight, and body height) (Haddad 2006; Tardif 2011; Levallois 2012). Finally, total internal dose accounted for all routes may be estimated. Because toxic properties for some substances may differ by incorporation route (e.g., inhaled or dermally absorbed chemicals enter directly in the portal circulation and are rapidly metabolized in the liver), this should be taken into account by PBTK models. Also, such models could be used to estimate the concentration of toxic metabolites at the target organs (Levesque 2002).

16.3.4 Approaches to Address Measurement Error

Exposure estimates with minimal measurement error are necessary to produce valid effect estimates. Misclassification of exposure is of particular concern at the low exposure range, as it tends, under most scenarios, to attenuate associations toward the null (Cantor 2007; Waller 2001) or reduce the precision of associations (Wright 2004). Strategies to minimize measurement error are necessary from study design to data analysis, and include for example the collection of repeated measures of individual water use over the relevant exposure period (Forssen 2009), assessing reliability of interviews to exclude unreliable questionnaires (Villanueva 2009), and statistical modeling the magnitude of the misclassification (e.g., through simulation extrapolation method, Simex).

16.4 RESEARCH NEEDS

16.4.1 Mixtures

Many chemicals occur simultaneously in drinking water and it is necessary to evaluate more globally the nature of the mixture and the impact on human biology. The evaluation of mixtures is a challenge beyond current methods, and new developments may contribute to understanding the health effects of chemical contaminants in drinking water (Villanueva 2014). The evaluation of chemicals in an isolated form may hide synergistic effects from mixtures of chemicals occurring at very low levels without observed effects individually (Silva 2002). The use of in vitro assays may be used to measure the global toxicity of chemical mixtures in water samples, and can be combined with chemical determinations. For example, the "effect-directed analysis" methodology combines toxicological evaluations with untargeted chemical analysis to identify putative substances from an agnostic perspective (Brack 2003; Weller 2012) and constitutes a promising tool in the evaluation of complex mixtures such as emerging contaminants in drinking water (Wagner 2013). In addition, the exposome paradigm may help to define adequate methods for evaluating such multiple exposures (Wild 2009; Rappaport 2011). Effects of different water exposures could be compared in terms of their biological impact using the new -omics biomarkers (Zhang 2011) when these tools become available for large epidemiologic studies (Scalbert 2009).

16.4.2 Long-Term Studies

Good exposure assessment is essential for epidemiological studies, especially when exposure levels are low. There is now a great interest to develop and follow cohort studies with biomarkers measurements using the exposome paradigm (Rappaport 2011; Vrijheid 2014). However, this would be useful for environmental health only if there is a clear link between internal and external measurements (Peters 2012). Major effort should be made to evaluate carefully the exposure to water contaminants of participants in ongoing cohort studies.

16.5 CONCLUSION

Accurate exposure assessment is essential for epidemiologic studies to evaluate health effects of water contaminants. Data on the levels of contaminants in the water consumed for the relevant period is essential. Personal habits on consumption of water and handlings before consumption (e.g., filtering) need to be collected. Showering and bathing frequency should be recorded when inhalation and dermal absorption are concerned. Combining the different routes of exposure is essential to construct a measure of the total internal dose, at least for home exposure. When possible, validated biomarkers should be used, but few are presently available. There is a need to develop methods to evaluate effects of mixtures. In addition, given the necessity for chronic diseases to collect exposure information over a long period of time, the exposure to waterborne chemicals should preferably be assessed in prospective study designs. Finally, there is a need for an improved coordination of researchers working on drinking water pollution to conduct studies to evaluate human health effects.

ACKNOWLEDGMENT

The contribution of Patrick Levallois is based on an initial work done during a sabbatical spent at the International Agency for Research on Cancer (IARC) in Lyon and the Centre for Research in Environmental Epidemiology (CREAL) in Barcelona.

REFERENCES

Aral, M. M., Guan, J., Maslia, M. L., Sautner, J. B., Gillig, R. E., Reyes, J. J., and Williams, R. C. (2004). Optimal reconstruction of historical water supply to a distribution system: A. Methodology. *Journal of Water and Health*, **2**, 123–136.

Aschebrook-Kilfoy, B. Heltshe, S. L., Nuckols, J. R., Sabra, M. M., Shuldiner, A. R., Mitchell, B. D., et al. (2012). Modeled nitrate levels in well water supplies and prevalence of abnormal thyroid conditions among the Old Order Amish in Pennsylvania. *Environmental Health*, **11**, 6.

Barbone, F., Valent, F., Brussi, V., Tomasella, L., Triassi, M., Di Lieto, A., et al. (2002). Assessing the exposure of pregnant women to drinking water disinfection byproducts. *Epidemiology*, **13**, 540–544.

Bessonneau. V, Derbez, M., Clement, M., and Thomas, O. (2011). Determinants of chlorination by-products in indoor swimming pools. *International Journal of Hygiene and Environmental Health*, **215**, 76–85.

Bond, T., Huang, J., Templeton, M. R., and Graham, N. (2011). Occurrence and control of nitrogenous disinfection by-products in drinking water—a review. *Water Research*, **45**, 4341–4354.

Brack, W. (2003). Effect-directed analysis: a promising tool for the identification of organic toxicants in complex mixtures? *Analytical and Bioanalytical Chemistry*, **377**, 397–407.

Burow, K. R., Nolan, B. T., Rupert, M. G., and Dubrovsky, N. M. (2010). Nitrate in groundwater of the United States, 1991-2003. *Environmental Science and Technology*, **44**, 4988–4997.

Cantor, K. P., and Lubin, J. H. (2007). Arsenic, internal cancers, and issues in inference from studies of low level exposures in human populations. *Toxicology and Applied Pharmacology*, **222**, 252–257.

Chu, H., and Nieuwenhuijsen, M. J. (2002). Distribution and determinants of trihalomethane concentrations in indoor swimming pools. *Occupational and Environmental Medicine*, **59**, 243–247.

Costet, N., Garlantezec, R., Monfort, C., Rouget, F., Gagniere, B., Chevrier, C., and Cordier, S. (2012). Environmental and urinary markers of prenatal exposure to drinking water disinfection by-products, fetal growth, and duration of gestation in the PELAGIE birth cohort (Brittany, France, 2002-2006). *American Journal of Epidemiology*, **175**, 263–275.

Erdinger, L., Kuhn, K. P., Kirsch, F., Feldhues, R., Frobel, T., Nohynek, B., and Gabrio, T. (2004). Pathways of trihalomethane uptake in swimming pools. *International Journal of Hygiene and Environmenetal Health*, **207**, 571–575.

Font-Ribera, L., Esplugues, A., Ballester, F., Martinez, B., Tardon, A., Freire, C., et al. (2010a). Trihalomethanes in swimming pool water in four areas in Spain participating in the INMA project. *Gaceta Sanitaria*, **24**, 483–486.

Font-Ribera, L., Kogevinas, M., Nieuwenhuijsen, M. J., Grimalt, J. O., and Villanueva, C. M. (2010b). Patterns of water use and exposure to trihalomethanes among children in Spain. *Environmental Research*, **110**, 571–579.

Font-Ribera, L., Kogevinas, M., Zock, J. P., Gomez, F. P., Barreiro, E., Nieuwenhuijsen, M. J., et al. (2010c). Short-term changes in respiratory biomarkers after swimming in a chlorinated pool. *Environmental Health Perspectives*, **118**, 1538–1544.

Forssen, U. M., Wright, J. M., Herring, A. H., Savitz, D. A., Nieuwenhuijsen, M. J., and Murphy, P. A. (2009). Variability and predictors of changes in water use during pregnancy. *Journal of Exposure Science and Environmental Epidemiology*, **19**, 593–602.

Gallagher, L. G., Vieira, V. M., Ozonoff, D., Webster, T. F., and Aschengrau, A. (2011). Risk of breast cancer following exposure to tetrachloroethylene-contaminated drinking water in Cape Cod, Massachusetts: reanalysis of a case-control study using a modified exposure assessment. *Environmental Health*, **10**, 47.

Haddad, S., Tardif, G. C., and Tardif, R. (2006). Development of physiologically based toxicokinetic models for improving the human indoor exposure assessment to water contaminants: Trichloroethylene and trihalomethanes. *Journal of Toxicology and Environmental Health A*, **69**, 2095–2136.

Hoffman, C. S., Mendola, P., Savitz, D. A., Herring, A. H., Loomis, D., Hartmann, K. E., et al. (2008). Drinking water disinfection by-product exposure and fetal growth. *Epidemiology*, **19**, 729–737.

IARC. (2010). *Ingested nitrate and nitrite, and cyanobacterial peptide toxins*. IARC monographs on the evaluation of carcinogenic risks to humans. Vol 94. IARC, Lyon.

Karagas, M. R., Tosteson, T. D., Morris, J. S., Demidenko, E., Mott, L. A., Heaney, J., and Schned, A. (2004). Incidence of transitional cell carcinoma of the bladder and arsenic exposure in New Hampshire. *Cancer Causes Control*, **15**, 465–472.

Kasim, K., Levallois, P., Johnson, K. C., Abdous, B., and Auger, P. (2006). Chlorination disinfection by-products in drinking water and the risk of adult leukemia in Canada. *American Journal of Epidemiology*, **163**, 116–126.

Kaur, S., Nieuwenhuijsen, M. J., Ferrier, H., and Steer, P. (2004). Exposure of pregnant women to tap water related activities. *Occupational and Environmental Medicine*, **61**, 454–460.

Kogevinas, M., Villanueva, C. M., Font-Ribera, L., Liviac D, Bustamante M, Espinoza F, et al. (2010). Genotoxic effects in swimmers exposed to disinfection by-products in indoor swimming pools. *Environmental Health Perspectives*, **118**, 1531–1537.

Lee, J., Jun, M. J., Lee, M. H., Lee, M. H., Eom, S. W., and Zoh, K. D. (2010). Production of various disinfection byproducts in indoor swimming pool waters treated with different disinfection methods. *International Journal of Hygiene and Environmenetal Health*, **213**, 465–474.

Levallois, P., Ayotte, P., Louchini, R., Desrosiers, T., Baribeau, H., Phaneuf, D., et al. (2000). Sources of nitrate exposure in residents of rural areas in Quebec, Canada. *Journal of Exposure Anaysis andl Environmental Epidemiology*, **10**, 188–195.

Levallois, P., Gingras, S., Marcoux, S., Legay, C., Catto, C., Rodriguez, M., and Tardif, R. (2012). Maternal exposure to drinking-water chlorination by-products and small-for-gestational-age neonates. *Epidemiology*, **23**, 267–276.

Levallois, P., Guevin, N., Gingras, S., Levesque, B., Weber, J. P., and Letarte, R. (1998). New patterns of drinking-water consumption: results of a pilot study. *Science of the Total Environment*, **209**, 233–241.

Levesque, B., Ayotte, P., LeBlanc, A., Dewailly, E., Prud'Homme, D., Lavoie, R., et al. (1994). Evaluation of dermal and respiratory chloroform exposure in humans. *Environmental Health Perspectives*, **102**, 1082–1087.

Levesque, B., Ayotte, P., Tardif, R., Ferron, L., Gingras, S., Schlouch, E., et al. (2002). Cancer risk associated with household exposure to chloroform. *Journal of Toxicology and Environmental Health A*, **65**, 489–502.

Levesque, S., Rodriguez, M. J., Serodes, J., Beaulieu, C., and Proulx, F. (2006). Effects of indoor drinking water handling on trihalomethanes and haloacetic acids. *Water Research*, **40**, 2921–2930.

Malde, M. K., Scheidegger, R., Julshamn, K., and Bader, H. P. (2011). Substance flow analysis: a case study of fluoride exposure through food and beverages in young children living in Ethiopia. *Environmental Health Perspectives*, **119**, 579–584.

Nieuwenhuijsen, M. J. (2003) Questionnaires. In *Exposure assessment in occupational and environmental epidemiology* (ed. M. J. Nieuwenhuijsen), 21–38. Oxford University Press, Oxford.

Nieuwenhuijsen, M. J., Toledano, M. B., and Elliott, P. (2000). Uptake of chlorination disinfection by-products: A review and a discussion of its implications for exposure assessment in epidemiological studies. *Journal of Exposure Analysis and Environmental Epidemiology*, **10**, 586–599.

Nuckols, J. R., Freeman, L. E., Lubin, J. H., Airola, M. S., Baris D, Ayotte, J. D., et al. (2011). Estimating water supply arsenic levels in the New England Bladder Cancer Study. *Environmental Health Perspectives*, **119**, 1279–1285.

Nuckols, J. R., Ward, M. H., and Jarup, L. (2004). Using geographic information systems for exposure assessment in environmental epidemiology studies. *Environ Health Perspect*, **112**, 1007–1015.

Payne M. (2008). Lead in drinking water. *Canadian Medical Association Journal*, **179**, 253–254.

Peters, A., Hoek, G., and Katsouyanni, K. (2012). Understanding the link between environmental exposures and health: Does the exposome promise too much? *Journal of Epidemiology and Community Health*, **66**, 103–105.

Prüss-Üstün, A., Bos, R., Gore, F. and Bartram, J. (2008). Safer water, better health: costs, benefits and sustainability of interventions to protect and promote health. Geneva. Available at: http://whqlibdoc.who.int/publications/2008/9789241596435_eng.pdf

Rabin, R. (2008). The lead industry and lead water pipes "a modest campaign." *American Journal of Public Health*, **98**, 1584–1592.

Rappaport, S. M. (2011). Implications of the exposome for exposure science. *Journal of Exposure Science and Environmental Epidemiology*, **21**, 5–9.

Riboli, E., Hunt, K. J., Slimani, N., Ferrari, P., Norat, T., Fahey, M., et al. (2002). European Prospective Investigation into Cancer and Nutrition (EPIC): Study populations and data collection. *Public Health Nutrition*, **5**, 1113–1124.

Richardson, S. D., and Ternes, T. A. (2011). Water analysis: emerging contaminants and current issues. *Analytical Chemistry*, **83**, 4614–4648.

Rivera-Nunez, Z., Wright, J. M., Blount, B. C., Silva, L. K., Jones, E., Chan, R. L., et al. (2012). Comparison of trihalomethanes in tap water and blood: A case study in the United States. *Environmental Health Perspectives*, **120**, 661–667.

Rodriguez, M. J., Serodes, J.B., and Levallois, P. (2004). Behavior of trihalomethanes and haloacetic acids in a drinking water distribution system. *Water Research*, **38**, 4367–4382.

Sadiq, R., and Rodriguez, M. J. (2004). Disinfection by-products (DBPs) in drinking water and predictive models for their occurrence: a review. *Science of the Total Environment*, **321**, 21–46.

Savitz, D. A. (2012). Invited commentary: biomarkers of exposure to drinking water disinfection by-products—are we ready yet? *American Journal of Epidemiology*, **175**, 276–278.

Savitz, D. A., Singer, P.C., Hartmann, K. E., Herring, A. H., Weinberg, H. S., Makarushka, C., et al. (2005). *Drinking water disinfection by-products and pregnancy outcome*. American Water Works Association Research Foundation and U.S. Environmental Protection Agency. Denver. Available at: http://www.waterrf.org/PublicReportLibrary/91088F.pdf

Scalbert, A., Brennan, L., Fiehn, O., Hankemeier, T., Kristal, B. S., van Ommen, B., et al. (2009). Mass-spectrometry-based metabolomics: Limitations and recommendations for future progress with particular focus on nutrition research. *Metabolomics*, **5**, 435–458.

Schwarzenbach, R. P., Escher, B. I., Fenner, K., Hofstetter, T. B., Johnson, C. A., von Gunten, U., and Wehrli, B. (2006). The challenge of micropollutants in aquatic systems. *Science*, **313**, 1072–1077.

Shimokura, G. H., Savitz, D. A., and Symanski, E. (1998). Assessment of water use for estimating exposure to tap water contaminants. *Environmental Health Perspectives*, **106**, 55–59.

Silva, E., Rajapakse, N., and Kortenkamp, A. (2002). Something from "nothing"—eight weak estrogenic chemicals combined at concentrations below NOECs produce significant mixture effects. *Environmental Science and Technology*, **36**, 1751–1756.

Singer, P. C. (2001). Variability and assessment of disinfection by-product concentrations in water distribution systems. In *Microbiological pathogens and disinfection by-products in drinking water: Health effects and management of risks* (eds. G. F. Craun, F. S. Hauchman, and D. E. Robinson), 211–223. International Life Sciences Institute Press, Washington, DC.

Smith, R. B., Nieuwenhuijsen, M. J., Wright, J., Raynor, P., Cocker, J., Jones, K., et al. (2013). Validation of trichloroacetic acid exposure via drinking water during pregnancy using a urinary TCAA biomarker. *Environmental Research*, **126**, 145–151.

Symanski, E., Savitz, D. A., and Singer, P. C. (2004). Assessing spatial fluctuations, temporal variability, and measurement error in estimated levels of disinfection by-products in tap water: implications for exposure assessment. *Occup Environ Med*, **61**, 65–72.

Tardif, R., Haddad, S., Catto, C., Hamelin, G., and Rodriguez, M. J. (2011). Modeling exposure to disinfection byproducts. In *Encyclopedia of environmental health* (ed. J. O. Nriagu), 810–819. Elsevier, Burlington, MA.

Templeton, M. R., Graham, N., and Voulvoulis, N. (2009). Emerging chemical contaminants in water and wastewater. *Philosophical Transactions. Series A, Mathematical, Physical, and Engineering Sciences*, **367**, 3873–3875.

Ternes, T. (2007). The occurrence of micopollutants in the aquatic environment: A new challenge for water management. *Water Sience and Technology*, **55**, 327–332.

Thompson,T., Fawell, J., Kunikane, S., Jackson, D., Appleyard, S., Callan,P., et al. (2007). *Chemical safety of drinking-water: Assessing priorities for risk management.* WHO, Geneva.

Toledano, M. B., Nieuwenhuijsen, M. J., Best, N., Whitaker, H., Hambly, P., de Hoogh, C., et al. (2005). Relation of trihalomethane concentrations in public water supplies to stillbirth and birth weight in three water regions in England. *Environmental Health Perspectives,* **113**, 225–232.

Villanueva, C. M., Castano-Vinyals, G., Moreno, V., Carrasco-Turigas, G., Aragones, N., Boldo, E., et al. (2012). Concentrations and correlations of disinfection by-products in municipal drinking water from an exposure assessment perspective. *Environmental Research,* **114**, 1–11.

Villanueva, C. M., Kogevinas, M., Cordier, S., Templeton, M. R., Vermeulen, R., Nuckols, J. R., et al. (2014). Assessing exposure and health consequences of chemicals in drinking water: current state of knowledge and research needs. *Environmental Health Perspectives,* **122**, 213–221.

Villanueva, C. M., Silverman, D. T., Malats, N., Tardon, A., Garcia-Closas, R., Serra, C., et al. (2009). Determinants of quality of interview and impact on risk estimates in a case-control study of bladder cancer. *American Journal of Epidemiology,* **170**, 237–243.

Vineis, P., and Perera, F. (2007). Molecular epidemiology and biomarkers in etiologic cancer research: the new in light of the old. *Cancer Epidemiology Biomarkers and Prevention,* **16**, 1954–1965.

Vineis, P., van Veldhoven, K., Chadeau-Hyam, M., and Athersuch, T. J. (2013). Advancing the application of omics-based biomarkers in environmental epidemiology. *Environmental and Molecular Mutagenesis,* **54**, 461–467.

Vrijheid, M., Slama, R., Robinson, O., Chatzi, L., Coen, M., van den Hazel, P., et al. (2014). The human early-life exposome (HELIX): Project rationale and design. *Environmental Health Perspectives,* **122**, 535–544.

Wagner, M., Schlusener, M. P., Ternes, T. A., and Oehlmann, J. (2013). Identification of putative steroid receptor antagonists in bottled water: combining bioassays and high-resolution mass spectrometry. *PLoS One,* **8**, e72472.

Waller, K., Swan, S. H., Windham, G. C., and Fenster, L. (2001). Influence of exposure assessment methods on risk estimates in an epidemiologic study of total trihalomethane exposure and spontaneous abortion. *Journal of Exposure Analysis and Environmental Epidemiology,* **11**, 522–531.

Walse, S. S., and Mitch, W. A. (2008). Nitrosamine carcinogens also swim in chlorinated pools. *Environmental Science and Technology,* **42**, 1032–1037.

Weaver, W. A., Li, J., Wen, Y., Johnston, J., Blatchley, M. R., and Blatchley, E. R., III. (2009). Volatile disinfection by-product analysis from chlorinated indoor swimming pools. *Water Research,* **43**, 3308–3318.

Weinberg, H. S, Pereira, V. R., Singer, P. C., and Savitz, D. A. (2006). Considerations for improving the accuracy of exposure to disinfection by-products by ingestion in epidemiologic studies. *Science of the Total Environment,* **354**, 35–42.

Weisel, C. P., and Jo, W. K. (1996). Ingestion, inhalation, and dermal exposures to chloroform and trichloroethene from tap water. *Environmental Health Perspectives,* **104**, 48–51.

Weller, M. G. (2012). A unifying review of bioassay-guided fractionation, effect-directed analysis and related techniques. *Sensors (Basel),* **12**, 9181–9209.

Weyer, P. J., Cerhan, J. R., Kross, B. C., Hallberg, G. R., Kantamneni, J., Breuer, G., et al. (2001). Municipal drinking water nitrate level and cancer risk in older women: the Iowa Women's Health Study. *Epidemiology*, **12**, 327–338.

WHO. (2012). Pharmaceuticals in drinking water. Available at: http://apps.who.int/iris/bitstream/10665/44630/1/9789241502085_eng.pdf?ua=1

Wild, C. P. (2005). Complementing the genome with an "exposome": The outstanding challenge of environmental exposure measurement in molecular epidemiology. *Cancer Epidemiol Biomarkers Prev*, **14**, 1847–1850.

Wild, C. P. (2009). Environmental exposure measurement in cancer epidemiology. *Mutagenesis*, **24**, 117–125.

Wilkes, C. R., Mason, A. D., and Hern, S. C. (2005). Probability distributions for showering and bathing water-use behavior for various U.S. subpopulations. *Risk Analysis*, **25**, 317–337.

Willet, W. (1998). *Nutritional epidemiology*. Oxford University Press, New York.

Wright, J. M., and Bateson, T. F. (2004). A sensitivity analysis of bias in relative risk estimates due to disinfection by-product exposure misclassification. *Journal of Exposure Analysis and Environmental Epidemiology*, **15**, 212–216.

Xie, S. H., Li, Y. F., Tan, Y. F., Zheng, D., Liu, A. L., Xie, H., and Lu, W. Q. (2011). Urinary trichloroacetic acid levels and semen quality: A hospital-based cross-sectional study in Wuhan, China. *Environmental Research*, **111**, 295–300.

Zhang, Y., Wu, B., Zhang, Z. Y., and Cheng, S. P. (2011). A metabonomic analysis on health effects of drinking water on male mice (Mus musculus). *Journal of Hazardous Material*, **190**, 515–519.

Zhou, W. S., Xu, L., Xie, S. H., Li, Y. L., Li, L., Zeng, Q., et al. (2012). Decreased birth weight in relation to maternal urinary trichloroacetic acid levels. *The Science of the Total Environment*, **416**, 105–110.

Zwiener, C., Richardson, S. D., De Marini, D. M., Grummt, T., Glauner, T., and Frimmel, F. H. (2007). Drowning in disinfection byproducts? Assessing swimming pool water. *Environmental Science and Technology*, **41**, 363–372.

17

THE DEVELOPMENT OF BIOMARKERS

Clifford P. Weisel

17.1 INTRODUCTION

Biomarkers are measures of chemical, physical, or biological agents in a body fluid. They have been used to assess exposures in occupational and environmental settings as well as in clinical medicine. Measurements of biomarkers have been an important to link toxicology and exposure science by providing insight into potential mechanisms of action, linking the metabolism of a toxicant in humans and animals, and understanding differences in susceptibility across populations and individuals. They provide a measure of internal exposure or dose. When linked with external exposure characterization, biomarker measurements can lead to quantitative risk analysis and effective risk management protocols.

Biomarkers fall into three broad classes (National Research Council, 1987):

1. *Biomarker of exposure*: A cellular, biochemical, chemical, or molecular measure in a biological medium indicative of or proportional to an external exposure.
2. *Biomarker of effect*: A specific physical, biochemical, or chemical response documenting that an agent is harming health, is related to a specific disease, or is an early biological event that can lead to a disease.
3. *Biomarker of susceptibility*: A specific trait in a person (e.g., genetic, physical, behavioral) that predisposes an individual to become ill from an exposure.

There is a continuum of these biomarkers along the pathway between an agent entering the body and it causing an adverse effect at a target organ or tissue (i.e., disease state). This chapter focuses on biomarkers of exposures to xenobiotic agents. Ideally, biomarkers of exposure are proportional to the external exposure levels. The US Environmental Protection Agency (http://www.epa.gov/pesticides/science/biomarker.html#table1) lists three broad categories of biomarkers of exposure:

1. *Chemical*: A direct measurement of the chemical of interest in a body fluid.
2. *Metabolite*: A measure of a stable product of the metabolism of a chemical that is part of the natural biochemical process for eliminating or degrading chemicals from the body.

3. *Endogenous surrogate*: A physiological or biochemical response within the body that is highly characteristic of the incorporation of a chemical or its metabolite at a cellular level.

Differences exist between measures of external exposure and that of a biomarker or internal exposure, which can provide complementary information. Biomarkers are typically an integration of exposures across all routes, whereas each exposure route is measured separately and summed to determine a total exposure. Biomarkers represent the concentration at a point in time in a body fluid that often changes over time post-exposure and whose levels may not be the same for equivalent exposures or across different exposure routes. Biomarker levels reflect an integrated or averaged exposure over time, even if the exposure varies, with the caveat that the estimate of total exposure is dependent upon an agent's biological half-life, that is, how long it takes for half the concentration in the body to be eliminated. This integration process can be beneficial for interpreting chronic exposure but may not provide information on peak exposures for agents with acute toxicity. Biomarker measurements rarely identify the environmental source of an exposure, which is a necessary component in risk management. They can indicate if all exposure routes have been evaluated when compared with an external exposure measurement. Compared with external exposure measurements and survey or questionnaire data, biomarkers have the advantages of being an objective assessment of exposure, can be precise, reliable, and have less bias, with a closer understanding of the exposure leading to disease. Their disadvantages include that the timing for collection is critical, the expense for collection and analysis, concerns of sample stability, laboratory errors, contamination, interferences from the sample matrix, the need for adequate detection limits, difficulties in interpreting the levels, and the burden it can present to subjects along with ethical considerations. For occupational exposure in which the sources of an agent are known due to an industrial process or job classification, biomarkers can help identify when exposures exceed levels of concern. Biomarkers can provide key information in exposure science, but are most useful when combined with information about external exposure and activities.

17.2 PROPERTIES OF BIOMARKERS

Ideally, an exposure biomarker should provide a quantitative assessment of an exposure with minimum misclassification. Properties of useful biomarkers include specificity, sensitivity, chemical stability, ease of analysis, acceptability of sample collection, and appropriate biological half-life for the exposure timeframe of interest. The collection and analysis of the biomarker should also be regarded as ethically acceptable, and guidelines for human subject review should be followed whenever human subjects are part of a research study. Even when biomarker measurements are made for clinical or occupational evaluations that do not require research consent, it is still critical to protect against releasing the biomarker levels linked to the personal information about the subject.

17.2.1 Specificity

Specificity relates the uniqueness of a biomarker to be associated with a specific exposure agent and the underlying quantitative relationship. Measurement of the actual exposure agent in a biological medium, if that agent is not formed in the body, is considered specific; for example, blood lead is a specific marker for lead exposure. Other biomarkers, such as some metabolites or body responses that can be derived by multiple agents, either a family of compounds or diverse agents, are not specific; for example, metabolites of pesticides span across ranges of specificity. Urinary 3,5,6-trichloro-2-pyridinol (TCPy) comes only from chlorpyrifos, and so has high specificity, whereas 3-phenoxybenzoic acid (3-PBA) is a metabolite from multiple pyrethroid moieties, indicating that a person has been exposed to that class of pesticide but not a specific pyrethroid. The inhibition of acetyl cholinesterase (AChE) activity, a critical enzyme in nerve function measured by the metabolite levels of cholinesterase in blood or AChE activity in red blood cells, has been used as a biomarker of exposure to organophosphate (OP) and carbamate pesticides. It is often used as a general clinical marker of OP poisoning, making it a useful marker of these classes of pesticide exposure. However, other agents can also inhibit AChE activity, making it a non-specific biomarker.

17.2.2 Sensitivity

Sensitivity should be sufficient so that the biomarker can be measured at exposure levels of health concern. This is governed by both the analytical sensitivity of the measurement and the levels in the body at the time of sample collection. Humans have biological mechanisms to excrete or metabolize most toxicants. Toxicants and their metabolites change with time. They increase during the exposure, and then decline once the exposure declines or ceases, though a time lag in the responses can occur. The rate of change is given by the biological half-life of the biomarker, which is the length of time for its concentration to decrease in the body by a factor of two. Some agents are metabolized by more than a single metabolic pathway. Sometimes one pathway can be more important at a low concentration and a second pathway at a higher concentration. In addition, other sources of metabolites could exist that may be relevant for only one of the pathways. For example, benzene is metabolized by a ring opening mechanism which can be monitored through the biomarkers of urinary *trans, trans* muconic acid and by a ring hydroxylation mechanism that produces phenol and S-phenylmercapturic acid. Phenol is the metabolite of choice for occupational exposure assessment (>10 ppm) but is not applicable for lower-level exposure because there is a background urinary phenol level from dietary sources, an example of how other sources contribute to a "biomarker." This has led to other metabolites or urinary benzene being used as biomarkers for low environmental exposures. In addition, the ring opening mechanism of benzene metabolism appears to be favored at lower exposures, whereas the ring hydroxylation mechanism metabolizes a greater percentage of the benzene at higher exposure levels (Weisel 1996; Rappaport 2013). Extrapolation of biomarkers from the different pathways across different concentrations can lead to underestimating exposure and health effects depending on which metabolism pathway leads to disease. Decision trees have been proposed for how to choose appropriate biomarkers of exposure (Zelenka 2011; LaKind 2014). Biomarkers that are endogenous in the body have a background concentration in body fluids. Thus, they have a threshold exposure level that needs to be exceeded before being useful as a biomarker. A quantitative relationship is desirable between the exposure and the biomarker levels.

17.2.3 Chemical Stability

The biomarker should be chemically stable from the time of its collection to its analysis using common storage conditions, which typically range from room temperature to being frozen at -80°C. In some case a stabilizing agent or pH adjustment needs to be done. Optimally, the biomarker should be amenable to analysis by common instrumentation with a minimum amount of sample preparation so that the analyses can be done in many different laboratories. Common instrumentation with necessary sensitivity for biomarker measurements include: 1) for metals, atomic absorption spectrometry (AAS) and inductively couple plasma with mass spectrometry or optical emission spectrometry (ICP-MS or ICP-OES); and 2) for organic compounds, gas chromatography/mass spectrometry (CG/MS) or GC, with other detectors sensitive to specific atoms (e.g., electronic capture detector for halogens, nitrogen phosphorus detector) and high performance liquid chromatography/mass spectrometry (HPLC/MS) or HPLC with other detectors, such as ultraviolet and fluorescent. The use of mass spectrometry as a detector provides confirmation of a compound's identity. Gas chromatography is used when the biomarker is volatile and thermally stable or can be derivatized to form compounds with those properties; otherwise, HPLC is used. Most metabolites are formed by the addition of polar groups to increase their solubility in urine, which tends to decrease their volatility. This results in volatility being a major consideration in selecting the analytical method. Multiple approaches have been used to prepare the sample for biomarker analysis. These include digestion in acid assisted by microwave heating or on hotplates to remove potentially interfering matrix constituents for metal analyses and some organic compounds. Gas chromatography preparation includes liquid/liquid extraction (LLE), solid phase extraction (SPE), solid phase microextraction (SPME), and purge and trap. If a metabolite can be derivatized making it amenable to GC analysis, this is typically done after extraction. Concentration of the biomarker is often needed as part the extraction protocols. Liquid/liquid extraction and SPE are common cleanup protocols to remove interfering matrix

Table 17.1 Examples of biological media and agents that are used for biomarkers

Biological media	Agent	Biological media	Agent
Urine	Metals Organic compounds Metabolites	Adipose tissue	SVOCs
Blood or Serum	Metals Organic compounds Metabolites Adducts	Breath condensate	Volatile agents
Breath	Volatile agents Metabolites Endogenous species	Sputum	Microbes Endogenous species
Hair	Metals	Bone	Lead
Feces	Metals Microbes	Fingernails/toenails	Metals
Breast milk	Metals Organic compounds Metabolites	Salvia	Metals Metabolites

species before HPLC analysis. Recent advances in new sensors have promise for direct reading methodologies being applied to biomarkers (NAS, 2012).

17.2.4 Acceptability of Sample Collection

The biological media should be relatively easy to obtain. Several common biological media and analytes determined are given in Table 17.1. Urine, breath, hair, and nails are typically easiest to collect from a large population. Blood or serum is also commonly used though its collection requires a trained phlebotomist and some individuals are reticent about providing blood samples. The amount of blood that can be collected is restricted, particularly from children. An additional consideration is when the sample is collected and whether the biomarker concentration needs to be normalized for matrix variations.

17.2.5 Appropriate Biological Half-Life

One major consideration for being able to interpret the biomarker levels is whether the time period between when the exposure occurred and when the sample was collected is appropriate relative to the biomarker's biological half-life. The decision should also consider whether an acute or chronic exposure is occurring and if the health effect is related to acute or chronic exposure. Biological half-lives can vary from seconds to years (Table 17.2). The half-life of a compound can vary dependent upon the tissue into which it has penetrated. For example, small molecule volatile

---

Table 17.2 Examples of Biological Half-Lives of Classes of Compounds

Seconds to Minutes

Small organic molecules in blood and breath for short exposures and pre-shift work samples

Examples: solvents—benzene, methyl ethyl ketone, trihalomethanes, trichloroethene

Hours

Small polar molecules in blood and breath

Example: carbon monoxide

Second phase elimination of small organic molecules (solvents) in blood and breath

Post-shift work solvents/their metabolites eliminated in urine

Examples: acetone, phenol, aromatic compound metabolites, TCAA

Days to Weeks

Lead in blood

Metals in urine (chromium, inorganic mercury)

Adducts (hemoglobin adducts, albumin adducts)

Years

Lead in bone

Cadmium in urine

Polybrominated biphenyl, polychlorinated biphenyl, dioxin, DDT in blood, fat and urine

---

organic compounds (VOCs) (e.g., hydrocarbons, both aliphatic and aromatic, halogenated hydrocarbons) are typically metabolized and expire/excreted rapidly with half-lives of minutes following a brief exposure. Sequential measurement of these compounds in an individual in blood or breath shows a rapid, exponential decline once an exposure ceases to near background levels within minutes (Xu 2004). However, if a longer exposure occurs, such as an 8-hour occupational exposure for a 5-day work week, the urinary metabolite levels of solvents in the pre-shift samples continually increase throughout the week. Different half-lives of a single compound can occur in different biological matrices, which represent different body compartments where the compound resides. A simplified approach to understanding these differences is to consider that the body is composed of several compartments through which toxicants and metabolites reside in and move (Figure 17.1). Each compartment would have a distinct half-life for a particular toxicant or metabolite. For short-duration exposure, solvents would remain primary in the systemic circulation (blood compartment) system, with only a small percentage transferred to rapidly perfused tissue or adipose (fatty) tissue where the biological half-lives are longer. The rapid removal from the circulation system is due to metabolism in the liver or expiration via the lung. For chronic or repetitive exposures much more of the VOC is transferred to adipose tissue, which would slowly transfer back to the systemic circulation system and be eliminated once the exposure ceased. Another

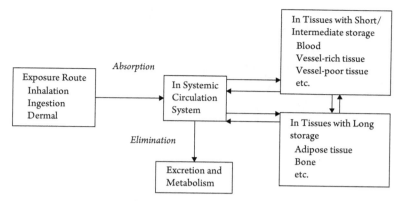

Figure 17.1 Schematic compartment model for distribution of toxicants into the body.

example of multiple compartments resulting in different biological half-lives for a toxicant is lead. Its biological half-life in blood is approximately 1 month, whereas that in the bone is years. Bone tissue serves as a reservoir for lead exposure, which subsequently can be mobilized when life cycles such as pregnancy release bone calcium along with lead. Therefore, measurement of lead in blood and bone provide information about different exposure periods.

The effect of biological half-life in interaction between exposure and biomarker concentration is illustrated in Figure 17.2 (Nieuwenhuijsen and Droz 2004). For a constant exposure scenario the time it takes for the biomarker to reach steady-state concentration in the body is much quicker for compounds with shorter half-lives than for those with longer half-lives. For scenarios that have long intermittent exposures, such as work place settings, the concentration of biomarkers with very short half-lives will mirror the exposure and return to background levels between exposure events. In contrast, the concentrations of biomarkers with longer half-lives will still be somewhat elevated at the start of subsequent exposures, resulting in increased body burdens each day until no exposure is present for an extended time period so that the body can recover and the body burden of the biomarker can return to a background level. In the occupational setting, samples collected pre-work shift often show continued increases in levels during the work week, with a return to lower baseline after a weekend or extended vacation. For compounds with a very long half-life, the body burden can continue to build up until a steady-state is reached in a manner similar to a constant exposure. The interpretation of the biomarker concentration in any biological matrix for repetitive exposures can be complex because different tissues in the body could have different biological half-lives for the same compound and there is an exchange of biomarkers throughout the body based on partitioning coefficients for the different tissues. To obtain a more complete interpretation of the distribution of compounds within the body over time the concept of the simple compartmental model can be extended to full physiologically based toxicokinetic (PBTK) or pharmacokinetic (PBPK) models. These

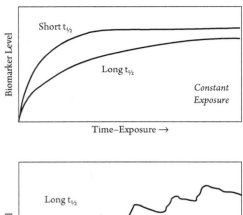

Figure 17.2 Effect of air exposure variability on biomarkers with short and long biological half-life ($t_{1/2}$).
Adapted from Nieuwenhuijsen, M., and Droz, P. (2004). *Biological monitoring. Exposure assessment in occupational and environmental epidemiology.* 167–180. Oxford Univrsity Press, London.

models describe the full distribution of toxicants in the body and how they change with time due to uptake, excretion, and metabolism (Dorman 2001; Georgopoulos 2007; Tan 2012). These models should be evaluated with biomarker data and once validated used with new biomarker data to better predict both the exposure and potential target tissue dose that might lead to a disease.

17.3 BIOLOGICAL MATRICES

Table 17.1 provides a list of media and types of exposure biomarkers commonly employed. The progression of biomarkers of exposure from the parent compound, to metabolites to DNA- or protein adducts also reflects a progression from internal exposure or dose to biologically effective or target dose and an understanding of the exposure level to the metabolism to the likelihood of adverse effects.

When reporting biomarkers levels, some biological media need to be normalized. Two of the most common media used, urine and blood/plasma/serum, are in this category.

17.3.1 Urine

Spot urine samples, the collection of a portion of a single urine void, is relatively easy to obtain from adults and older children, and sampling protocols have been designed to collect urine from very young children who wear diapers (Hu 2004). Urine has been analyzed for the exposure toxicant, commonly referred to as the parent agent, for example, metals (mercury, cadmium, chromium, arsenic) and poorly or partially metabolized organic species with some aqueous solubility (chlorinated hydrocarbons, aromatic compounds, cotinine, nitroso compounds), and for metabolites of organic compounds (aldehydes and ketones, pesticides, herbicides, polyaromatic hydrocarbon, phthalates). However, spot urine samples do not provide excretion rate because urine voids occur at various time intervals, typically hours apart, and the volume of the voids vary with hydration status of the individual. Urine samples provide a measure of the integrated exposure over at a minimum, the time period between voids, though it often represents accumulation over longer time periods. Some studies have collected all urine voids over 24 hours for one or more days to determine the actual excretion rate. However, this presents a burden to the participants because it requires collection, storage, and transport of all urine excreted in all locales an individual moves through during the day. The more usual approach is the collection of a spot sample from a first morning void, which can be collected at an individual's residence and can be stored cold, as is commonly done as part of a medical exam, a procedure with which a subject may be familiar. Toxicant levels have been reported as the concentration in the urine, as a creatinine corrected level, and as normalized to specific gravity. The latter two values can account for dilution or concentration of the urine associated with varying liquid intakes or degree of exercise that can cause loss of water through perspiration. Creatinine, a breakdown product of creatinine phosphate in muscle, can be readily measured by ultraviolet spectroscopy. Its production rate has been proposed to be constant in a sedentary individual and was originally developed to monitor kidney function of patients in hospital settings. Because people are generally sedentary overnight, normalization by creatinine in first morning urine may be appropriate. It has also been used for samples collected at other times of the day and has been commonly adapted to compare urinary concentrations of toxicants across subjects. The biomarker would be reported as the ratio of the mass of the biomarker to the mass of urinary creatinine (UCr) (e.g., µg/mg UCr). A second common approach is to normalize the concentration to the specific gravity of the urine (ratio of the density of urine to the density of water), which is related to the concentration of excreted waste in the urine. If the waste elimination rate is constant, then the specific gravity can be used to normalize the urine to the volume of urine excreted and provide a rationale for comparing the ratio of toxicant levels to specific gravity across individuals (Aylward 2014). The normal range for specific gravity of urine is 1.003 to 1.03.

Selecting urine as the sampling media should consider the biomarker's solubility in urine, whether the biological half-life is appropriate for the clearance rate of the biomarker by the kidneys and whether other sources of the biomarkers exist besides the target compound.

17.3.2 Blood, Plasma, and Serum

Blood is a biomonitoring matrix that reflects what is currently circulating through the body and connects the portals of entry into the body (lungs–inhalation, gastrointestinal tract–ingestion, dermis–dermal), the portals for excretion from the body (kidney–urine, lung–expiration, liver–detoxification via metabolism), and body tissue where biomarkers are stored and accumulated in the body (e.g., adipose tissue, bone). Blood also transports agents to potential target organs; this is often referred to as the *biologically effective dose*. Blood levels can reflect recent exposures or releases of stored biomarkers from tissues (e.g., adipose or fatty tissues, bones, perfuse tissue). Blood is a composite of plasma and cells (red blood cells, white blood cells, and platelets). Biomarkers are measured in whole blood, plasma, or serum (plasma without clotting factors such as fibrin). Common constituents measured include metals; volatile organic compounds such as chlorinated, aromatic, and aliphatic hydrocarbons (parent and metabolites); and semi-volatile compounds such as dioxins and furans, polychlorinated hydrocarbons, and brominated flame retardants. When blood is drawn into a collection tube, stabilizing agents are sometimes added to keep the blood from clotting or to preserve it. These, as well as the rubber in the cap, can contaminate or alter the biomarkers. For example, rubber caps need to be heated and cleaned before collecting blood for volatile organic compounds analysis (Ashley 1994). In whole blood the concentrations are measured on a wet-weight basis. The lipid present in the blood can alter the amount of lipophilic compounds in the blood as the lipid concentration can change over the course of the day, such as following a meal or if the blood sample was taken after fasting, which is required for some clinical blood tests. Some biomarkers, especially lipophilic organic compounds, are reported on as lipid-adjusted concentrations in serum or blood. In addition to lipids, some proteins in blood can bind specific compounds (e.g., perfluorinated), introducing errors when comparing unadjusted levels across individuals (Aylward 2014). When measuring metals that bind to red blood cells it may be necessary to adjust the hemoglobin concentration for hematocrit. The volume of blood that can be collected is considerably less than urine and has a more concentrated matrix. Thus, the analyses can be challenging. However, the sensitivity of many of the instruments available today, GC/MS, HPLC/MS, and ICP/MS, makes blood an effective medium to measure a wide range of biomarkers when done with care to avoid contamination. Biomonitoring in blood has been adopted by a number of countries for large surveys.

17.3.3 Exhaled Breath

Exhaled breath can be used to evaluate gaseous (e.g., CO, NO) and volatile organic compounds that are expired. The underlying principle for exhaled breath as a biological media for biomarkers is based on the steady-state exchange that exists between the blood and the air within the alveolar sacs of the lung. When air is expired it contains breath in the top portion of the respiratory tract in addition to the air from the alveolar. Several different approaches have been used to collect or measure levels in breath. These include real-time instrumentation that continually monitors the concentrations expired, sampling bags that collect whole breath, and arrangements that partition the breath based on the order in which it is expired so that primarily alveolar breath is collected. For the last sampling approach, the initial portion of the breath containing the tidal volume is discarded and the latter portion of the breath from the alveolar is sampled or collected. Volatile organic compounds have been collected from breath using samplers designed to sample ambient air (e.g., stainless steel canisters, adsorbent traps) and subsequently analyzed by GC/MS. Exhaled breath samples have the advantage of being non-invasive and the option to collect time series samples. This provides the opportunity to evaluate rapid changes in concentrations of biomarkers that should be proportional to blood concentration. Those changes can be used to evaluate PBTK models. An example of the application of exhaled breath analysis is the monitoring of trihalomethane (THMs) concentrations, a disinfection by-product present in chlorinated drinking water (Roy 1996).

17.3.4 Other Biological Matrices

Hair and nails have had limited use in measuring specific metals. These media incorporate metals over time and can be subsampled to provide a historic exposure evaluation over their growth periods, from weeks to years, if the hair is very long or samples of the nails or hair have been save or archived. Contamination of hair and nails is a potential concern because they are exposed to the environment and can be colored or treated. Complete removal of external contamination without altering the levels incorporated during their growth is a challenge. Evaluation of hair or nails from different parts of the body can help determine if the sample was contaminated but have different growth rates. The other media given in Table 17.1 have had much more limited applications because of the greater difficulty for collection and limited number of biomarker agents for which they can be analyzed.

17.4 USES OF BIOMARKERS

Biomontoring has been used to evaluate spatial and temporal trends of body burden of toxicants and to provide exposure estimates in epidemiological studies. The US National Health and Nutritional Examination Survey (NHANES) has reported blood levels of a plethora of environmental toxicants across the United States for several decades using a population-based study design (Centers for Disease Control and Prevention, 2014). A similar program has been conducted in Canada: the Human Biomonitoring of Environmental Chemicals in Canada (Haines 2011). A number of human biomonitoring initiatives have been reported in Europe: the Consortium to Perform Human Biomonitoring on a European Scale (COPHES) (Joas 2012), the German Environmental Survey (GES) (Kolossa-Gehring 2012), and the French Nutrition and Health Survey (Fréry 2012). These have been used to evaluate trends in body burden, although, with the exception of a limited num-ber of special projects, they do not include information on external exposure. Thus, although biomonitoring survey data can document trends in body burden, the source of toxicants associated with the biomarker levels usually cannot be definitively identified based solely on that measurement. For example, lead blood in children in the United States declined in the general population staring in the mid-1970s through the 1990s (Pirkle 1994). To understand the reason, the poten-tial actions that affected exposure needed to be known, that is, the banning of lead from gasoline and solder in food cans in the early 1970s.

Once a biomarker has been sufficiently evaluated, that is, a definable relation-ship has been documented between the environmental exposure level (e.g., per-sonal air concentration, surface wipe loading, concentration in food or liquid) and the biomarker concentration, inter-individual differences in that relationship can still exist. These differences can result from variability in activity patterns among individuals that alter the level of contact with the environment (e.g., breathing rate for inhalation exposure, frequency/duration of contact and percent of exposed skin for dermal exposure, difference in diet and food preparation for direct ingestion, and frequency of hand-to-mouth activity for inadvertent ingestion exposure), phys-iological differences that affect uptake rate into the body, and metabolism rate and genetics that alter the removal and excretion of the exposure agent and biomarker from the bodies. The last items control the biological half-life. These processes are studied as part of PBTK modeling. Knowledge of these factors can improve the design and interpretation of biomarker data and their use in epidemiological studies.

17.5 APPLICATION OF BIOMARKERS

Exposure to disinfection by-products in drinking water is prevalent across popu-lations throughout the world and occurs through all three exposure routes, inges-tion, inhalation, and dermal contact. Trihalomethanes (THMs) and haloacetic acids (HAAs) are the two groups of disinfection products produced at the great-est concentrations and their concentrations are currently regulated in drinking water in a number of countries. Biomarkers have been used to evaluate multi-route exposures and to add to our understanding of population exposures to these agents, which have been linked to bladder cancer and adverse reproductive out-comes (Nieuwenhuijsen 2000; Villanueva 2003). A number of these studies can be illustrative of the strengths and the caution in using biomarkers and the benefit of combining biomarker measurements with external information about exposures. Trihalomethane levels in alveolar expired breath and blood have been used to understand the relative importance of exposure routes and how different water uses contribute to THM exposures. Showering and bathing result in inhalation THM exposure because THMs volatilize into the air within a shower stall and to dermal exposure because water continually contacts the skin while showering and bathing. Water is consumed directly, resulting in ingestion exposure. Controlled exposure studies in which individuals showered for a set time, stood next to the shower streams but avoided getting wet (inhalation only exposure), or took a bath while breathing purified air (dermal exposure) resulted in elevated breath THM concentrations in a linear fashion to the water concentration (Jo 1990a,b). The breath concentrations following a normal shower were approximately twice that measured during the inhalation-only exposure in the shower stall, indicating approximately equivalent uptake between inhalation and dermal exposure routes. It was further determined that the chloroform internal exposure or dose from a 10-minute shower was approximately equivalent to that from consuming 2 liters of water, the upper daily consumption rate. These results document that THM exhaled breath levels are biomarkers of inhalation and dermal exposure.

When sequential THM breath concentrations were measured before, during, and after an individual took a bath that contained 10 µg/l of four THMs, the rise in breath THM levels were evident during the bath exposure followed by a decline that could be fit by three exponential functions (Figure 17.3) (Trabaris 2009). However, the four THMs breath concentrations were not equivalent, suggesting that there were differences in exposures, uptake, and/or metabolism rates for the fours THMs that would affect the ability to interpret these biomarkers if only a single point measurement was made. For the inhalation exposure, the air concentrations differ based on Henry's Law coefficients. The highest air and breath concentrations were measured for chloroform and the lowest for bromoform, consistent with the Henry's Law coefficients. Although the water concentrations and therefore the dermal exposures were equivalent, the penetration through the skin as estimated by the water octanol coefficient (K_{ow}) differed. This contributes to different internal exposures

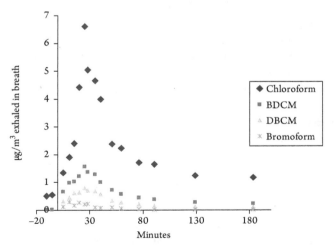

Figure 17.3 Trihalomethane breath concentrations after dermal only (bath) exposure (each THM at 10 µg/l).

Adapted from Trabaris, M. (2009). *Dermal and inhalation exposure to trihalomethanes, haloacetonitriles and chloral hydrate during showering and bathing activities.* Ph.D. thesis. Rutgers University, New Brunswick, NJ.

or doses and breath concentrations for equivalent water concentrations. In addition, the metabolism rates of the THMs vary, with bromoform >> dibromochloromethane >> bromodichloromethane >> chloroform. Thus, the predicted rise and decline in breath concentrations with time would differ across the four THMs.

When THM breath concentrations were measured after ingesting water with THM concentrations similar to that used in the showering and bathing studies, there was no measurable increase. This is not due to a lack of intake of THM, but rather to differences in the distribution of agents within the body based on exposure routes, a crucial consideration when evaluating biomarkers. Inhaled agents cross a very thin boundary in the lung and then directly enter the systemic blood circulation system where they can be distributed to all parts of the body. For dermal exposure, compounds cross the thicker skin boundary before entering the systemic blood circulation system. The difference in the thickness of the boundary that a compound must penetrate before reaching the blood capillaries for the lung and skin results in a longer time lag between the exposure and the increase in blood concentration following the dermal exposure. The skin layer is also a reservoir for additional uptake into the blood after the exposure ceases. Thus, slightly different breath time profiles can be observed for the dermal and inhalation exposures. However, following ingestion exposure the THMs along with other substances ingested are directed through the portal vein to the liver, where the majority of the body's metabolism occurs. At the exposure levels studied, the THMs were very efficiently metabolized, so little of the parent THMs entered the blood circulation system and was subsequently expired. Thus, breath THMs are not valid biomarkers for low-level THM ingestion exposures.

A study of THM levels in blood collected from individuals after they participate in various activities using water, such as showering, hand washing, washing dishes, using a washing machine, and consuming hot and cold beverages, showed similar results to the breath studies. Activities that included potential inhalation or dermal exposure, but not ingestion of cold water, resulted in increased blood THM levels (Nuckols 2005; Gordon 2006).

The role of biomarkers in defining the importance of multi-route exposure to disinfection by-products from chlorinated water, particularly THMs, was used to better evaluate the relationship between bladder cancer and DBP exposures (Villanueva 2007). The odds ratio for bladder cancer with THM exposure increased when shower/bath frequently was included in the exposure estimate in addition to average ingestion exposure as the decreased exposure misclassification (Table 17.3).

Another series of studies measuring urinary dichloroacetic acid (DCAA) and trichloroacetic acid (TCAA) illustrate the role in biological half-life and multiple exposures that can confound their utility as biomarkers (Kim 1998; Froese 2002). These two DBPs have low volatility and are ionic at the pH of tap water. Thus, they have low inhalation exposure and dermal absorption, resulting in ingestion being the primary exposure route for most individuals. Both compounds are also metabolites of trichloroethene and tetrachloroethylene, common dry cleaning fluid and

Table 17.3 Odds Ratio of Bladder Cancer with Trihalomethane Exposure from Drinking Water

Exposure	Odds ratio	95% Confidence interval
Ave ingestion 0 ≥ μg/day	1.0	
<1–10	0.88	0.61–1.27
>10–35	1.17	0.80–1.71
>35	1.35 ($P_{trend} = 0.09$)	1.09–1.99
Shower/bath <50 min/day* μg/l	1.0	
50–167	1.30	0.90–1.87
167–<333	1.38	0.90–2.13
≥333	1.83 ($P_{trend} < 0.01$)	1.17–2.87

Adapted from Villanueva, C. M., Cantor, K. P., Grimalt, J. O., Malats, N., Silverman, D., Tardon, A., et al. (2007). Bladder cancer and exposure to water disinfection by-products through ingestion, bathing, showering, and swimming in pools. *American Journal of Epidemiology*, **165**(2), 148–156.

degreasing agents. If an individual consumes chlorinated tap water, he or she is expected to be exposed to DCAA and TCAA daily, which would be excreted in urine. However, the applicability of urinary DCAA or TCAA as a biomarker needs to consider their biological half-lives and other exposures that could lead to their excretion in urine. The biological half-lives TCAAs and DCAAs are estimated to be 70 to 120 hours and 0.9 to 1.6 hours, respectively. Thus, for daily exposures, TCAA body burden should increase until it reaches steady-state, whereas urinary DCAA levels would reflect exposures that occurred between urinary voids. A study of subjects in New Jersey was done to assess exposure to DCAA and TCAA from residential tap water using measurements of their urinary levels (Kim 1998). The initial evaluation found no relationship between TCAA and DCAA water concentration, and either the urinary excretion rates or their concentrations normalized to creatinine in first morning voids for individuals. This may suggest that neither urinary TCAA nor DCAA is a valid biomarker of water ingestion exposure. However, it must be realized that water concentration is only one component of the exposure calculation. The other factors to include are the amount of tap water consumed (either as cold water or in beverages and foods), whether the water was filtered, removing the TCAA and DCAA, and whether chlorinated tap water was consumed at locations other than the home. To account for this, a 48-hour ingestion exposure estimate was calculated based on the amount of water consumed at home multiplied by the water concentration measured during a home visit adjusted for use of a water filter. A statistically significant association was then identified for 42 individuals in the study for TCAA excretion rate ($r^2 = 0.306$ $p < 0.001$) and urine concentrations normalized to creatinine ($r^2 = 0.149$ $p = 0.012$). These correlations improved for a subset of 25 participants who only consumed tap water at home for TCAA excretion rate ($r^2 = 0.575$ $p < 0.00001$) and urine concentrations normalized to creatinine ($r^2 = 0.603$ $p < 0.00001$). This is consistent with urinary TCAA being a biomarker of ingestion exposure because the biological half-life and exposure time frame were compatible. However, for the same populations no statistically significant relationship was found for first morning urinary DCAA excretion rate or concentration and the 48-hour ingestion exposure index. The lack of validation of urinary DCAA as an exposure biomarker for ingestion of tap water is consistent with the short biological half-life of DCAA. The utility of urinary TCAA as a useful biomarker of ingestion exposure has been replicated in further studies (Zhang 2009).

An examination of the scatter plot of TCAA normalized to creatinine and the TCAA ingestion exposure indicate that although there is a correlation, individual urinary levels were elevated compared with the expected calculated from the ingestion exposure (Figure 17.4). This suggests additional sources of urinary TCAA. Thus, understanding other sources of urinary TCAA, whether they are ingestion of chlorinated water at other locations or exposure to chlorinated solvents that are metabolized to TCAA and excreted, need to be accounted for when predicting the exposure based solely on urinary TCAA concentration or excretion rate. Not doing so would lead to exposure misclassification because urinary TCAA has multiple sources.

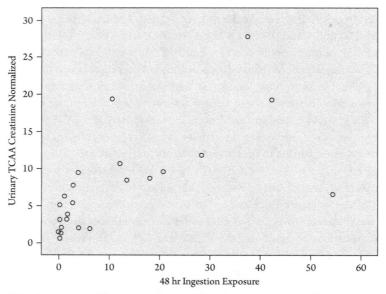

Figure 17.4 Comparison of first morning urine TCAA concentration normalized to creatinine levels with 48-hour ingestion exposure for 25 subjects who did not work outside of home. Data from Kim, H. (1997). *Human exposure and dichloroacetic Acid and trichloroacetic acid from chlorinated water during household use and swimming.* Ph.D. thesis. Rutgers University, New Brunswick, NJ.

17.6 METABOLOMICS AND THE EXPOSOME AS EXPOSURE BIOMARKERS

The biomarkers discussed in the preceding focused on exposure to a single agent or a family of compounds. However, people are exposed to a wide range of environmental agents and stressors continuously throughout their lifetime. Two methodologies have been proposed as potential biomarkers to understand the range of exposures that people encountered and their linkage to health. They are:

1. *Metabolomics*: The measurement of the profile or fingerprint of small molecule metabolites in body fluid (urine and blood are most common) to assess the interaction of the human biological system and the environment. An individual's metabolome profile is influenced by both environmental and genetic factors, and changes in the profile can be linked to environmental exposures. Understanding those changes can provide information on both the exposure and the body's mechanistic response to exposure and stressors and how the body detoxifies the exposure agents.
2. *Exposome*: A characterization of all lifetime events that define an individual's cumulative environmental exposures starting from conception. The goal of determining the exposome is to illuminate non-genetic factors that contribute to disease. It encompasses the external domain (general—social factors, education, financial status, psychological and mental stress, urban–rural environment, climate, etc.; and specific—exposure to chemical contaminants, biological agents, radiation, diet, lifestyle, occupation, medical treatment, etc.) and the internal domain (e.g., metabolism, hormones, physical activity, microbiome, inflammation, lipid peroxidation, oxidative stress, aging, etc.) (Wild 2013). Conceptually, it is the -omic equivalent for exposure that genomics is for genetics.

The proper interpretation of metabolomics and the exposome data relative to exposure requires understanding/characterizing external exposures in addition to the biomarker measurements. These techniques are being developed with the advent of robust, highly sensitive instrumentation that can analyze large numbers of samples and statistical analysis techniques applicable to large datasets.

Metabolomics, as is the case for each of the -omic techniques (e.g., proteomics, genomics), generates large datasets by measuring many metabolites simultaneously. The measurements of endogenous and exogenous metabolites in an unbiased fashion are done using different instrumentation, for example, GC/MS, HPLC/MS and nuclear magnetic resonance (NMR) spectroscopy. The output of these techniques generates a metabolic profile for each sample. These are being developed for use in high-throughput approaches leading to large dataset generation. The data analysis requires sophisticated/powerful statistical methodologies to achieve a physically and biologically valid interpretation. Data analyses considerations include dealing with missing data points, data normalization, detection of outliers, and a combination of basic statistical tests followed by higher-order analyses such as cluster analysis, discriminant function analysis, principal component analysis, and decision trees. The basic statistics are used to evaluate overall differences in abundances among the different exposure groups and associations among the metabolites. The higher-order analyses can be conducted as part of an exploratory analysis to provide insight into which group of metabolites can discriminate among exposures and explain the most amount of variation within the dataset. The overall goals of data analysis are to explore the data to determine underlying trends in the data, identify differences and similarities between groups, and develop predictive power of the variables for use in future analyses. Ideally, the relationships among the metabolites associated with different exposures can be placed in a biological context through visualization, enrichment, and network analysis to connect the exposure to a biological response and the mechanism leading to that response. Biological systems are highly complex, often with multiple pathways and reactions to individual exposure, which can vary across individuals due to genetic differences. Thus, the changes in the metabolome with differential exposures can be subtle and require multivariate analyses to determine how an exposure changes responses on the molecular level and the interconnectivity between cellular components reflected in the metabolomic analyses. The tools developed for genomic analysis that preceded the development of this field are being applied.

The application of the exposome attempts to identify a lifetime of exposures and stressors using a single point in time biological profile. The profile could include not only the metabolites in the metabolome, but also protein expressions, DNA and protein adduct formation, RNA transcriptome, general biochemical constituent such as sugars, nucleotides, amino acids, lipids, and so on. Although the levels and individual components can be perturbed as a cell goes through its typical physiological and pathological states, the exposome seeks to understand how lifetime, rather than only recent, exposures produce the current profile. Daily cellular activities and responses can cause the exposome to be highly variable and dynamic throughout an individual's lifetime and across a population. The assessment of exposure early in life on health and potentially the exposome can vary greatly. For example, lead exposure during young age can be highly impactful, leading to demonstrated cognitive deficiencies. Other early exposure could be manifested as more subtle effects, such as increasing the predisposition to chronic diseases. The linkage between the gene and the environment needs to be incorporated in any evaluation of the exposome. It has been proposed that the approach developed for the genome-wide association studies (GWAS) to generate hypotheses linking gene and disease be applied to exposure by analyzing data collected as part of exposure-wide association studies (EWAS). Exposure-wide association studies should facilitate identification of associations between health outcomes and patterns of biomarkers of exposure and responses.

As discussed for individual biomarkers, the application of metabolomics and the exposome are complementary to external measures of exposures. Using biomarker-based exposure evaluations as the starting point can be thought of as a top-down approach, whereas starting with external exposure (concentrations at the body's boundary and activity patterns) is a bottom-up approach (Lioy 2011). When both external and internal exposure evaluations are incorporated, there is the potential to identify the relationship between a disease and exposure and prevent hazardous exposures that could cause disease.

REFERENCES

Ashley, D. L., Bonin, M. A., Cardinali, F. L., McCraw, J. M., and Wooten, J. V. (1994). Blood concentrations of volatile organic compounds in a nonoccupationally exposed US population and in groups with suspected exposure. *Clinical Chemistry,* **40**(7 Pt 2), 1401–1404.

Aylward, L. L., Hays, S. M., Smolders, R., Koch, H. M., Cocker, J., Jones, K., et al. (2014). Sources of variability in biomarker concentrations. *Journal of Toxicology & Environmental Health Part B: Critical Reviews,* **17**(1), 45–61.

Centers for Disease Control and Prevention. (2014). *National Health and Nutrition Examination Survey.* Retrieved August 25, 2014. http://wwwn.cdc.gov/nchs/nhanes/search/nhanes13_14.aspx.

Dorman, D. C., Allen, S. L., Byczkowski, J. Z., Claudio, L., Fisher J. E. Jr., Fisher, J. W., et al. (2001). Methods to identify and characterize developmental neurotoxicity for human health risk assessment. III: pharmacokinetic and pharmacodynamic considerations. *Environmental Health Perspectives,* **109**(Suppl 1), 101–111.

Fréry, N., Vandentorren, S., Etchevers, A., and Fillol, C. (2012). Highlights of recent studies and future plans for the French human biomonitoring (HBM) programme. *International Journal of Hygiene and Environmental Health,* **215**(2), 127–132.

Froese, K. L., Sinclair, M. I., and Hrudey, S. E. (2002). Trichloroacetic acid as a biomarker of exposure to disinfection by-products in drinking water: A human exposure trial in Adelaide, Australia. *Environmental Health Perspectives,* **110**(7), 679–687.

Georgopoulos, P. G., Wang, S.-W., Yang, Y.-C., Xue, J., Zartarian, V. G., McCurdy, T., and Ozkaynak, H. (2007). Biologically based modeling of multimedia, multipathway, multiroute population exposures to arsenic. *Journal of Exposure Science and Environmental Epidemiology,* **18**(5), 462–476.

Gordon, S. M., Brinkman, M. C., Ashley, D. L., Blount, B. C., Lyu, C., Masters, J., and Singer, P. C. (2006). Changes in breath trihalomethane levels resulting from household water-use activities. *Environmental Health Perspectives,* **114**(4), 514–521.

Haines, D. A., Arbuckle, T. E., Lye, E., Legrand, M., Fisher, M., Langlois, R., and Fraser, W. (2011). Reporting results of human biomonitoring of environmental chemicals to study participants: A comparison of approaches followed in two Canadian studies. *Journal of Epidemiology and Community Health,* **65**(3), 191–198.

Hu, Y., Beach, J., Raymer, J., and Gardner, M. (2004). Disposable diaper to collect urine samples from young children for pyrethroid pesticide studies. *Journal of Exposure Analysis and Environmental Epidemiology,* **14**(5), 378–384.

Jo, W. K., Weisel, C. P., and Lioy, P. J. (1990a). Chloroform exposure and the health risk associated with multiple uses of chlorinated tap water. *Risk Analysis,* **10**(4), 581–585.

Jo, W. K., Weisel, C. P., and Lioy, P. J. (1990b). Routes of chloroform exposure and body burden from showering with chlorinated tap water. *Risk Analysis,* **10**(4), 575–580.

Joas, R., Casteleyn, L., Biot, P., Kolossa-Gehring, M., Castano, A., Angerer, J., et al (2012). Harmonised human biomonitoring in Europe: Activities towards an EU HBM framework. *International Journal of Hygiene and Environmental Health*, **215**(2), 172–175.

Kim, H., and Weisel, C. P. (1998). Dermal absorption of dichloro- and trichloroacetic acids from chlorinated water. *Journal of Exposure Analysis and Environmental Epidemiology*, **8**(4), 555–575.

Kolossa-Gehring, M., Becker, K., Conrad, A., Schroter-Kermani, C., Schulz, C., and Seiwert, M. (2012). Environmental surveys, specimen bank and health related environmental monitoring in Germany. *International Journal of Hygiene and Environmental Health*, **215**(2), 120–126.

LaKind, J. S., Sobus, J. R., Goodman, M., Barr, D. B., Fürst, P., Albertini, R. J., et al. (2014). A proposal for assessing study quality: Biomonitoring, Environmental Epidemiology, and Short-lived Chemicals (BEES-C) instrument. *Environment International*, **73**, 195–207.

Lioy, P. J., and Rappaport, S. M. (2011). Exposure science and the exposome: An opportunity for coherence in the environmental health sciences. *Environmental Health Perspectives*, **119**(11), A466–A467.

National Academies Press. (2012). *Exposure science in the 21st century: A vision and a strategy.* The National Academies Press, Washington, DC.

Nieuwenhuijsen, M., and Droz, P. (2004). *Biological monitoring. Exposure assessment in occupational and environmental epidemiology.* 167–180. Oxford Univrsity Press, London.

Nieuwenhuijsen, M. J., Toledano, M. B., Eaton, N. E., Fawell, J., and Elliott, P. (2000). Chlorination disinfection byproducts in water and their association with adverse reproductive outcomes: A review. *Occupational and Environmental Medicine*, **57**(2), 73–85.

National Research Council. (1987). Biological markers in environmental health research. Committee on Biological Markers of the National Research Council. *Environmental Health Perspectives*, **74**, 3–9.

Nuckols, J. R., Ashley, D. L., Lyu, C., Gordon, S. M., Hinckley, A. F., and Singer, P. (2005). Influence of tap water quality and household water use activities on indoor air and internal dose levels of trihalomethanes. *Environmental Health Perspectives*, **113**(7), 863–870.

Pirkle, J. L., Brody, D. J., Gunter, E. W., Kramer, R. A., Paschal, D. C., Flegal, K. M., and Matte, T. D. (1994). The decline in blood lead levels in the United States. The National Health and Nutrition Examination Surveys (NHANES). *Journal of the American Medical Association*, **272**(4), 284–291.

Rappaport, S. M., Kim, S., Thomas, R., Johnson, B. A., Bois, F. Y., and Kupper, L. L. (2013). Low-dose metabolism of benzene in humans: Science and obfuscation. *Carcinogenesis*, **34**(1), 2–9.

Roy, A., Weisel, C. P., Lioy, P. J., and Georgopoulos, P. G. (1996). A distributed parameter physiologically-based pharmacokinetic model for dermal and inhalation exposure to volatile organic compounds. *Risk Analysis*, **16**(2), 147–160.

Tan, Y. M., Sobus, J., Chang, D., Tornero-Velez, R., Goldsmith, M., Pleil, J., and Dary, C. (2012). Reconstructing human exposures using biomarkers and other "clues". *Journal of Toxicology & Environmental Health Part B: Critical Reviews*, **15**(1), 22–38.

Trabaris, M. (2009). *Dermal and inhalation exposure to trihalomethanes, haloacetonitriles and chloral hydrate during showering and bathing activities.* Ph.D. thesis. Rutgers University, New Brunswick, NJ.

Villanueva, C. M., Cantor, K. P., Grimalt, J. O., Malats, N., Silverman, D., Tardon, A., et al. (2007). Bladder cancer and exposure to water disinfection by-products through ingestion, bathing, showering, and swimming in pools. *American Journal of Epidemiology,* **165**(2), 148–156.

Villanueva, C. M., Fernández, F., Malats, N., Grimalt, J. O., and Kogevinas, M. (2003). Meta-analysis of studies on individual consumption of chlorinated drinking water and bladder cancer. *Journal of Epidemiology and Community Health,* **57**(3), 166–173.

Weisel, C., Yu, R., Roy, A., and Georgopoulos, P. (1996). Biomarkers of environmental benzene exposure. *Environmental Health Perspectives,* **104**(Suppl 6), 1141–1146.

Wild, C. P., Scalbert, A., and Herceg, Z. (2013). Measuring the exposome: A powerful basis for evaluating environmental exposures and cancer risk. *Environmental & Molecular Mutagenesis,* **54**(7), 480–499.

Xu, X., and Weisel, C. P. (2004). Dermal uptake of chloroform and haloketones during bathing. *Journal of Exposure Analysis and Environmental Epidemiology,* **15**(4), 289–296.

Zelenka, M. P., Barr, D. B., Nicolich, M. J., Lewis, R. J., Bird, M. G., Letinski, D. J., et al. (2011). A weight of evidence approach for selecting exposure biomarkers for biomonitoring. *Biomarkers,* **16**(1), 65–73.

Zhang, W., Gabos, S., Schopflocher, D., Li, X.-F., Gati, W. P., and Hrudey, S. E. (2009). Reliability of using urinary and blood trichloroacetic acid as a biomarker of exposure to chlorinated drinking water disinfection byproducts. *Biomarkers,* **14**(6), 355–365.

18

RADIOFREQUENCY EXPOSURE:
MEASUREMENTS AND HEALTH EFFECTS

Frank de Vocht and Martie van Tongeren

18.1 INTRODUCTION

One of the important new agents to which human populations got ubiquitously exposed in the twentieth century was electromagnetic radiation (EMR). Human exposure to electromagnetic fields (EMF) has always occurred. For example, the earth's static magnetic field ranges from about 0.25 to 0.65 Gauss. Humans are exposed to low-frequency EMR from the sun, and as a result of thunderstorms, as well as from the earth itself (~50 picotesla), while visible light is also a form of EMR. In addition, people are further exposed to about 2 milliSievert per year of ionizing radiation from natural sources such as radon and cosmic radiation (detailed, recent data for Europe [Tollefsen et al. 2014]). Nonetheless, in the last 100 years exposure to electromagnetic fields has dramatically increased, whereas the spectrum of the EMF exposure has also changed. The use of electricity in nearly all aspects of modern life results in ubiquitous exposure in the developed world, and near ubiquitous exposure in the developing world to extremely low frequency (ELF) 50 to 60 Hz electromagnetic fields. The more recent introduction in the 1990s of mobile technology similarly exposes nearly everyone regularly, if not almost continuously, to radiofrequency EMF. Other applications also result in human exposure to EMF, such as health care (e.g., MRI scanning), manufacturing (e.g., dielectric heaters), cooking (microwave ovens, induction heaters), and broadcasting.

18.2 ELECTROMAGNETIC SPECTRUM AND RADIOFREQUENCY RADIATION

Electromagnetic radiation is characterized by waves of specific shape, amplitude, and wavelength or frequency. The electromagnetic spectrum is the range of all possible frequencies and the associated wavelength of this radiation, and is generally used to characterize a particular EMF exposure. For example, the earth's magnetic field is static, electrical power supply in Europe and in the US is based on alternating currents with a frequency of 50 Hz and 60 Hz, respectively, resulting in an electromagnetic field of the same frequency, and FM radio operates at 88 to 108 megahertz (Mhz). An overview of the electromagnetic spectrum is shown in Table 18.1.

Table 18.1 The electromagnetic spectrum and overview of bioeffects

Radiation type	Class	Frequency*	Wavelength (meter)*	Bioeffects
Extremely low frequency	Static	0 Hz		Nonthermal
	Extremely low	3–30 Hz	10–100 Mm	
	Super low	30–300 Hz	1–10 Mm	
	Ultra low	300 Hz–3 kHz	100 km–1 Mm	
Radiofrequency	Very low	3 kHz–30 kHz	10–100 km	Thermal
	Low	30 kHz–300 kHz	1–10 km	
	Medium	300 kHz–3 MHz	100 m–1 km	
	High	3 MHz–30 MHz	10–100 m	
	Very high	30 MHz–300 MHz	1–10 m	
	Ultra high	300 MHz–3 GHz	1 dm–1 m	
	Super high	3 GHz–30 GHz	1 cm–1 dm	
	Extremely high	30 GHz–300 GHz	1 mm–1 cm	
Infrared	Far infrared	300 GHz–3 THz	100 μm–1 mm	Photochemical
	Mid infrared	3 THz–30 THz	10–100 μm	
	Near infrared	30 THz–300 THz	1–10 μm	
Visible (400–700 nm)	Near ultraviolet	300 THz–3 PHz	100 nm–1 μm	
Ultraviolet	Extreme ultraviolet	3 PHz–30 PHz	10–100 nm	Damages DNA
X rays	Soft X-rays	30 PHz–300 PHz	100 pm–1 nm	
	Hard X-rays	300 PHz–30 EHz	10–100 pm	
Gamma radiation	Gamma rays	30 Ehz–300 EHz	1–10 pm	

White is non-ionizing and grey is ionizing radiation. *: p(ico) 10^{-12}; n(ano) 10^{-9}; μ(micro) 10^{-6}; m(illi) 10^{-3}; c(enti) 10^{-2}; d(eci) 10^{-1}; K(ilo) 10^3; M(ega) 10^6; G(iga) 10^9; T(era) 10^{12}; P(eta) 10^{15}; E(xa) 10^{18}.

Radiofrequency (RF) radiation is defined by electromagnetic radiation ranging from 3 kHz up to 300 GHz, with wavelengths between 1 mm and 100 km. From a frequency of about 10^{16} Hz the energy of radiation is high enough to directly damage DNA (about 10^2 electron volts) and cause mutations. Below this frequency the established biological effects of RF radiation are (primarily) of a thermal nature and are the result of the absorption of energy by the tissue and the currents induced in the body. It is these thermal effects, resulting in measurable increases of temperature in biological matter, that are the basis for protection guidelines in Europe and elsewhere. However, a range of other effects have been associated with exposure to RF radiation, including sensory effects (hearing and vision), effects on central nervous, neuroendocrine, reproductive, hematopoietic and immunologic systems.

18.3 HUMAN EXPOSURE TO RADIOFREQUENCIES

In human history and evolution exposure to RF has only occurred relatively recent. The invention of radio exposed humans to RF, but only to a relatively limited amount. The first significant exposure occurred during the Second World War among military staff working with radar. After the Second World War, data from US Navy radar-exposed workers indicated increased incidence of several cancers, including leukemia; evidence which has subsequently been reproduced in other populations (Goldsmith 1995).

Aside from medical applications, RF exposure of the general population mainly occurred as a result of radio and television; either from using these or from living in the vicinity of transmitter masts. Significant RF exposure in terms of frequency, duration, and intensity until fairly recently remained limited to the occupational environment, and included, for example, those involved in the design, manufacture, repair, or installation of electrical or electronic equipment (Thomas et al. 1987). This changed significantly with the introduction of mobile phones in the 1990s, which led to an overall increase in RF exposure; mobile phone use (and subsequently the exposure to RF) is now ubiquitous in the developed as well as in the developing world (ITU 2010; de Vocht, Burstyn, and Cherrie 2011). In the general, outdoor environment, exposure has similarly increased because of the requirement for cell towers for relaying RF signals from and to mobile phones (Urbinello et al. 2014).

18.4 EXPOSURE LIMITS

Existing exposure limits are predominantly set to prevent thermal effects, although nonthermal effects as a result of RF exposure are also reported (Vijayalaxmi and Scarfi 2014). The absorption rate of energy in the tissues is expressed in specific energy absorption rates (SAR), which is a measure of the power absorbed in the body per unit mass of tissue and is expressed in watts per kilogram (W/kg). The limits are set at 0.08 W kg for the general population and 0.4 W kg for the occupational environment (International Commission on

Table 18.2 Specific absorption rate in Watts per Kilogram

Whole body	Exposed body part	Head	Local SAR*		
			Head	Trunk	Extremities
2	2–10	3.2	10	10	20

SAR, specific absorption rate.

* Local SAR is determined over the mass of 10 g.

Non-Ionizing Radiation Protection (ICNIRP) 2009). Because the susceptibility to thermal injury differs between different tissues, with for example the testes and lens of the eye being very susceptible, SARs are also calculated specifically for different tissues. For example, to ensure patient safety during magnetic resonance imaging (MRI) limit values have been defined for RF in the MRI normal operating mode (IEC 2010) (Table 18.2).

Although we often refer to electromagnetic fields, they are in fact made up of two distinct components: the electric and the magnetic fields, which are linked through the Maxwell-Faraday equation (where ∇ relates to a change in E, E is the electric field, B is the magnetic field, and t denotes time):

$$\nabla \times E = -\frac{\partial B}{\partial t}$$

Because it is generally very difficult to measure or accurately estimate the SAR (in areas that are less controlled than an MRI environment), indirect reference levels have also been issued specifically for the external electric fields and for the magnetic field strength individually (ICNIRP 1998).

18.5 HEALTH EFFECTS

18.5.1 Adults

The main concern with respect to health effects of RF is whether it may be carcinogenic to humans. The World Health Organisation's International Agency for Research on Cancer has classified RF as "possibly carcinogenic to humans (class 2B)" in its Monograph programme, based on all the scientific evidence available at the time (IARC 2013).

Because the most important contemporary exposure source for the general population is the use of mobile phones, which are now almost ubiquitously used everywhere in the world, important data to date are provided by the INTERPHONE study. INTERPHONE was a large, international study conducted in 13 countries (Australia, Canada, Denmark, Finland, France, Germany, Israel, Italy, Japan,

New Zealand, Norway, Sweden, and the United Kingdom) and consisted of a set of case-control studies (Cardis et al. 2007). It focused specifically on four types of tumors and included 2765 glioma and 2425 meningioma (tumors of the brain) cases, 1121 acoustic neuroma (schwannoma), and 109 malignant parotid gland tumor cases and 7658 controls; it is currently the largest published study looking at the association between RF exposure from mobile phones and cancer (Wild 2011). The study was finished in 2011 and concluded that although increased risks for tumors in the temporal lobe compared to other lobes of the brain were observed, overall no plausible increased risks were observed for glioma and meningioma, and also no increased risks were observed for acoustic neuroma. Increased risks were observed in the highest exposure groups (e.g., regular use of a mobile phone for 10 years or more or reported accumulated use of 1640 hours or more), but the INTERPHONE researchers indicated these may have been the result of biases and errors rather than being causal associations. However, because the follow-up was relatively short, especially for a slow-growing tumor like acoustic neuroma, cancer incidence trends should continue to be monitored (Wild 2011).

Because of the importance of the study and the ambiguity of the results, INTERPHONE generated much scientific debate on how the results should be interpreted (Saracci and Samet 2010; Olsen 2011; Swerdlow et al. 2011). The main problem was that it had a retrospective design and exposure was self-reported by participants based on memory rather than prospectively measured (although it is known how well people can recall their use of mobile phones and whether this differs between cases and controls) (Vrijheid et al. 2006; Vrijheid, Armstrong, et al. 2009). A recent meta-analysis, taking into account all published studies including INTERPHONE, suggested an increased risk for glioma in the most exposed part of the brain, the temporal lobe, with an odds ratio of 1.71 and a 95% confidence interval (CI) of 1.04 to 2.81 when a latency of at least 10 years was considered, and an increased risk (OR = 2.29, CI = 1.56–3.37) for cumulative ipsilateral mobile phone use of at least 1640 hours (Hardell et al. 2013). The meta-analysis further indicated no increased meningioma risk and an increased risk for acoustic neuroma associated with high cumulative hours of ipsilateral mobile phone use (OR = 2.55, 95% CI = 1.50–4.40). Summarizing all available evidence, a recent meta-analysis further indicated increased risk of acoustic neuroma in relation to mobile phone use (De Vocht 2014).

Nonetheless, despite some evidence that RF exposure may be carcinogenic to humans (IARC 2013), analyses of cancer time trends in relation to increased mobile phone use for various cancer sites have not provided complimentary evidence of increased cancer risk (Deltour et al. 2009; Inskip, Hoover, and Devesa 2010; de Vocht 2011; de Vocht, Burstyn, and Cherrie 2011; Aydin et al. 2012; Little et al. 2012; Shu, Ahlbom, and Feychting 2012), with the exception of one study in one country (Barchana, Margaliot, and Liphshitz 2012). Although this may point to an absence of cancer risk, the relatively short lag time since the introduction of mobile phones has been suggested as a reason why increased cancer risks may not have not been observed yet in cancer incidence statistics (Kundi 2011).

In addition to cancer, exposure to RF has been linked to a wide variety of other outcomes. Most notably, RF exposure (from carrying and using a mobile phone) has been linked to male reproductive health and may effect sperm concentration, motility, and viability, and may be lead to morphometric abnormalities and increased oxidative stress (La Vignera et al. 2012; Adams et al. 2014). Outcomes for which less evidence is available, include dermatitis (Rajpara and Feldman 2010), neurological effects (Hocking and Westerman 2003; Westerman and Hocking 2004), cardiovascular outcomes (Jauchem 1997), and a variety of biological effects for which it is unclear whether they result in adverse health outcomes (Hardell and Sage 2008; Vijayalaxmi and Scarfi 2014).

18.5.2 Children

There are some indications that children may be more vulnerable to the potential effects of cell phones and other RF-emitting technologies (Kheifets et al. 2005; Rosenberg 2013) because of their developing nervous system (Mead 2008), and effects on well-being, cognition, and behavior (Feychting 2011), as well as increased cancer risks have been observed (Li et al. 2012), although not consistently (Aydin et al. 2011). It has also been suggested that, whereas RF energy absorption from cell phone use is generally underestimated, this is especially pronounced in children because of smaller head sizes and tissue properties compared to adults (Gandhi et al. 2012).

To address these concerns, a multicenter epidemiological study has been initiated that will specifically look at mobile phone use and brain cancer risk in children (MOBI-Kids) (Sadetzki et al. 2014). At the time of writing of this chapter, the study is still ongoing.

18.6 EXPOSURE MEASUREMENT AND ASSESSMENT

Similar to other epidemiological studies, ideally measurements of personal exposure should be collected for the duration of the etiologically relevant time period. Exposure assessment of RF is complicated due to the need to characterize frequency and intensity of the exposure, as well as modulation. In addition, the temporal as well as spatial variability is generally considerable. Ideally, a measure of internal exposure should be obtained at the anatomical site of interest; which may or may not be correlated with external exposure. Because the main biological effects are thought to result from thermal absorption, site-specific absorption rates should ideally be obtained as the measure of dose that the target tissue receives. Unfortunately, under normal circumstances these cannot be directly measured and have to be inferred from measured body currents or from external measurements of electric and magnetic fields. The use of body currents, although possible, is not that useful for epidemiology because the measurements currently can not be done for large numbers of participants for extended time periods. Nonetheless, for relatively stationary situations, such as for plastic welders but also for patients who undergo an MRI scan, tissue-specific SAR values can be estimated using computational dosimetry (e.g., Jin et al. 2012).

Instead of resorting to computational dosimetry to accurately calculate (tissue-specific) heating resulting from an RF dose over a certain time period, "external" RF exposure can be measured using personal dosimeters ("exposimeters") worn by individuals. Although these give estimates of personal RF exposure, important limitations are that they need to be worn for long periods of time (to account for spatial and temporal variability) to provide reasonably good estimates of true long-term exposure, and also the location of the personal dosimeters (for example at the waist) generally does not correspond to the biological site of interest (for example the brain). Nonetheless, if done correctly the use of personal dosimeters can provide reasonable approximations of true exposure (Roosli et al. 2010; Lauer et al. 2012), and they have been used accordingly to provide estimates of the general, urban environment (Frei et al. 2009; Joseph et al. 2010; Urbinello et al. 2014), in the occupational environment (Cooper et al. 2004; Alanko and Hietanen 2008; Tanaka et al. 2012), and to estimate childrens' exposure (Thomas et al. 2010; Juhasz et al. 2011).

Because of the complexity of accurately measuring personal RF exposure (at the target anatomical site and for the aetiologically relevant time period), especially for large populations required for epidemiological studies, researchers are often forced to rely on proxy measures and infer exposure from these. Although the different proxy measures are of varying quality, the underlying assumption of all of these is that the exposure received by every person in the same group is comparable. For example, in occupational epidemiology people are often grouped based on their occupation, assuming that people with the same occupation received comparable RF exposure. An example of such an exposure assessment strategy for RF is work by Karipidis et al., who used the Finnish general-population job-exposure matrix FINJEM to estimate RF exposure in a case-control study of non-Hodgkin lymphoma (incidentally, no convincing evidence of an association was observed in this study) (Karipidis et al. 2007). More recent work by Vila et al. (2014) aimed at better characterization of RF exposure variability by developing a source-based measurement database for occupational exposure to electromagnetic fields as part of the INTEROCC project. Data from the literature was extracted using a standard protocol that included an assessment of the quality of the measurement data, and results of the measurements were linked to common sources of RF and ELF exposure based on the responses on the questionnaires from the INTERPHONE study. The database consists of 1602 measurements for 273 EMF sources. This database can be used in epidemiological studies of RF and ELF exposure but requires information on sources of exposure rather than jobs.

In addition to RF exposure directly from mobile phones, the use of mobile phones also requires cell towers, which expose the population to RF even in the event they do not have a phone on them themselves, and this exposure has also been suggested to result in increased risk of cancer and neurobehavioral symptoms (Khurana et al. 2010). RF exposure from these base stations has been estimated by using personal dosimeters worn in the outdoor environment (Viel et al. 2009; Urbinello et al. 2014), or by using modelling approaches (Meyer et al. 2003; van Wyk, Bingle, and Meyer 2005; Beekhuizen et al. 2014). If none of these methods were possible, instead proximity measures to indicate RF exposure have also been used (Kundi and Hutter 2009; Khurana et al. 2010).

Because of the importance of assessing effects of RF exposure from the use of mobile phones for population health, attempts have been made to better characterize mobile phone use (and type of phone) and infer exposure from that, while also modeling the actual dose to the brain (Ghanmi et al. 2014). For example, this has been done for INTERPHONE (Cardis et al. 2011). The INTERPHONE study relied on self-reported years since first use, duration of use of mobile phones, and an estimate of cumulative hours of use. Of course this method has limitations, and to quantify these the INTERPHONE study conducted several validation studies. An assumption underlying the use of duration and hours of use to estimate exposure is that all mobile phone handsets generate the same exposure. The RF exposure of the handsets is directly related to the phone's output power, and data from over 60,000 calls from 12 countries indicated two- to threefold differences between INTERPHONE study center and network operators (Vrijheid, Mann, et al. 2009); thus introducing differences between individuals despite their usage being comparable. More importantly, usage was self-reported, which could result in recall bias. Two validation studies were conducted, both indicating that self-reported mobile phone use resulted in substantial random recall error compared with network operators' data of phone use (Vrijheid et al. 2006; Vrijheid, Armstrong, et al. 2009). Additionally, these studies indicated that users generally underestimated the number of calls but overestimated the duration (Vrijheid et al. 2006), and they also indicated that although for short-term recall the error was random, people overestimated their mobile phone usage in more distant time periods, thus giving rise to positive bias of the study outcomes (Vrijheid, Armstrong, et al. 2009).

As a result of these sources of random error, as well as bias as a result of the exposure assessment methodology used, interpretation of the results of studies on adverse effects of RF remains difficult. Nonetheless, new studies have developed better assessment methods that do not (solely) rely on self-reported use of mobile phones anymore (e.g., Sadetzki et al. 2014), which is expected to have an important impact on the conclusions on adverse effects from RF on humans and will hopefully provide stronger evidence for causality (or the absence thereof).

REFERENCES

Adams, J. A., Galloway, T. S., Mondal, D., Esteves, S. C., and Mathews, F. (2014). Effect of mobile telephones on sperm quality: A systematic review and meta-analysis. *Environmental International*, **70**, 106–112.

Alanko, T., and Hietanen, M. (2008). A practical method to evaluate radiofrequency exposure of mast workers. *Radiation Protection Dosimetry*, **132**, 324–327.

Aydin, D., Feychting, M., Schuz, J., Roosli, M., and Team, C. S. (2012). Childhood brain tumours and use of mobile phones: Comparison of a case-control study with incidence data. *Environmental Health,* **11,** 35.

Aydin, D., Feychting, M., Schuz, J., Tynes, T., Andersen, T. V., Schmidt, L. S., et al. (2011). Mobile phone use and brain tumors in children and adolescents: A multicenter case-control study. *Journal of the National Cancer Institute,* **103,** 1264–1276.

Barchana, M., Margaliot, M., and Liphshitz, I. (2012). Changes in brain glioma incidence and laterality correlates with use of mobile phones—a nationwide population based study in Israel. *Asian Pacific Journal of Cancer Prevention,* **13,** 5857–5863.

Beekhuizen, J., Vermeulen, R., van Eijsden, M., van Strien, R., Burgi, A., Loomans, E., et al. (2014). Modelling indoor electromagnetic fields (EMF) from mobile phone base stations for epidemiological studies. *Environmental International,* **67,** 22–26.

Cardis, E., Richardson, L., Deltour, I., Armstrong, B., Feychting, M., Johansen, C., et al. (2007). The INTERPHONE study: Design, epidemiological methods, and description of the study population. *European Journal of Epidemiology,* **22,** 647–664.

Cardis, E., Varsier, N., Bowman, J. D., Deltour, I., Figuerola, J., Mann, S., et al. (2011). Estimation of RF energy absorbed in the brain from mobile phones in the Interphone Study. *Occupational and Environmental Medicine,* **68,** 686–693.

Cooper, T. G., Allen, S. G., Blackwell, R. P., Litchfield, I., Mann, S. M., Pope, J. M., and van Tongeren, M. J. (2004). Assessment of occupational exposure to radiofrequency fields and radiation. *Radiation Protection Dosimetry,* **111,** 191–203.

de Vocht, F. (2011). Cell phones and parotid cancer trends in England. *Epidemiology,* **22,** 608–609.

de Vocht, F. (2014). The case of acoustic neuroma: Comment on: mobile phone use and risk of brain neoplasms and other cancers. *International Journal of Epidemiology,* **43,** 273–274.

de Vocht, F., Burstyn, I., and Cherrie, J. W. (2011). Time trends (1998-2007) in brain cancer incidence rates in relation to mobile phone use in England. *Bioelectromagnetics,* **32,** 334–339.

Deltour, I., Johansen, C., Auvinen, A., Feychting, M., Klaeboe, L., and Schuz, J. (2009). Time trends in brain tumor incidence rates in Denmark, Finland, Norway, and Sweden, 1974-2003. *Journal of the National Cancer Institute,* **101,** 1721–1724.

Feychting, M. (2011). Mobile phones, radiofrequency fields, and health effects in children—epidemiological studies. *Progress in Biophysical Molecular Biology,* **107,** 343–348.

Frei, P., Mohler, E., Neubauer, G., Theis, G., Burgi, A., Frohlich, J., et al. (2009). Temporal and spatial variability of personal exposure to radio frequency electromagnetic fields. *Environmental Research,* **109,** 779–785.

Gandhi, O. P., Morgan, L. L., de Salles, A. A., Han, Y. Y., Herberman, R. B., Davis, D. L. (2012). Exposure limits: The underestimation of absorbed cell phone radiation, especially in children. *Electromagnetic Biological Medicine,* **31,** 34–51.

Ghanmi, A., Varsier, N., Hadjem, A., Conil, E., Picon, O., and Wiart, J. (2014). Analysis of the influence of handset phone position on RF exposure of brain tissue. *Bioelectromagnetics,* **35,** 568–579.

Goldsmith, J. R. (1995). Epidemiologic evidence of radiofrequency radiation (microwave) effects on health in military, broadcasting, and occupational studies. *International Journal of Occupational and Environmental Health*, 1, 47–57.

Hardell, L., Carlberg, M., and Hansson Mild, K. (2013). Use of mobile phones and cordless phones is associated with increased risk for glioma and acoustic neuroma. *Pathophysiology*, 20, 85–110.

Hardell, L., and Sage, C. (2008). Biological effects from electromagnetic field exposure and public exposure standards. *Biomedical Pharmacother*, 62, 104–109.

Hocking, B., and Westerman, R. (2003). Neurological effects of radiofrequency radiation. *Occupational Medicine (London)*, 53, 123–127.

IARC. (2013). *IARC monographs on the evaluation of carcinogenic risks to humans.* Volume 102. Non-Ionising Radiation, Part 2: Radiofrequency Electromagnetic Fields. IARC, Lyon, France.

ICNIRP. (1998). Guidelines for limiting exposure to time-varying electric, magnetic, and electromagnetic fields (up to 300 GHz). International Commission on Non-Ionizing Radiation Protection. *Health Physics*, 74, 494–522.

IEC. (2010). IEC 60601-2-33 ed3.0. Medical electrical equipment—Part 2-33: Particular requirements for the basic safety and essential performance of magnetic resonance equipment for medical diagnosis. http://webstore.iec.ch/Webstore/webstore.nsf/artnum/043851?opendocument

Inskip, P. D., Hoover, R. N., and Devesa, S. S. (2010). Brain cancer incidence trends in relation to cellular telephone use in the United States. *Neuro Oncology*, 12, 1147–1151.

International Commission on Non-Ionizing Radiation P. (2009). ICNIRP statement on the "Guidelines for limiting exposure to time-varying electric, magnetic, and electromagnetic fields (up to 300 GHz)." *Health Physics*, 97, 257–258.

ITU. (2010). World Telecommunications/ICT Indicators Database.

Jauchem, J. R. (1997). Exposure to extremely-low-frequency electromagnetic fields and radiofrequency radiation: Cardiovascular effects in humans. *International Archives of Occupational and Environmental Health*, 70, 9–21.

Jin, J., Liu, F., Weber, E., and Crozier, S. (2012). Improving SAR estimations in MRI using subject-specific models. *Physics and Medical Biology*, 57, 8153–8171.

Joseph, W., Frei, P., Roosli, M., Thuroczy, G., Gajsek, P., Trcek, T., et al. (2010). Comparison of personal radio frequency electromagnetic field exposure in different urban areas across Europe. *Environmental Research*, 110, 658–663.

Juhasz, P., Bakos, J., Nagy, N., Janossy, G., Finta, V., and Thuroczy, G. (2011). RF personal exposimetry on employees of elementary schools, kindergartens and day nurseries as a proxy for child exposures. *Progress in Biophysical and Molecular Biology*, 107, 449–455.

Karipidis, K. K., Benke, G., Sim, M. R., Kauppinen, T., Kricker, A., Hughes, A. M., et al. (2007). Occupational exposure to ionizing and non-ionizing radiation and risk of non-Hodgkin lymphoma. *International Archives of Occupational and Environmental Health*, 80, 663–670.

Kheifets, L., Repacholi, M., Saunders, R., and van Deventer, E. (2005). The sensitivity of children to electromagnetic fields. *Pediatrics*, 116, e303–313.

Khurana, V. G., Hardell, L., Everaert, J., Bortkiewicz, A., Carlberg, M., and Ahonen, M. (2010). Epidemiological evidence for a health risk from mobile phone base stations. *International Journal of Occupational and Environmental Health*, 16, 263–267.

Kundi, M. (2011). Comments on de Vocht et al. "Time trends (1998-2007) in brain cancer incidence rates in relation to mobile phone use in England." *Bioelectromagnetics*, **32**, 673–674; author reply 75–76.

Kundi, M., and Hutter, H. P. (2009). Mobile phone base stations: Effects on wellbeing and health. *Pathophysiology*, **16**, 123–135.

La Vignera, S., Condorelli, R. A., Vicari, E., D'Agata, R., and Calogero, A. E. (2012). Effects of the exposure to mobile phones on male reproduction: A review of the literature. *Journal of Andrology*, **33**, 350–356.

Lauer, O., Neubauer, G., Roosli, M., Riederer, M., Frei, P., Mohler, E., and Frohlich, J. (2012). Measurement setup and protocol for characterizing and testing radio frequency personal exposure meters. *Bioelectromagnetics*, **33**, 75–85.

Li, C. Y., Liu, C. C., Chang, Y. H., Chou, L. P., and Ko, M. C. (2012). A population-based case-control study of radiofrequency exposure in relation to childhood neoplasm. *Science of the Total Environment*, 435–436, 472–478.

Little, M. P., Rajaraman, P., Curtis, R. E., Devesa, S. S., Inskip, P. D., Check, D. P., and Linet, M. S. (2012). Mobile phone use and glioma risk: Comparison of epidemiological study results with incidence trends in the United States. *British Medical Journal*, **344**, e1147.

Mead, M. N. (2008). Strong signal for cell phone effects. *Environmental Health Perspectives*, **116**, A422.

Meyer, F. J., Davidson, D. B., Jakobus, U., and Stuchly, M. A. (2003). Human exposure assessment in the near field of GSM base-station antennas using a hybrid finite element/method of moments technique. *IEEE Trans Biomedical Engineering*, **50**, 224–233.

Olsen, J. (2011). The interphone study: Brain cancer and beyond. *Bioelectromagnetics*, **32**, 164–167.

Rajpara, A., and Feldman, S. R. (2010). Cell phone allergic contact dermatitis: Case report and review. *Dermatology Online Journal*, **16**, 9.

Roosli, M., Frei, P., Bolte, J., Neubauer, G., Cardis, E., Feychting, M., et al. (2010). Conduct of a personal radiofrequency electromagnetic field measurement study: Proposed study protocol. *Environmental Health*, **9**, 23.

Rosenberg, S. (2013). Cell phones and children: Follow the precautionary road. *Pediatric Nursing*, **39**, 65–70.

Sadetzki, S., Langer, C. E., Bruchim, R., Kundi, M., Merletti, F., Vermeulen, R., et al. (2014). The MOBI-Kids Study Protocol: Challenges in assessing childhood and adolescent exposure to electromagnetic fields from wireless telecommunication technologies and possible association with brain tumor risk. *Frontiers in Public Health*, **2**, 124.

Saracci, R., and Samet, J. (2010). Commentary: Call me on my mobile phone. . . or better not?—a look at the INTERPHONE study results. *International Journal Epidemiology*, **39**, 695–698.

Shu, X., Ahlbom, A., and Feychting, M. (2012). Incidence trends of malignant parotid gland tumors in Swedish and Nordic adults 1970 to 2009. *Epidemiology*, **23**, 766–767.

Swerdlow, A. J., Feychting, M., Green, A. C., Leeka Kheifets, L. K., Savitz, D. A., International Commission for Non-Ionizing Radiation Protection Standing Committee on E. (2011). Mobile phones, brain tumors, and the interphone study: Where are we now? *Environmental Health Perspectives*, **119**, 1534–1538.

Tanaka, M., Uda, T., Wang, J., and Fujiwara, O. (2012). Performance test of personal RF monitor for area monitoring at magnetic confinement fusion facility. *Radiation Protection Dosimetry*, **148**, 277–283.

Thomas, S., Heinrich, S., von Kries, R., and Radon, K. (2010). Exposure to radio-frequency electromagnetic fields and behavioural problems in Bavarian children and adolescents. *European Journal of Epidemiology*, **25**, 135–141.

Thomas, T. L., Stolley, P. D., Stemhagen, A., Fontham, E. T., Bleecker, M. L., Stewart, P. A., and Hoover, R. N. (1987). Brain tumor mortality risk among men with electrical and electronics jobs: A case-control study. *Journal of National Cancer Institute*, **79**, 233–238.

Tollefsen, T., Cinelli, G., Bossew, P., Gruber, V., and De Cort, M. (2014). From the European indoor radon map towards an atlas of natural radiation. *Radiation Protection Dosimetry*. doi: 10.1093/rpd/ncu244

Urbinello, D., Joseph, W., Verloock, L., Martens, L., and Roosli, M. (2014). Temporal trends of radio-frequency electromagnetic field (RF-EMF) exposure in everyday environments across European cities. *Environmental Research*, **134C**, 134–142.

van Wyk, M. J., Bingle, M., and Meyer, F. J. (2005). Antenna modeling considerations for accurate SAR calculations in human phantoms in close proximity to GSM cellular base station antennas. *Bioelectromagnetics*, **26**, 502–509.

Viel, J. F., Clerc, S., Barrera, C., Rymzhanova, R., Moissonnier, M., Hours, M., and Cardis, E. (2009). Residential exposure to radiofrequency fields from mobile phone base stations, and broadcast transmitters: A population-based survey with personal meter. *Occupational Environmental Medicine*, **66**, 550–556.

Vijayalaxmi, V., and Scarfi, M. R. (2014). International and national expert group evaluations: Biological/health effects of radiofrequency fields. *International Journal of Environmental Research and Public Health*, **11**, 9376–9408.

Vila, J., Bowman, J. D., Kincl, L., Conover, D. L., van Tongeren, M., Figuerola, J., et al. (2014). Development of a source-based approach to assessing occupational exposure to electromagnetic fields in the INTEROCC study. Conference abstract at the International Conference on Epidemiology in Occupational Health (EPICOH); Chicago, USA: *Occup Environ Med*, **71**(Suppl 1), A35–6.

Vrijheid, M., Armstrong, B. K., Bedard, D., Brown, J., Deltour, I., Iavarone, I., et al. (2009). Recall bias in the assessment of exposure to mobile phones. *Journal of Exposure Science Environmental Epidemiology*, **19**, 369–381.

Vrijheid, M., Cardis, E., Armstrong, B. K., Auvinen, A., Berg, G., Blaasaas, K. G., et al. (2006). Validation of short term recall of mobile phone use for the Interphone study. *Occupational Environmental Medicine*, **63**, 237–243.

Vrijheid, M., Mann, S., Vecchia, P., Wiart, J., Taki, M., Ardoino, L., et al. (2009). Determinants of mobile phone output power in a multinational study: Implications for exposure assessment. *Occupational Environmental Medicine*, **66**, 664–671.

Westerman, R., and Hocking, B. (2004). Diseases of modern living: neurological changes associated with mobile phones and radiofrequency radiation in humans. *Neuroscience Letter*, **361**, 13–16.

Wild, C. (2011). IARC Report to the Union for International Cancer Control (UICC) on the Interphone Study. http://interphone.iarc.fr/UICC_Report_Final_03102011.pdf

INDEX